Out of Assa: Heart of the Congo

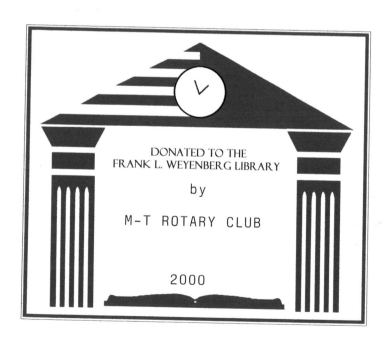

Out of Assa: Heart of the Congo
Medical Adventures in Central Africa

Glenn W. Geelhoed, M.D.
Professor of Surgery
Professor of International Medical Education
The George Washington University
School of Medicine
Washington, D.C.

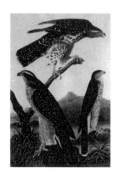

Three Hawks Publishing LC, Alexandria, Virginia

Front Cover: Author with lepromatous woman with her only surviving daughter of her 10 live births. This daughter is a mature cretin, deaf-mute and mentally retarded.

Inside Front Cover: Author and Jean Marco with bushbuck, a source of much-needed protein, secured by well-practiced hunting skills in an enviromental awareness that is necessary for survival.

Composition and Layout: Goodway Graphics
Editing and Cover Design: Kurt E. Johnson, Ph.D.
Printing Supervisor: Robert Perotti, Jr.
Printing: Goodway Graphics of Virginia, Inc., Springfield, VA

Library of Congress Catalog Card Number 99-074543

ISBN 0-9669305-0-9

Frontispiece

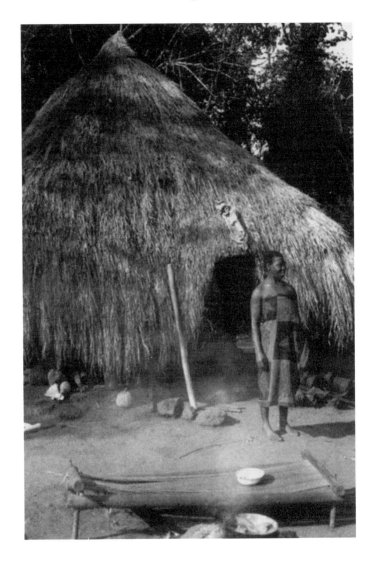

Ex Africa semper aliquid novi.
Pliny the Elder (A.D. 23-79)

Dedication

For my friends in Assa, in Africa,
and for all who try to adapt to inflicted suffering,
and have the courage to still keep on trying.

Acknowledgements

The author would like to acknowledge Kurt E. Johnson, Ph. D. for his tireless editorial effort. Without his support and encouragement, this book would not have been published. He also provided some of his photographs for use in this book. David C. Campbell, Ph.D. also made important editorial contributions. Gary Douglas kindly supplied some valuable information on flora and fauna. Diane Downing provided helpful corrections of names and places in and around Assa.

CONTENTS

PART III ZIM/ZAM: SAFARI FROM HARARE

PART IV OUT OF AFRICA

I first met Glenn W. Geelhoed, M.D. when I was his patient. I went to him for a minor but annoying lipoma on my arm. I signed up at the George Washington University (GWU) Medical Center's In-and-Out Surgery clinic and waited briefly for Dr. Geelhoed's entrance. I had seen him around GWU (where we are faculty colleagues) but didn't know him well. I made a minor joke about my essentially trivial surgical case being the culmination of his otherwise undistinguished surgical career. He got the joke and played along. I noticed that he was cheerful, funny, upbeat, and relentlessly energetic. He had a high-speed motor running inside of him. Little did I know!

Years later, I recruited him to write a surgery book for my small medical publishing company. We were tending to some minor editing when I casually mentioned that I was planning my second birding trip to Venezuela. This set him off on a long (but interesting) dissertation about Venezuela wherein he mentioned a surgeon friend, Luis Arturo Ayala, M.D., in Caracas. Luis has his own airplane and enjoys adventure travel. Coincidentally, Luis and Glenn were in the midst of planning a trip to explore several tepuys in Venezuela's Amazonas Territory. Arthur Conan Doyle had called this region *The Lost World* in his novel.

Tepuys are mesas scattered across Guyana, Venezuela, and Brazil on the Guyana Shield. This biogeographic zone is a hotbed of endemism. Tepuys are isolated islands in a sea of rainforest. They are exceedingly old geologic formations with hard rock caps overlying sandstone. They were formed over millennia by erosion. The plant life on the tepuys is highly specialized, consisting of exotic and unique bromeliads, ferns, mushrooms, and carnivorous plants probably found nowhere else on earth. The surrounding jungle is largely uninhabited and essentially virgin, a birder's paradise by any measure.

Before I knew it, Glenn invited me on the trip. When Glenn filled me in on the details of the trip, I assumed he was harmlessly nuts but would be fun to travel with anyway. He and Luis had arranged plan "A" but I also had plan "B" well in hand with my detailed Venezuelan road map, American Express card, and a wad of colorful bolivares. Plan "A" was a trip via light plane from Caracas to Puerto Ayachuco and then on to a remote base camp/airstrip near Yutaje, about two hours east of Puerto Ayachuco, followed by helicopter ascent to the tops of two tepuys. Right! Plan "B" was renting a car in Caracas and then driving down the Grand Escelera toward Brazil for bird watching, hoping to see among other birds, the Guianan Cock-of-the-Rock (*Rupicola rupicola*). My Spanish is barely above the "¿Donde est el baño?"- "Dos cervecas, por favor." level. In contrast, Glenn's Spanish is quite good so he would be a plus in the countryside and could drive while I looked for likely stopping places for birds. Miraculously (I thought at the time), plan "A" unfolded without a hitch and plan "B" was soon forgotten.

I saw some fabulous birds and got to thrash around (carefully) in some incredible cloud forest on the top of Yavi and Yutaje tepuys. What fun!

Glenn's planning, guts, and good connections made it the trip of a lifetime, or so I thought at the time. After returning from the tepuys expedition to our base camp at Yutaje, we spent an evening and early morning hunting lapas (local name for the agouti, a large jungle rodent) with some Yutaje Indians. Glenn shared a written report of this night hunt on a tributary of the Orinoco River in the rainforest. I was blown away. The report was so evocative of our trip that I was able to relive its magic. Glenn wrote up our later adventures. The stories were incredible but true. I had been there with him. I realized that he could write. We decided to form a collaborative venture to publish his work and, in our dreams, fund further trips.

In conversations with Glenn, I realized that he was obsessed with Africa but I didn't understand this obsession until the summer of 1996 when I lost my "African virginity." My book business took me to the Zimbabwe International Bookfair in Harare and then on to safari camps in Mana Pools National Park in the Zambezi River Valley in northern Zimbabwe. I discovered that Africa really is different from other places I had traveled to. After my first African experience, I was already making plans to go back, and, I had a visceral understanding of Glenn's obsession.

From a vast array of what Glenn immodestly calls "photojournalism," we have selected a few (in focus) images to give the reader glimpses of his work in Assa in the Congo and our naturalist's safari to Zambia in the summer of 1998. The maps will clarify the geographical issues relevant to the book. The tales in this book represent Glenn's thoughts, opinions, and observations. The superficial reader might be upset by Glenn's apparent flippancy regarding the plight of impoverished people in the underdeveloped world. While you are reading about the grim realities of daily life for African bush people, realize that in many instances, Glenn was giving his surgical training and experience to patients who often have never had benefit of any kind of medical intervention other than that provided by the local traditional healers. Furthermore, Glenn's work as surgeon and mentor to indigenous personnel was donated, as was most of his cash and clothing, through the generosity of the "Geelhoed Foundation," an informal arrangement where he gives away cash and personal possessions to the most needy. His serious attempts to train a local medical cadre using techniques that were appropriate for local conditions have had a multiplicative effect after the departure of the "white medicine man from America." He is not cynical but rather experienced and realistic. Glenn is compassionate, committed to helping and gives back much more to his fellow human beings than he takes from them, and maintains his sense of balance and humor while doing all this. We should all be so caring.

Glenn's web site contains all manner of goodies (http://gwis2.circ.gwu/edu/~gwg). This web site offers a bit of a running reportage on Glenn's adventures. Don't give him your e-mail address. YOU HAVE BEEN WARNED! I require him to send all e-mail to my George Washington University (GWU) address, where the server has an effectively unlimited capacity. Once when he was in Africa, he sent me enough information to choke my e-mail. It only had a capacity of several megabytes! After what seemed like hours on hold at the Netcom "Help Desk," I got some relentlessly cheerful nerd who explained to me how to clean out my mailbox so that I could continue to receive hot tips on stocks, X-rated spam, and even important messages.

About a week before Glenn departed for one of his frequent trips to Africa, we were sitting in a sidewalk cafe in Washington, D.C. having a veggie burger for lunch. I am an obligate carnivore but have become more aware of the propaganda of the "eating-meat-causes-cancer" crowd—so—we eat veggie burgers, doing something kind for our colons, and tell lies. A good-looking woman walked by as we ate and talked. She had one physical defect, made all the more remarkable because she was otherwise stunning. She had thick ankles. I said to Glenn, "You don't often see women with legs thicker at the bottom than the top." thinking that this was clever and funny.

He automatically shot back, "Alley Oop's girlfriend!" without missing a beat. This was funny—brilliant even—in a twisted "guy" way. I hadn't thought about Alley Oop for years, although often as a child I had tried to understand this daily comic strip because my now deceased father thought it was funny. To this day, I have never understood Alley Oop. How had Glenn made this connection? I was flabbergasted and not a little impressed by the metaphorical quality of the joke. I wanted to call this book *Alley Oop's Girlfriend* but realized that this title would be meaningless to all but ourselves and a few other poor demented souls, more liable to be found sleeping in the winter on grates near the State Department; and, therefore, clearly unlikely to buy our books. So, *Out of Assa: Heart of the Congo* was chosen as a title. Clear away your preconceived notions. This is the real Africa, warts and all, from different vantage-points in several kinds of jungles.

Glenn loves to tell stories of his adventures. I hope you will agree that he has succeeded in conveying the excitement of his mission in this book. While editing his book, I read Conrad's *Heart of Darkness* and found a passage that appropriately described Glenn and my thoughts about his adventures. "He surely wanted nothing from the wilderness but space to breathe in and to push on through. His need was to exist, and to move onwards at the greatest possible risk, and with a maximum of privation. If the absolutely pure, uncalculating, unpractical spirit of adventure had ever ruled a human being, it ruled this be-patched youth. I almost envied him the possession of this modest and clear flame. It seemed to have consumed all thought of self so completely, that, even while he was talking to you,

you forgot that it was he – the man before your eyes – who had gone through these things."

Kurt E. Johnson, Ph.D.
President and Publisher
Three Hawks Publishing Company
March, 2000

INTRODUCTION

AND, HERE, MY STORY MIGHT HAVE ENDED

The rogue bull elephant ran at me swiftly in a silent deadly charge. When I turned and saw him closing on me in a cloud of dust, I could not believe anything that big moving that fast could be so silent. But his intent was unmistakable. It was no bluff. In a "mock charge" an elephant warns by a noisy and intimidating shuffle with ears flapping wide and trunk raised up, making himself look even bigger and more threatening than he already is. He had already done that earlier to a group of Africans who had been walking down the road, and they were still watching when he turned to come at me. He could not bluff again, so this time he had to make good the threat in closing on the target he had locked on to, which, unfortunately, happened to be me. I was in a wide open savanna near a small acacia (thorn) tree when I looked over my shoulder to get a very impressive and unobstructed view of this cantankerous, one-tusked, belligerent, five-ton beast, swiftly and silently bearing down on me.

PART III OF THE STORY WAS ALMOST OVER
AT THE BEGINNING

I saw the worrisome signs that this was a deadly charge with lethal intent. As he came on, the bull had lowered his head and had fixed me with his rheumy eye with ears folded back flat along his sides. Then he *curled back the tip of his trunk and withdrew it into the protective open mouth behind his upper lip.* This is the position in which a charging elephant prepares for the collision by reflexly protecting the sensitive tip of his trunk from the impact of the charge that will be struck with the massive front of his head. He was intent on collision and could not bluff again, since the group of men he had recently threatened was still watching, and he had to carry through on this threat against the lone man walking away toward the thorn tree.

I heard a shout as I paused for a moment, since I knew I could not outrun him, and then jumped back behind the small thorn tree as he closed within one body length. As he veered around the small tree, he vented his rage, noisily stamping his feet in the dust and flapping his ears, then raising his trunk and letting out a trumpeting scream. He crab-walked around the far side of the tree as I sidled around opposite him. The tree would not have been much of a barrier for long, since he had just torn down a thorn tree twice the size of this one when he had threatened the group of men walking the road toward the airstrip earlier. I heard Gary Douglas start up the Toyota Diesel Hi-Lux and drive from the airstrip over behind me where I backed up and got into the vehicle on the side opposite the elephant as Gary sped the vehicle away along Lake Kariba.

xv

Only later did we learn that this same "problem elephant" had killed a person here earlier in the week, and that the rangers had been notified to come for him. This one-tusked rogue bull had become habituated to being too close to people around the Kariba airstrip in the Zambezi watershed, and then, possibly acquiring the unique "road rage" elephants can undergo in the behavior change called "must," or for no apparent reason currently known to man that remains no match for this king of beasts in this Zimbabwean valley, he can turn killer.

It might have been me. In that case, this story might have stopped, at least at the point after Parts I, *Into Africa* and II, *Out of Assa*, and you would have had to read a sad summary from the other eyewitnesses of this event which begins Part III, *Zim/Zam: Safari from Harare*. Fortunately, I continued to live and experience Africa, and write about these adventures all the way through Part IV, *Out of Africa* from Umtata, Transkei. You can not only read the account of the adventures within the four parts of this most recent African excursion, but also see for yourself the principal actors in the drama—the people, the birds, and the beasts, complete with a photographic record of the elephant charge!

PART II OF THE STORY MIGHT NEVER HAVE REACHED YOU IF AN EXPLOSION IN NAIROBI'S US EMBASSY HAD OCCURRED ONLY HOURS EARLIER

Out of Assa: Heart of the Congo might have ended after emerging out of Assa, but still in East Africa. The events of the story from my experiences in Assa were carefully recorded against considerable odds, but I had completed the manuscript draft and reduced it to computer discs which I wanted to be sure came back to America. As security against the possible accidental or deliberate loss of the computer or any of my other equipment which held much of the story of Assa and its people, I made sure the discs were separated from the hardware, which carried the risk of the possible disappearance of the attractive electronics. This loss of computer equipment, tape recorder, camera and notepads had happened to me earlier in my travels in 1996 in Mozambique at bayonette-point, so worries about any loss along the way did not represent exaggerated paranoia. I made copies and mailed them from the US Embassy in Nairobi, the most secure place I could imagine in East Africa on emergence through the mendacious gauntlet of the Congo and the hazards of official loss of valuables.

As I went forward into Part III of the itinerary of this African excursion, from what would pass for "work" to a "holiday in the bush," I was on a safari into remote Zambian bush, out of touch with what the "wired-in world" considers news. I was unaware that the same US Embassy in Nairobi I had visited to post my manuscript and correspondence with security had blown up just behind me. On return to Washington DC on the long flights back from South Africa at the end of this journey, I found the discs of my journals I had sent back to my office waiting for me—most probably the last mailing to be posted out of the doomed embassy.

**EVEN PART I WOULD NOT HAVE BEEN RELAYED BACK
IF I HAD BEEN ENTERING ASSA A BIT EARLIER, OR LEFT
A BIT LATER, SINCE THE CONTINUING CIVIL WAR
IS OVERRUNNING CENTRAL AFRICA, AND I MIGHT HAVE
SUFFEREDTHE SAME FATE AS SEVERAL ASSA RESIDENTS HAD
AT THE HANDS OF WARRING FACTIONS PLUNDERING
ZANDELAND**

The story might have ended before it had got started. Central Africa has experienced incredible and under-reported carnage from the civil wars and deprivation resulting from ethnic and politico-economic struggles spilling over into the countryside and onto its residents from which the armed bands forage and pillage. I witnessed first hand the rogue bands of warring factions, and saw the graves of those they had used for demonstrations of their terrorism.

My story might have ended for me in Central Africa, but it did not. That happy outcome was not true for several Central Africans I learned about during my visit to Assa and someone must tell their story as well. I have come out alive, and can do that for them.

**PART IV IN UMTATA, TRANSKEI
AT UNITRA AND UMTATA GENERAL HOSPITAL
MIGHT NOT HAVE BEEN REPORTED FOR REASONS OF ILLNESS,
VIOLENCE, POVERTY, IF ONLY BECAUSE THE INDIGENOUS
PEOPLE WERE THE VOICELESS SUFFERERS WHOSE STORY
DOES NOT CARRY VERY FAR OUTSIDE THEIR VILLAGE**

The story might have stopped in Umtata, Transkei, but for the fact that I did not contract malaria, suffer violent criminal attack, get bitten by a black mamba, or miss much of what went on around me because of malnutrition, febrile illness, diarrhea, pneumonia, or each of these on top of a prodigious rate of AIDS. My story did not stop, but many of theirs did. This book may furnish a voice for the litany of unfinished works cut short through untimely death in much of Africa.

In chapter 10, I will describe my three part agenda in Assa: (1) the medical/surgical health care and training mission; (2) linguistic anthropology research in attempting to measure results in the humanitarian benefit of prior hypothyroidism control; (3) the author-in-Africa function of producing this book *Out of Assa: Heart of the Congo*. Throughout the book in the very different venues of what is still the "real Africa," this reality may take several metaphoric tropes: the birds, such as the turaco, or particularly the raptors, such as the Crowned Eagle; the beasts, such as predators, e.g., the leopard, the Green Mamba, and most especially, the elephant.

But, I have not gone back repeatedly to Africa as an outdoor zoo. As fascinating as the natural history of this continent is to me, and as complex and intricate are the poorly understood relationships between species and the environment, Africa is also home to people. These people have problems and potentials of their own, and even more complex relationships with their environment and each other. I am one of those "others". There remains a fascinating and ambiguous relationship and it is still not understood completely by either side.

Every good adventure into the unknown is an exploration of self. How to sustain this ambiguity and still not be incapacitated by it in trying to understand, assist, and learn from others, is a challenge that is focused particularly sharply in Africa. I have had heroes who dedicated their lives to attempts to assist and understand Africa. They came to the end of their lives with many of those ambiguities unresolved. Dr. David Livingstone sought to abolish slavery, save souls and explore the interior of Central Africa. Richard Burton was also an inveterate adventurer who had several obsessions, from the origin of the Nile, the Mountains of the Moon, the Rift Valley lakes, and a prodigious capacity to absorb the languages, cultures and mores of Africans.

My story might have stopped here, but did not. It had not stopped with writers who had tried to summarize Africa before, and the story will not stop with this, or the next excursion into Africa. Many of these African adventurers spent lifetimes exploring and the more they learned, their questions became more sophisticated and the obvious answers became rarer. Africa is like that. It is big and tough enough to expand any man or woman. Joseph Conrad had Marlowe find in the agent Kurtz a simple approach to this unknown darkness: "The Horror!" I would hope to look into this massive and complex continent and forever come out with a differing perspective: "The Wonder!" Africa is a mirror that allows us to see in this glass, but reflects darkly at best the scrutiny we apply to our own souls. As Sir Thomas Browne wrote in *Religio Medici* (1643):

"We carry within us the wonders we seek without us:
There is all Africa and her prodigies in us."

PART I

INTO AFRICA

1 INTO AFRICA

AIRBORNE: THE FIRST STEP IN A LONG JOURNEY—
INTO AFRICA

July 1-3, 1998

My journey was not a simple trip from Washington to the Congo and back. Assa, my ultimate destination, is an isolated village in a country that is not high on the carefree jet-setters' list of chic destinations. Shortly before I left, a well-meaning acquaintance told me about an article on Africa in *Vanity Fair,* you know, where to buy jewelry in South Africa, art galleries in Johannesburg, the best restaurants and hotels in the wine district. I was not destined for *that* Africa. My journey began in Washington and took me through London, Johannesburg (for a reunion with friends), and Nairobi. Then I continued on from Nairobi by light plane in several flights through intermediate Congolese towns before arriving in Assa in the remote bush of the "Heart of Darkness."

I flew to the world's local airport, London's Heathrow on British Air (BA), the "world's favorite airline." I have accumulated so many miles on BA (as well as quite a few other of the "world's favorite airlines") that I am a member of their Executive Club. That may have contributed to the minor miracle that had just occurred at check-in at Washington's Dulles Airport, where I presented my blue Executive Club card, without calling direct attention to it, at the same time making a "small request." Would they mind terribly "if I checked these three pieces of luggage, since—you see—the one is actually divisible into two, since it is a very large container of medicines that I am transporting to Central Africa. Oh, and while you are about it, would it be too much trouble to check it all the way through to Nairobi?"

❧ OUT OF ASSA: HEART OF THE CONGO

LUCKED OUT IN CHECK-IN: IF ONLY I COULD CONTINUE TO BE SO LUCKY AS ON MY HOME TURF!

While crossing my fingers, I talked the agent at check-in into accepting my luggage, without any mention of excess baggage fees. He protested that I leave Washington on July 1 and London on July 2 and I do not arrive in Nairobi until July 4, which appears to be a greater than 24 hour layover in South Africa. He wanted me to claim all three of the heavy bags, filled with medicines and surgical instruments for the Congo, at every intermediate stop. I surely don't want to carry these through too many entrepôts with their suspicious and greedy customs agents. I pointed out that, yes, the flight from London did take-off on July 2, and I *did* arrive in Nairobi on July 4, but it did not *arrive* in Jo'burgh until July 3, so that it was essentially just one, continuing, out-of-the-ordinary, long, circuitous trip, with many of those hours coming off time zone changes. Even though Kenya Airways is the carrier to Nairobi, this diversion through the winter of South Africa is only in order for me to fly the world's favorite airline for such a long haul, so "be a dear, now, won't you?"

Perhaps I did not resort to such flagrant Briticisms, but I did talk with him, as I invariably do, about where he was from. It turned out to be Bangalore. We got to talking about which languages he speaks in India and my upcoming trips, later in the year, on other medical missions to Himachal and Ladakh in Nepal. While we were distracted him with talk about familiar places in India, the *three* bags were checked all the way through to Nairobi. If only I could have extended this luck for all my air-freight all the way to Assa, thus bypassing the rampant kleptocracy of Bunia, my Congolese entrepôt!

ABOARD BRITISH AIWAYS FLIGHT 222 FROM DULLES TO HEATHROW

I am sandwiched in the "world class" (read steerage) while all of the first class section is empty. I am trying to stuff the things I am going to have with me for the next few days into my carry-on luggage. My other bags and all their medical supplies are in the cargo hold at this moment. I hope the collection of clothes (I dare not call it a wardrobe) is warm enough for the South African winter yet light enough for the warm, humid Central African jungle during the rainy season. Will my clothes be comfortable in the daytime heat and night-time cold of the dry woodlands of a Zambian vacation safari and still appropriate for rubbing shoulders with other physicians at the Health Volunteers Overseas evaluation stint in South Africa on my way home in autumn? A proper missionary-explorer of the last century would have had the appropriate wardrobe carefully ironed and folded in huge leather and brass trunks and a band of bearers to carry it around for him. Times have changed and since I was going to be the bearer as well as the wearer, I chose my wardrobe carefully. As you might imagine, there wasn't much left of my wardrobe (or me, for that matter), by the time all this was done.

There is a small movie of British style, a sort of "Woody Allen-wannabe" film, called *Sliding Doors* (a film about alternate endings, starring Gwyneth Paltrow) in progress during the flight. It is about psychological shake-ups over broken relationships in a snooty accent. I bagged the film, and the writing, and napped before arrival in London, my European hometown.

A LONG DAY IN HEATHROW

I have not moved out of the arrival area of Heathrow. My original plan was to go out to visit some place in a city I know well. Once I had used up some time in Heathrow by running around the entire perimeter of the airport but then I had a shower and hotel room available. Hoping to locate an inexpensive hotel, I went to the Executive Club where they explained "...terribly sorry, chap..." and all that. It seems that the British are forever apologizing that the world they once controlled has fallen to rack and ruin, and there is jolly little they can do about it except to "...fear that they are terribly sorry, but there we are...." Ninety pounds and up for a few hours sleep and a shower seemed steep. Anyway, I was going to need to get used to being uncomfortable, unwashed, and tired.

Oh, well, I will send a postcard. I find that it will cost me 74 P for two stamps. Naturally, that must be paid in sterling. To exchange any money entails a fee of 2 pounds and they could only give me change in sterling again, so once again I heard: "I am terribly sorry about that, but I am awfully afraid there is nothing I can do that would make it worth that much of a pinch." I addressed one card and put an airmail sticker where the stamp should be to see how close the surveillance is in Her Majesty's Royal Mail. It arrived flawlessly. This is a considerably better record than previous cards sent with the 74 P stamps.

Fatigue was overcoming me, so I found a row of seats together off the beaten path and lay out across from two other lost souls snoring nearby. I tried to find a seat next to an electrical outlet to charge up my portable PC batteries. Charged batteries will allow me to write some part of this experience on the long haul across the whole Dark Continent. I assembled four adapters to get me into the electrical power here. The first two outlets had no power in them. Finally, exhausted, I just spread out and tried to take a brief nap. My residency training in surgery had taught me to sleep whenever and wherever I could. Unfortunately, a group of middle European immigrants came in with several kids. They all were carrying on in a language I do not believe I have ever heard. So, I got up, shaved in the loo, and found a working outlet to charge my computer batteries and began writing. I will see if I can get to bang away on the primary work I had planned to do when I was not 7 hours jet-lagged and needing catch-up sleep in this Noah's Ark of a zoo.

AND NOW, ALOFT OVER THE LENGTH OF AFRICA

With a freshened battery in the computer and a slightly less refreshed author at his usual altitude of 30,000 feet over trackless lands in moonlight, I am winging away, again into Africa. What number trip would this be? I have made nearly annual excursions into and through Africa since my first arrival on my birthday in 1968, now thirty years ago. As always, the familiar tingle of anticipation makes this flight feel like a homecoming. My first flight was in a BOAC VC-10. Neither the company nor the aircraft are flying any more, but neither is the Pan Am of my next several trips. I had made my first transatlantic flight to the Old World, visiting the half-millennium-old imperial capitals of Portugal and Spain to explore their early records of African coastal cruising. I then visited Rome before catching the BOAC flight destined for Kano in the Nigerian north. We never made it to Kano, since the harmattan had blotted out visibility with wind-blown Sahara sand, so we had to overfly it to land in Lagos, then the port capital of Nigeria.

Except for the costly civil war focused in Biafra province, in 1968, Nigeria appeared poised to prosper. Nigeria is the most populous African nation. It had an educated population relative to most other new states. Its farmers grew abundant crops and large deposits of oil had been recently discovered and were being developed. Nevertheless, I learned first hand what this transition into what passed for African modernity meant. I was "wawaed" in Lagos airport for three days before finally getting to Kano, where I was awaited by the pilot of the single engine bush plane that would take me farther into the interior of Nigeria's Benue River State. I worked for four months in 1968 in a remote mission hospital, an experience that influenced much of my life and career. I heard the term WAWA many times in the Lagos airport, in trying to make alternate arrangements to continue my journey, but did not ask for translation. When I finally *did* arrive in Kano three days late, the bush pilot, Ray Browneye, waved off my explanatory apologies: "It is just WAWA." he smiled.

"What's that?" I asked.

"West Africa Wins Again!" he responded cheerfully.

So, this African entry marks my graduation from my third decade in experiencing this continent. I learned up front what I would need to know later;

namely, things never unfold precisely as planned. The single requirement for my international excursions and medical adventures in the African bush is simple: have an infinitely high threshold for tolerance of frustration. This is said to be an era of modernity. On my first African entry, thirty years ago, I had paused to reflect on the half-millennium of exploration beginning in Iberia, and the two millennia of Roman civilization, and now I would deplane from the jet age into a continent where pockets of the Bronze Age were contemporary. I developed the habit of viewing people with a question in my mind. I didn't wonder what language do they speak, what religion do they follow, or what nationality do they claim? Instead, I wondered what century are they living in?

So I welcomed myself, once again, to the heart of Africa. Let's see what surprises are in store for me on this incursion to begin my fourth decade of visits. I'm ready and eager to have at it. Come on along; I am ready if you are.

2 SOUTH AFRICA

FROM JOHANNESBURG TO NAIROBI OVER THE GREAT RIFT

July 4, 1998

MY ARRIVAL AND BRIEF STAY IN JO'BURG AND RIEPAN PARK

In 1986, I made my first visit to South Africa as an honored James IVtth Surgical Association Scholar, awarded by a group of surgical leaders from the English-speaking world. Gordon and Maeve Hersman hosted me during part of my initial visit at the University of the Witwatersrand (affectionately known as "Wits" throughout South Africa). Gordon was a surgeon at Hillbrow Hospital, and Maeve was the administrator of the Department of Medicine at Wits. Gordon is a talented painter and playwright in addition to his surgical skills. His many portraits made their home one of the more interesting galleries I had visited in South Africa. I visited the Hersmans each subsequent visit to Jo'burg, and especially during my last extended visit as Senior Fulbright Scholar for Africa in 1996, when I had visited them regularly for half of the year. They had been preparing for a transition in going to work in Abu Dhabi the following year. Before this 1998 trip, I heard from mutual friends that they had returned from the Middle East to South Africa and purchased a new apartment in Riepan Park. I had arranged through fax, post and e-mail (only one of the three typically makes it through) to visit them upon my arrival in Jo'burg at the beginning and near the end of my current African mission.

I should also tell a story about Gordon's application of his artistic talents. On one occasion he had said to me: "Whilst you are making up your mind on whether you are willing to take the chair of surgery at Wits, I will do your portrait in oils to prepare it to hang along the hall where the other prior chairmen are so honored." I was flattered but was not certain he was serious.

We spent long evenings talking about many things, but prominent among them were the insatiable appetite among South Africans of that era for stories about my travels through other parts of Africa. Back then, the apartheid government of South Africa was isolated and its citizens were forbidden to visit other parts of black Africa. This isolation fed a curiosity for reports of other parts of Africa that were off limits to them and which were familiar to me from repeated visits.

Gordon had taken a few photographs of me while we were strolling through the garden in their previous home in Parktown "to get the eyes right," but I had not thought more of it until one day when a visitor came calling at my GWU office. Students surrounded me at the time, and they watched as I unrolled the canvas with the oil portrait sent to me as a gift by the Hersmans. It portrays me posed in front of a map of all Africa, not just of South Africa, with a bookcase in which I can even recognize the spines of my own surgical books as well as those of prior African explorers and heroes of mine such as Richard Burton and David Livingstone. The students immediately said, "It must be hung along the portrait walls of the GWU School of Medicine's Himmelfarb Library!"

I responded "Don't you have to be dead first before they hang your portrait in that group? (I was remembering the *Time* magazine cover portrait of GWU alumnus Dr. Paul Carlson, a medical volunteer killed in the Congo.) But for the honor, I really would rather keep going for a while longer!"

I was eager to revisit the Hersmans to catch up on their lives. I wanted to compare notes on Abu Dhabi, on which I coached them from many visits before they went there, and to hear about their reactions to return to Jo'burg in the era of a change brought about by the new government. I arrived in Jo'burg at mid-morning, and went into a bustle of activity, stopping first to buy a few rands and some stamps, use the mail, and attend to some details of rearranging flights. I had begun traveling from Maryland in mid-afternoon and now arrived in mid-morning two days later, adding the eastbound 9 hours to the new time zone. If this is not disorienting enough, the further transition from mid-summer to mid-winter in the antipodes should muddle one's mind further than jet lag and sleeplessness already have. But, in this dizzy state, I had to begin making calculations, connections, and transitions.

As I attended to my errands, I noticed a sign: *SHOWERS AVAILABLE TO INTERNATIONAL PASSENGERS ONLY*. Wonderful! I ducked in. It turns out a fellow named Enoch was standing guard with his African Zionist Church badge in place as he blocked access to a locked shower stall. Now, I do not know if "Enoch walked with God" but, more like Peter, he was the keeper of the keys, so I arranged with him to get it unlocked. There were only two things missing—soap and a towel—each elements I have found to be somewhat useful in showers

I have taken in the past, so I cut a deal with Enoch. He found a towel—used—but this is Africa, and one can never be too fussy. I found fragments of soap trapped in the drain filter and washed as well as possible. Then I stood in the hot water as long as I could, as a substitute for two missed nights without a bed or shower—reminding me of my days in surgical training.

I then tidied up at the sink—where a sign urged: *SOUTH AFRICAN WATER IS PRECIOUS-DO NOT WASTE IT.* I did not. But I was relieved that it did not say what the sign said in the Heathrow loo, in which I had last shaved and cleaned up and drunk a fair amount of it—to see the sign on leaving: *NO DRINKING WATER.* Sigh—what an irony! If I come down with some gastrointestinal crud, I will know it is a disease from the underdevelopment of Heathrow Terminal Four rather than the cholera for which the warnings are now being issued for the whole of eastern region of the Democratic Republic of the Congo (DRC).

After I finished these ablutions and details regarding my return arrangements, I walked out into the bright cold winter sun, adding my sweater made by my sister Martheen to my less than elegant outfit. I hailed a taxi, which for 125 rand (about $20.00) brought me past my 1996 Wits flat for sentimental reasons, and delivered me to Wits Medical School. I made my way along the long corridors of Jo'burg General which were familiar to me, to the Trauma Ward, where I recognized Lynette, the secretary, who said that Gordon had been looking for me but had gone home already.

We called him at home and I went down to see Maeve who is in a temporary office called the "Internal Truth and Reconciliation Council" for Jo'burg General, which unlike the "temporary TRC," headed by Bishop Desmond Tutu, did *not* get an extension on life beyond its two month office. These Councils are designed to exorcise apartheid, but they also lead to the airing of grievances and the public humiliation of many people, some of whom were officials of the former government. Dredging up all the evils of apartheid also has the added benefit of giving a smoke-and-mirrors distraction from the major evils of the day in postapartheid South Africa.

I heard plenty of gossip about a number of academic scandals, especially about the head of University of Venda, a black professor with a Ph.D. from Yale University. As it was told to me, this degree was revoked because it was founded on a thesis that was plagiarized. I was told that he had packed the university with cronies and spent more than all of the collective departments' salaries in personal global travel and perks, while accusing everyone around him of racial prejudice. It was reported to me that he had essentially been selling degrees to applicants based on race since taking office. He was also accused of firing, demoting or relieving of salary all who opposed or even questioned him.

A black editor asked in the newspaper, if the recent South African revolution was not designed to eliminate pass laws (which he had essentially reinstated, except that the color was reversed), special privilege, and cronyism. The injustices appear to be scandalously like the corruption and insider deals of all the rest of Africa. I didn't hear any hard facts to back up this gossip but didn't have any reason to doubt it either.

ACADEMIC SCANDALS AND RACIAL TENSIONS

Fierce debates are raging at Wits regarding the postapartheid control of medical institutions. Now, Lewis Levian, holding the prestigious title of the Chairman of Wits Surgery Department, is resigning this month. The vacant chair will be filled by one of two black candidates. It is difficult to find good candidates from the applicant pool of those who had been suppressed, and some have presented curriculum vitae that are, shall we say charitably, enhanced. Some of the newly promoted leaders are amazed to learn that the electric power would be turned off at their private homes since they had not paid utility bills. Why should they pay now, in this postapartheid era? Many had not paid before out of protest when they lived in Soweto. Their protests against the government (you remember, the apartheid government that was voted out of office some four years ago now) continue. One does not ever give up advantage easily obtained, and one never voluntarily relinquishes privilege. The Afrikaners claim to be the unique exception to this maxim. They voluntarily relinquished state control only when it became obvious that it was insupportable. So, there is nothing new in these aspects of Africa, from which "*Ex Africa semper aliquid novi*" is otherwise still true.

I have developed the habit of writing serial letters on aerogrammes that I can then post from a reliable postal system to family back home, to recollect this parallel track of recording these adventures. NASA refers to such back-up systems as "redundancy in depth." I have recorded adventure travels on audiotape, posted serial letters, and computer disc, transmitted by e-mail when possible. It has been helpful in the past when I have retained only one of these three parallel means of recording part of my experiences due to errant baggage, accidental or deliberate destruction of equipment, or theft. Three decades of exposure to "Africana" have made me not necessarily more cynical, but a wiser adventurer.

No one has received any of the packages of pictures, letters, books and goodies I have mailed here since the new government has been put in place. The postal service is getting to be every bit as good as the DRC's. More surprising is that Gordon's nomination of me for the Nobel Peace Prize did get submitted, although I do not know if the committee received it. Also, he received none of my dozen packages posted to Abu Dhabi. I tried to e-mail home to tell all I had arrived and forward the first chapter of this book. I will try to do the same for this message en route to Kenya if I can find a server somewhere between Nairobi and Nyankunde.

So, for now, I leave Southern Africa and go on into East Africa, while heading for Central Africa—and it is getting more and more African with each passing mile.

"MY MOVEMENTS" AS THE BRITICISM HAS IT FOR MY TRAVELS IN AFRICA

I hoped to be traveling exactly according to the itinerary I had prepared and sent forward to friends, colleagues, and family, many months ago. My schedule nearly came a cropper today, since I impressed the Hersmans that I was not nervous about being the requisite two hours ahead of any international check-in. Gordon said that they had the habit of "pitching up" about four to six hours in advance. I had no luggage since mine had been through checked and I am as casual about such affairs as anyone, so long as I have running room, and can catch the flight even when it is in motion already. Fine, said Gordon, "We will leave at 1:00 PM for your 2:15 PM flight." We did not get away until 1:30, and I "pitched up" at the counter of Kenya Airways (fortunately run by KLM!) after the flight had already closed at 2:00 PM. We managed to reopen it, and call down my numbers for the three bags that I discovered by reading the claim forms were 35 kg. That excess would be expensive at charges based on a total per nautical mile per kg when I check in at African Inland Mission (AIM) Air at Wilson Field, in Nairobi. I hope I will not have to pay more since they are already checked into the custody of Kenya Airways.

The KLM ground staff was reasonable in recognizing that if they held me up for the excess baggage surcharge at the Jo'burg gate, I would miss the flight altogether. It was in one way fortunate that I was late, since I have almost twice the 20 kg allowance, even without counting my three personal carry-on items—my only personal effects, including this laptop computer I am using to record these events. I borrowed a battery recharge from Gordon's house after making a Rube Goldberg extravagant contraption of every one of my adapters to get a rig that would finally trickle the electricity through all the step-downs and AC/DC conversions to make up for the battery that I flattened in flight. I did make it onto the plane to Nairobi with plenty of battery power in my ThinkPad even if somewhat short of a time cushion.

ORIENTATION

Go ahead, make my day! Ask me if I know where I am! Now I know, and can give it back to you with some precision, since I have learned how to reprogram my portable global positioning system (GPS). On arrival in Jo'burg, I could not raise a single satellite. I had to wait until I was on this Kenya Airways flight to play randomly with the device while sitting in a window seat. I was holding the antenna to the window at this mile-high elevation above the highveld when I discovered, more or less by accident, how to focus on the Southern Hemisphere, Africa, and then South Africa. Johannesburg is at 26° 68.93′ S, and 28° 14.96′ E exactly 8,117 miles on bearing 320° from home in Derwood, Maryland or 8,108 miles at bearing 320 ° from work at my GWU office at Ross Hall marked at the bust of George Washington by Foggy Bottom/GWU Metro station.

I need to practice shakedown runs of my GPS. I established many locations in North America that were important to me as I carried this new tool to "get my bearings" in Africa. Precision location has become important to me, and is nowhere as critical as in Africa. I can not rely on maps, signs, or local landmarks very often since much of this continent is covered in a trackless bush. Where I happen to be at any time can make the difference between working where I am needed or intruding into a neighboring war.

It is unlikely that a glance around any unfamiliar jungle at any time could orient the unaided nonresident. In the Congolese rainy season, even the equatorial sun can not be clearly seen. The bush often has a mind-numbing sameness. It is easy to get lost there. The droll Peter Tetlow (a guide for the later safari in Zambia) was fond of saying colorfully, "Look! That's Africa! Miles and miles of bloody fuck-all."

So, with practice, it is possible to determine your exact location on earth, wherever you happen to be. I am currently flying over Lake Victoria. Richard Burton, the nineteenth-century British explorer, never had such an aid to his European discovery of this body of water in his successful identification (with Speke) of the long-sought source of the mysterious Nile. I will need this device when I am tramping along in the 15-foot high elephant grass at this height of the rainy season in the depths of the rainforest's darkness. So, I might stay somewhat less lost than I sometimes am even in such remote and landmarkless places as Assa in the heart of the Congo. My GPS will give me a precise localization of where it is that I am lost! Remind me to record home in Assa when I get there. I am over Zambia now, looking down on areas where I will be tramping late in July, on holiday safari, following my work in Central Africa on the far side of the Great Rift Valley that is now visible along its escarpment below.

OFF TO NAIROBI, AMID THE PARTY ABOUT ME

I wanted to work to avoid the monotony of the flight but was foiled by the party atmosphere of this flight. The overweight and sumptuously gowned women of the nouveau African upper class around me were rapidly becoming drunk and disorderly. They had had at the Duty Free and liquor trolley until they were hooting with laughter and singing drunken songs interchanging English and Kiswahili words with snores and slurs, while dumping the contents of their glasses over the aisle in my direction. Concentration was impossible, so I switched off my machines and watched the abrupt falling curtain of equatorial sunset. It seemed early, but on the equator, equinox is perpetual.

I have celebrated the last several (American) Independence Days in interesting ways, typically at some altitude almost as high as I am now. In 1996 it was the summit of Mt. Kilimanjaro. In 1997, it was the summit of Mt. Rainier on the glacial ice slopes and then into the icy volcanic cone. This year it is over the Great Rift Valley right at the equator. Many of the other passengers on this raucous flight got a little higher than I did on this holiday. Undaunted, I am pressing on, leaving South Africa for Kenya, heading toward the rainforests of the Congo.

3 KENYA

EAST AFRICAN ARRIVAL AS I CONSOLIDATE AND PREPARE FOR THE CONGO

July 4-6, 1998

I arrived in Nairobi and made it through both Kenyan customs and the bank to exchange money. I bought Kenyan stamps because the Kenyan post is the one to be used for the serial letters and cards from my Congolese outpost. Finally, I struggled through the queue of taxi drivers and phalanx of touts.

I looked around and did not see Rufus, who is the driver the African Inland Mission (AIM) often uses. I hired a driver who turned out to be a real go-getter named Allen Njenga (the name means "cracked, broken maize," similar to the "mealie pop" that I had for breakfast this morning). I received 2,700 KS for a US $50.00 traveler's check, so I was surprised to hear that the ride to AIM's Mayfield Guest House would cost me 1,100 KS. I learned a lot from Allen Njenga, about his warrior group of Kikuyu tribes who lived along the Navasha Road who cut their teeth battling the nomadic Masai for the land that they then settled. I also learned that the world-class Kenyan runners went out to the Ngong Hills out in the Karen District, where the air is less polluted and another 1,000 feet higher and thinner than Nairobi. I resolved to try to go 18 km out the Ngong Road tomorrow morning for a long run, hoping that some of the strengths of the world-class Kenyan distance runners will rub off on me.

I paid Allen and told him that if anyone is around who wants to do an afternoon safari, I will volunteer as an amateur guide. If not, I may just call up Allen and arrange my own. I met Debbie Wolcott, who was managing the desk at the Mayfield Guest House with her husband Steve. There was a note on the board assigning me to Room #6 for the next two nights and even confirming the reservation for July 24 upon my return from Assa. She knew about my interests in goiter management. As soon as I mentioned Assa, she said, "Steve told me that Assa was just hit again last week."

I said that they had been stripped bare according to my reading of a report from a few months ago, and she said they had been plundered again. Mawa was the nurse who was there at my last visit, but he is gone now. Inikpio is back there with his nurse-wife Tasamu, after advanced anesthetist training in Centre Médical Évangélique (CME) in Nyankunde, DRC. If they are trying to work after being pillaged again, it is a good thing I have brought all the materials I could carry, all 35 kg of drugs and instruments.

When I went through Kenyan Customs, I was courteous to the inspector. He thought I was with the High Commissioner, when I had mentioned the mission, and he had waved me through, even before I could take out the bill of lading and packing slip for the antibiotics and other drugs. So, I now have heard that Steve Wolcott had just returned from Bunia, so I will look for him tomorrow for more news after arrival and repacking. I have only the infamous Congolese border crossing at Bunia to decimate my stock of *matériel* brought along. I plan on leaving a few things in "left luggage" that I do not want stolen before I get a chance to use them in my safari through Zimbabwe and Zambia. I am leaving two thirds of my film so as not to draw the curiosity of the Bunia bloodsuckers in "customs." I will leave the few clothes that I will need on my Zambian vacation safari and in Umtata, Transkei in South Africa where I will be evaluating a surgical training program. Maybe I will even have something to wear home after all this is done.

BEARINGS IN NAIROBI, ORIENTING TOWARD ASSA

I am now in Nairobi, along the Great Rift Valley, in the Thika Highlands just below the equator. I have stepped outside at midnight, out behind my Room #6 in Mayfield Guest House, so as not to arouse the suspicions of the guards posted out in front, and raised four satellites at the equator to fix my bearings here in what is now landmarked as "NAIR." I am at 01° 17.88′ S and 036° 48.18′ E, which is 7,514 nautical miles from home on bearing 342°. My actual distance covered is more like 2.5 times that distance in the flights I took from Dulles Airport near home via Europe and South Africa to Nairobi. I calculated distances and bearings to other locations already stored in my GPS.

NOW, ABOUT THE ORIENTATION TO ASSA IN THE CONGO, MY ULTIMATE DESTINATION

I used the bearings and landmarked the readings I had taken off the Cessna's GPS on one of my earlier flights into Assa in the Congo. This was one of my first exposures to the GPS and its potential for what it could mean in orienteering on ground level. I had the longitude and latitude plugged in for the airstrip below the house at Assa. Using that landmark as "ASSA," I can now explain that in Nairobi, I am almost due east of Assa, and it is just above the equator by about as much as I am now below it. In more precise terms, I read off the GPS that I am 850 nautical miles from Assa at NAIR toward which I must head on bearing 299°.

The single engine aircraft I will be chartering does not go quite as fast as the airliners that delivered me to Heathrow, Jo'burg, and then Nairobi. I will not be able to go directly to Assa since the flight plan filed with Wilson Field air controllers must follow a few rules on the navigation over Nairobi and around military restrictions toward the west without entering the disputed airspace around Uganda. Who knows what new and changing restrictions apply for the paranoid people of the Kabila military government of the ironically named Democratic Republic of the Congo? This is Zaïre's new name. I will abbreviate the name changes as "the DRC" or "the Congo" for simplicity. Kabila closed all airfields except for military operations as recently as last month. That may change even while I am in the air.

Further, we have to go into Bunia to clear their extortion called "customs formalities." In preparation for customs, I am repacking here in Mayfield Guest House. Most of my film and the computer case will be kept here in "left luggage" for my July 24 return overnight before flying out of Nairobi to Harare.

I will use my GPS to keep me oriented while trekking around in the Congo, through elephant grass. This can hide all manner of ill-tempered creatures that have sophisticated olfactory capabilities. Cape buffalo are the worst threat. Elephants, and further down the list, carnivores such as the big cats and the hyenas, are also a concern. So, it will be important to have precise orienteering data for such landmarks. I will mark ZALA, the waterhole in the middle of an immense swamp at this time in the rainy season.

This would be my seventh trip to Assa, but the first time carrying this additional orienteering device. I hope I can continue to use the GPS and put it through its paces for purposes beyond telling you how far away I happen to be on what bearing. I will need to know how far I am from the front door of whatever is left at Assa's station when I am trekking through the deep "Green Hell" described in the *Heart of Darkness*. Who knows, I may even need to find my way back from the Congo through Banda, Bunia, all the way back to Nairobi! My GPS would be more than handy then.

The first thing I heard from Debbie Wolcott when she heard I was going to Assa, was that "Assa was hit again last week and stripped bare." Steve had just returned from Bunia with news that another mission station at Nepopo had been sacked and destroyed. Who knows what I will encounter in Assa, where

15

Mawa had been working as a nurse and Inikpio and Tasamu had just returned from CME-Nyankunde, now probably with no equipment or even basic supplies. And Bunia, here I come, a walking extortion target loaded with the supplies that may not even have to go so far as Assa to be looted and plundered!

Well, we will see how far I get and what I have after I get through whatever other barriers they plan to throw up in my way. I have just repacked the *"apparat"* they were so eager to find last time, when the film made them smell camera and the AC adapter made them search desperately for this very computer. *"Ou est l'apparat?"* they kept asking repeatedly. I may have passed the French exams as part of my now-stalled Ph.D. dissertation work, but I was completely unable to understand what they meant or what they were after!

[Editors Note: The following information arrived about a week after Glenn left for Africa. He had up-dated his will and gave me documents transferring his interests in Three Hawks Publishing, LC to his estate. He had dinner at my house the night before flying out to the Congo. I took him to Dulles Airport for his outbound flight and had an eerie sense that he was flying off into fatal danger. I gave him a manly hug and told him to be careful. I was already missing him and wondering how he was making out when the following arrived via e-mail.]

CONTACT POINTS AND NUMBERS
FOR INTERCEPT ALONG MY AFRICAN SAFARI

July 5-6, 1998

MAYFIELD GUEST HOUSE, NAIROBI, KENYA

Tomorrow, I go from Wilson Field (General Aviation) by AIM Air charter from Kenya into the Congo. After I pass through Bunia to Nyankunde, on July 7, I leave by MAF charter into remote Zandeland, and will be incommunicado for the next three weeks in the central Heart of Darkness. I should emerge, it is hoped, therefrom with a return via CME (Centre Médical Évangélique, which apparently has just got a phone for the first time and a fax, which may even work, but is hardly to be counted on). I will back up through the same channel through which I entered. This gives several potential points of contact, and I am listing them here, if needed, and the dates that would be the "windows" at which I might intercept any message so delivered. I will also list a series of potential e-mail addresses for folk who might wish to have such information or who might have a need to reach me for some reason whether or not a response is expected.

[Editor's Note: I have moved the rest of the particulars to Appendix 1. The potential contacts and requests for e-mail forwarding amounted to two pages. I wondered if this was really all necessary and worried a bit about the potential dangers of this trip. Glenn ended his message with what follows.]

Thank You! And Cheers, before my disappearance from the ether net incommunicado in the Congo's Heart of Darkness! I have heard a lot about those who have "gone missing" recently along similar routes into conditions of instability, filled with unknowns. If you don't hear from me again, at least after a month or more, you will know that I went missing somewhere near one of these locations from which I have last signed out.

GWG

4 TO THE CONGO

FINAL PREPEARATIONS FOR THE "NEW" CONGO

July 6, 1998

And, now, I am underway toward my "destination travel"—the Heart of the Congo here I come! Move over, Marlowe, and "Pass the Bottle!" This is *the* signature line of one of the greatest novels in English literature (written by a Polish immigrant who had not learned the English language until age 40). It marks a break in the story, with this transition in the tale. In my case, it would be more like the situation would have been if the agent Kurtz himself were getting back to where he belongs. Or, to update this from Joseph Conrad's time, it is like the quote from one of New York City Fire Department's finest: "My job is to run into a burning building every other sane person has been running out of."

MY LAST COMMUNIQUÉ FROM MAYFIELD HOUSE

I have spent the entire day in the Mayfield Guest House, sorting film, tapes, serial letters and other mailings, and typing a list of contact points along my journey. I wanted to e-mail this information home. I packed my bag to look very down-market to reinforce reality. After all, I am a visiting professor with nothing really worth stealing. I packed the computer and the camera equipment and stuffed them into a cloth bag with a lunch on top. The computer carry-on case is going into "left luggage" along with almost everything that looks like it was bought for more than 10 dollars and worth more than 5 dollars now. That leaves the troublesome matter of a lot of surgical instruments and medicine where the "Professeur's Rolex" should have been. Although not precisely understood by customs agents, these supplies could be used for maximum profit on a smaller number of people, all of them forthcoming for this distinction on the Bunia airstrip. None of them have ever been salaried, by either the new or the old government. The purpose for bribing someone to get this unpaid and unpleasant "civil service" job, is the same as that which comes from many American lawyers. It is a license to eat what you kill!

I walked the grimy streets of Nairobi with the smoke-belching buses and grit-throwing lorries along the roadways crowded with pedestrians and *matatus* very close together and each heedless of the other. Trash is piled around. Some young men come with an obsequious bow, with hands outstretched and a smile. The smile turns to a scowl when I wave off their begging. They are all certainly dressed better than I look. They can apparently see through my disguise of the clothes that I have taken on their one-way trip to Africa.

I went to get a photocopy made in a back alley, and posted my letters in the Yaya Center's Post Office. I remembered where the office of the Medical Assistance Program, Inc. (MAP) was and walked to it. The guard unlocked the gate saying there *was* someone up there and to just tap on the office door. There was, but the curtain stayed drawn, and after I rang the bell, I made a note on the back of my card saying I had stopped to call, and that I was carrying into remote Zandeland the MAP Travel Paks with a complete MASH unit of supplies for these plundered peoples. I remembered that when I had trekked around Nairobi on foot, I had traveled all the way out Ardwing Kodhek Road to the Mission Aviation Fellowship (MAF) office to send e-mails. As I now recall, this effort failed at that time. I forgot how far it was (or was I younger then?) but arrived a few miles farther than I had recalled.

I checked around the building in the back and tapped on the MAF door. A young and pretty woman came to the door, presumably the MAF pilot's wife. The MAF pilot himself appeared later to eye me suspiciously, since his wife seemed to want to be too enthusiastic in her help. She accompanied me to a few of the other buildings where the occupants were out. Her name, I learned later, was Eloisa Stohl. She said, "Yes, this was the building that had housed the e-mail office, but that was two years ago and now it is just my home."

MAF had built an office in a hangar at Wilson Field. She suggested that I might check there about the disc I was carrying in my pocket prior to the next morning's flight. Right! Walk around the Kenyan officials at 6:30 AM with messages to give a heads-up alert to the folk at CME Nyankunde that I had some highly valuable cargo that I might need help getting through Congolese customs at Bunia. The Kenyans could easily relieve me of the worry of having something too valuable on the plane. I thanked her, and walked all the way back to Mayfield with the disc still in my pocket.

On arrival at Mayfield, I still wanted to send my e-mail. I found a woman from Edinburg named Georgi Orme and asked for her help. She said she did not know how to do that but that there was another woman there who knew about such matters. Unfortunately, she did not know her name and therefore was unable to introduce me to the technologically savvy potential helper. Georgi said to me, "You Americans have a way of just walking up to someone you don't know, so why don't you do that, then I will know her too!"

I soon introduced myself to Linda Stryker a nurse midwife. She formerly worked in Mwanza in Tanzania. She had been in Bukavu, Congo, just last week. She was revisiting there after being evacuated because of civil unrest. She could instantly relate to the vagaries of the Congolese kleptocracy. We could not figure how to send messages to my entire list, but for the princely sum of 25 KS she could send a message to two of the addressees for forwarding to all the others. So, we picked two, and sent the list. While I was at it for the same 40 cents US, why not attach the chapters that I had already written? Within a twinkling, the files went winging to a Harvard colleague in Boston and my sister in Jenison, MI. I hoped that they would be forwarded to such as my protégé and recent GWU medical graduate, Eric Sarin, who was waiting to hear from me before starting out toward CME/Nyankunde to meet me. Maybe Kurt Johnson, my friend, editor, and world-traveler wannabe would need contacts where I might be reached with last minute details before he flew to Harare for our rendezvous in late July. We planned on going together on a vacation safari to Zambia. I also sent the message to a lot of people who wanted to know what I was doing. I could recall some of their e-mail addresses from memory. Many may even be correct. I sent my last messages to them for where I would be until after I emerge from Zandeland, hoping that something would get through and that they would be able to open them.

I wondered if the rusting hulk of a Bronco remains in Assa. I hoped it might have a battery, if it is still there, battery and all, I might plug an adapter into its cigarette lighter to charge the ThinkPad. Even in its decrepit condition, the soldiers who raided Assa last week might steal it. With everything else they had to carry, they could even load up the Bronco, and, if necessary, push it! I will soon head into the unknown on westward flights toward Assa, around the vast Ituri Rainforest. Hitch along for the ride. It is a less hazardous adventure for you, the hitchhiker in retrospect, than for me, the real life, real time traveler!

OVER THE GREAT RIFT TYPING FROM THE COPILOT'S SEAT

Good afternoon! After loading the medical supplies and my luggage into a charter plane (**Figure 1**), we left Nairobi, but not uneventfully. We are now flying over the Rift Valley of Africa at 01° 16.98′ S and 036° 27.46′ E (**Figure 2**). The Rift is the large chasm that just opened beneath our plane, "Echo Alpha One Alpha" Stationair. Mt. Sutra looms ahead. Below me now I see red-robed Masai in their acacia thorn *manyattas*, and a large volcanic cone up ahead in this geological sunderance.

I am now looking down some 500 feet, a small comfort. Earlier, we were at 200 feet and even down to 50 feet above those same thorny umbrella trees, too close by any measure. We were forced to fly under an opaque ceiling of clouds because we are in a Visual Flying Rules (VFR) situation where we need to see to fly. So much so, in fact, that when we were at Wilson Field early this morning, they required us to remain and see whether visibility improved. The delay was all right with me, since we were picking up one more passenger. The plane was already dangerously close to overload with me and my 67 kg of medical freight. I am allowed 20 kg and am surcharged for the extra 47 kg, an amount equivalent to an extra passenger's fare, which I already paid. This new passenger is a 54-kg Congolese linguistic informant for the Summer Institute of Linguistics (SIL) of the Wycliffe Bible Translators. A pair of SIL folk accompanied him to Wilson Field, one of whom was named Rob McKee, an expert in Congolese linguistics. I was eager to have a chat with him, looking for information that might facilitate my own linguistic work.

Rob had heard of my medical and linguistic efforts far afield at the remote Assa station in Zandeland. He earned his Ph.D. in anthropology from the University of Rochester with a dissertation entitled *Death Rituals and the Role of Languages*. He promised to send me some information on it and I will send him an outline of my dissertation proposal.

In conversation with Rob, I also dropped the name of Richard Grinker. He was involved in Harvard's Ituri Project studying the Lhese people. Rob had visited Grinker at the Ituri Project. Grinker had been working with a Korean psychiatrist, now his wife, and he had given Rob a copy of his book *Houses in the Rainforest*, because of their common interests in the Lhese people. Richard went to Rochester for an interview to get a faculty job and Rob took him to dinner. At about the same time, Richard had come to GWU and interviewed for a job, fresh from his first post-Harvard appointment at Carlton College. I attended Grinker's seminar before his appointment at GWU as a now full-time colleague of mine. I will carry a letter from Rob back to Grinker in doing some anthropological networking here.

As we chatted, suddenly the sky cleared. Our enjoyable conversation ended abruptly when the tower called us. We were instructed to take-off quickly, which we did. I strapped into the copilot's seat next to a handsome young Dutch MAF pilot named Fromme. The Congolese passenger and the precious medical cargo were in back. I had my trusty GPS in hand figuring the location of the "WILS" and the "RIFT" headed toward the Lake "VICT."

ABORT THE MISSION ON THE FIRST TRY

We took off from Wilson Field, overflying Nairobi National Park, but quickly flew into weather. We bobbed and weaved around low hanging clouds. We had to clear 6,200-foot mountains, but could not go above 6,000 feet. We corkscrewed around for 30 minutes. It looked like we were going to be scraping acacia thorns, so the pilot decided to abort the mission. It was left to me to explain to our Congolese linguistic informant that we were going to be landing in Nairobi again—a process that he understood less well even than my bad French or worse Bangala.

For an hour we waited looking at old *National Geographics*. Then I wrote one of my serial letters. Without much visible change in the weather, we tried again. Fromme is a nice guy who is stationed in Nairobi because his 8-year-old son has a serious medical condition. Thus, the family could not be in the Congo where any potential problem, for which he would need anything more sophisticated than a Band-Aid, would be untreatable.

On the second take-off, I pulled out my ThinkPad as soon as I saw more than 100 feet of air beneath us. The flight would take nearly all of the 3.75 hours we had programmed, particularly if we have another "go" at it *"la deuxieme fois."* I saw an empty cigarette lighter socket in the cockpit dash ahead of me and pulled out my new "1-800-BATTERY" D/C adapter charger, and *mirabile dictu*! It works! So, I am in an aircraft that only weighs 740 kg empty, but has more conveniences for me than the 747s that brought me along this far. I do have to prop my ThinkPad up on the steering yoke of the plane and avoid kicking the ailerons, while still periodically making notes on the avionics.

With the opening up of the Rift Valley and a drop-off beneath us making up for what we could not get by going up, we made a "carrier take-off." I noted landmarks on my GPS in this long and bouncy flight. I also did a few calculations on the GPS, now programmed with reference to Uganda, with the hope that we would not be landing in Entebbe, at least today. I had called and notified the people who should be meeting us that I may need help in Bunia with the claims they are going to make against me for the medicines and instruments I am carrying. I hoped that I had alerted the "good guys" without giving a "heads up" to the "bad guys."

Well, we will all just be able to see and find out later, what is at the end of this (not yellow brick road, but) bouncy cloudy fluff between (one form of) the Promised Land and us. After all, I had promised that I would be coming.

OVER GREAT LAKE VICTORIA

My wonder machine, the hand-held GPS, and my faithful (when charged up) ThinkPad are working so well in this flight that I am getting worried. Both have a tendency to attract a crowd, since they are very portable pieces of the developed world, and we "sure would wannabe just like you—perhaps seizing these will help!" It is not enough that I am transporting at my own expense a highly valuable gift to people who have been plundered, it is not just the plundered who are anxiously waiting for me in hopeful lip-smacking anticipation—so are their plunderers.

In my imagination, the border guard would say, "Sure, you have come to help people, and here right now in front of you is the first and foremost person you are here to help. I have no salary, but I do have a position obtained by expensive bribery. I can wield arbitrary and capricious power over fat cats like you, who are sent to me like a perfectly done standing rib roast set before a starving man, perfectly ready for immediate consumption."

FOCUS ON THE REAL CONGOLESE

These are thoughts about what may yet be coming. Rather than worrying about having my tools stolen by Congolese customs in Bunia, it was easier for me to look down and see the native fishermen. They are plying the waters of this great Lake Victoria. They are just trying to wrest some kind of living out of diminishing resources. These people are a better prototype of the Congolese. The ordinary folk of the Congo are the first and foremost victims of officialdom, waiting for me to recognize their firstness and foremostness.

Now I will tuck away my toys. I will hide them as best as I can until they too are discovered and raise the price for my entry, not just in dollars, but in the effort expended. "The cost of doing business" is how they see it, and that business, as I see it, is "life, on the run, on the margin."

5 ARRIVAL IN THE CONGO

THROUGH BUNIA RIPOFFS TO NYANKUNDE, NEWS FROM THE ASSA FRONT

July 6, 1998

I am here, and furthermore. I am on my way. After the second try, we got through the clouds. over the Rift. and crossed Lake Victoria. I happily typed my last message. dropped my GPS and computer into my bag. and covered them with a sweatshirt. I arrived in the (now militarized) Bunia Airport as the sole subject of customs scrutiny. There were no other planes there. The officials were waiting for me. They were cheered by my arrival. more so when they saw the big boxes and full suitcase. So intent were they on the wonders that emerged from the boxes that they never did find the carry-on bag. So. the good news is that my computer, cameras. and even the GPS made it in. Best of all. I did not have to ransom them twice over.

"You are a surgeon, right?" was the border guard's question. once translated. I speak no French at all for customs office purposes, remember? "And what might these be for?" was his next question. My camouflage hat, shorts, and shirt were immediately confiscated with an official stamped letter which stated my misdeeds in trying to import military *matériel*. Then the carefully-packed boxes of medical supplies were split open. The great gold embossed seal on the packing slip was passed around and admired. The inspector brandished one after another drug packet, asking, "What is this for?"

I told them a lot of stories I made up in English, and listened to their (sometimes funny) translation into French or native languages. I kept the precious antimalarial drugs, more valuable than gold, in my computer "lunch bag." They had lots of fun, and did figure out that I had valuables, although they had a real problem determining how much all this was worth. They especially liked the packing slip, since it had numbers with it, including various shipping charges, totaling $1350.00. This number was neatly doubled and *voilà*, they had the customs charge for importing a gift I have already paid for repeatedly.

While they continued discussing other ways to hold me up, they filled out countless forms, giving me the worthless carbon copies. I joked with them about my stupidity not knowing that they spoke some other language here, "I would have thought they spoke French in France, "*n'est ce pas?*" Fortunately, they never saw the color linguistics kit, which might blow that cover quickly. I had two interested pilots looking on, Tim from Bunia, who came to see me, alerted by the calls, and Fromme whose last trip this was before he goes back to Holland for his furlough.

I told Tim an estimate of the approximate value. He said the customs clerks would have to hit me up for some charges as well as some drug supplies, for "assay" no doubt. They filled out another fifteen minutes worth of forms (with carbons) and puzzled over all the English text with weird drug names on the bill of lading. Finally, they took the direct approach and asked how much US currency I had on me. The big man took most of it, officially stuffing it into one filthy shirt pocket. I interpreted the ransom I paid for the gift of free medical supplies to their poorest people as blood money for not finding my toys in the bag they never checked.

THE NEWS FROM ASSA

Lary Strietzel, the MAF pilot for the rest of the trip, flew over from Nyankunde as quickly as he could. I learned that my old friend and assistant Ahuka will not be coming to Assa with us as planned. Instead, Ahuka's friend Dr. Sonny Mwembo, a surgeon from Kisangani, will be his substitute. Ahuka left for South Africa this afternoon. He will return after I am gone into Zimbabwe, on July 27, when my student Eric Sarin should be in to help him. I also learned that last week, Assa was stripped bare by a marauding renegade band of Kabila's troops. So, MAF would not fly in there, and my friends in Assa fled into the bush. The troops ordered the local chief to dig his own grave, but he escaped into the bush when Kabila's mavericks got distracted.

And, now the better news. The distraction was the deployment of a second band of Kabila's regulars who apprehended and presumably killed the renegades. My friends in Assa (like Jean Marco and Inikpio perhaps?) have reappeared from the bush in time to send this news. They apparently know I am coming and they will try to be present to receive whatever medical supplies they can get from me. The one constant of all the coups and countercoups is that nothing looted from Assa had been returned.

This message was enough to reassure MAF pilot Lary so that he felt safe making the flight to Assa. He also needs an official medical examination before his FAA license expires in a few months. My credentials as an Aviation Medical Examiner give me an opportunity for an important service to Lary and the other MAF pilots. If I have any chance of getting to Assa, I had better do it ASAP, such as at 6:00 AM tomorrow as soon as there is enough light in Nyankunde. CME has been without power for three weeks. I will use the evening to pull the stuff together by the romance of candlelight and get moving. *Banzai!* Assa, here I come, *directement*.

IN THE CME GUEST HOUSE

I am in the CME Guest House, hosted by Antonio and Milly from Argentina. They have two young sons, Ezekiel and David. A steady diet of Spanish ("the language of heaven," say my Argentine friends) will ruin my ear for weeks for French, so that I will in fact speak and understand French almost as badly as I pretended in Bunia. My hosts are telling stories about Father Flanigan's visit here.

Kevin Flanigan is an ordained Franciscan priest who lived in a monastery in Washington DC while a student and resident at GWU School of Medicine. He is now a rising senior surgical resident. Dr. Joseph Giordano, GWU's current Chairman of Surgery, sent Kevin to me. Joe and I were colleagues through residency, rose together through the academic ranks, and are close friends. My stories about my African experiences (completed in 1996 while I was a Senior Fulbright Fellow) made Father Flanigan enthusiastic and curious about the continent.

When at the juncture in his surgical residency when he had the option of a year in the research laboratory, he asked if he could substitute instead a year of surgical mission work, since he would never be a test-tube researcher, given his background and future plans. So, we worked out the retracing of the steps I had taken in 1996, in Swaziland, Mozambique, and the Congo. During the time he spent at CME in 1997, the community was so devastated by the war and supplies were so depleted, that operations were infrequent. He spent considerable time at the CME Guest House, making himself useful, entertaining the children, and celebrating mass daily, in the tolerant hospitality of a Protestant mission station. Given the unpredictable and tense circumstances of the Congo, religious differences that have launched blood-baths elsewhere, seemed unimportant.

There is no electricity at CME tonight to recharge my computer batteries. There will be even less likelihood of electrical power 7.8 Cessna hours from here in my landfall in Assa tomorrow as I greet surviving returnees from internal exile as they re-emerge from the bush. So, I am signing this note off, and hope it can be relayed to those whom it may concern. I am on my way to where I am badly needed. What more can life offer anyone than this?

6 A NIGHT IN THE RAINFOREST

A NIGHT IN THE RAINFOREST IN RAINY SEASON, AN EARLY DEPARTURE FROM CME GUEST HOUSE, AND A "WEATHER WAIT" AT MAF HANGAR IN NYANKUNDE

July 7, 1998

I am here in the hangar of the Mission Aviation Fellowship (MAF) with aircraft maintenance workers. My computer sips gratefully from the wonderful electricity that their generator provides for their mechanical work. It was not easy marrying three adapters in series for a connection, but I am most happy to have this time and place to recharge what would have been an otherwise flattened battery. I had hoped to charge up at the Guest House, from which I would mail the last of my messages, and then shove off into the green mass of the Central African Rainforest. This is almost what happened.

IN SEARCH OF POWER

There has been no electricity in Nyankunde for the last three weeks. It usually has intermittent electricity from the hydroelectric generators run to power gold mines near the adjacent river. I arrived at dusk, a time when the sun sets with a definitive crash here on the equator, and was quickly in the dark. I was trying to repack the large medicine kits, ransacked in the inspection in Bunia. I also wanted to organize my papers for the onward travel, another light-dependent task. Candlelight may be very romantic, but is not quite efficient for this process.

The gang of my medical assistants and their "deputies" had gathered to speak to me and waited patiently in the dark on the porch. They were reluctant to disturb what would have been my dinner-time. As a last resort, we cranked up the Guest House generator. I got to sort out stuff quickly, most of which will go with us into Assa, the furthest spot reached by MAF in these parts, 5.8 Cessna air hours away on a direct line from our next stop, Nebobongo. I then typed up several e-mail messages that I figured I would send while the generator was cooking. The messages were intended to assure anyone interested that I was alive and well in Nyankunde, on my way into Assa, and would be passing back through CME according to plan within the next few weeks. On return to Nyankunde, I also planned to e-mail out the largest part of the manuscript for this book.

I know you are wondering why this nutcase is obsessed with communicating his deathless prose back to a wider, uncaring world. So what if everything he has carried and is generating gets ripped off and all plans go awry. This is Africa and that is SOP. It is true that this state of affairs is the rule and that is why these people are unknown to the outside world or forgotten in the first place. This communication link may be one of the first sustained to support concern, if not compassion. As much as I complain about getting, or expecting to be ripped off, I care about these isolated people in Zandeland. Many of them are friends of mine and they are all my patients. I have skills that they need and I intend to help them. When we graduated from medical school, all medical doctors took an oath to help people in need. Many have continued from that day forward in a comfortable career in the developed world in search of patients. The world is full of patients seeking help, but it is not always comfortable helping them, however rewarding otherwise. If anyone in health care tells me they are seeking more patients, I could tell them they might have a virtual corner on one of the world's largest growth industries—if only they are willing to go where the need is, and treat anyone, anywhere, without regard to payment for their services. My work in Assa is such an example of a moral obligation.

If I were to draw the most likely scenario of what would become of the computer, cameras, recorders or the media they are used to generate, it would be that they would be destroyed, lost, or stolen en route. If I can get to any working phone, functional post box, or outward bound traveler for hand delivery, I will try to download or deliver these messages back, whatever may become of the messenger, machines, and media later.

The phone at CME works only intermittently, but while it was working, for ten dollars, I sent some messages home. I will try to save files to a disc and to carry them back with me to the US Embassy in Nairobi, the only secure place in Central or East Africa for e-mailing or posting back to the US. *Never*, in all of my trying on many different consecutive visits, has any card or letter *ever* entrusted to a Congolese *boîte aux lettres* been delivered. Thus, all of the missionary personnel in the Congo have a Nairobi post-office box at AIM, and all messages are hand-carried by travelers such as I. I will e-mail what I have written so far from Nyankunde, if the phone is working, and post my saved discs from Nairobi before I move on to Southern Africa. Like the Cheshire cat's smile, the message may linger behind, even if the messenger disappears.

In the past, I have recharged computer batteries in the cigarette lighter socket in MAF aircraft. Unfortunately, an "Airworthiness Directive" had ordered the cigarette lighters removed from all MAF Cessnas. They were considered a fire hazard. Further, there has been radio silence from Assa since their storage battery went dead and we are going to have to carry a big battery, the heaviest piece of our freight. We may be forced to leave some items out to make room for it. Things do not look good for a power source in Assa for the computer, but we will see what can be improvised. It may be time for that solar power supply I have salivated over in the 1-800-BATTERY catalog.

It had been a long and busy day. I enjoyed some evening banter in Spanish with my CME host, whose e-mail address name is "Tony Africa." This must be the one of the more remote outposts of the *conquistadores*. I then went to bed by candlelight and even slept for a few hours.

SO, THIS IS WHAT IT IS LIKE TO BE IN THE RAINFOREST! HOW SOON WE FORGET!

About midnight, I saw what I thought were lights, but turned out to be lightning preceding a drenching downpour, the kind that cannot be seen through even *with* a light. Normally, the soft patter of rainfall makes for good sleeping when rain hits the pan roof. This rain was so hard that it sounded more like cannonade. I couldn't fall back into a sound sleep.

It rained very hard until 2:30 AM and then let up. Now bizarre changes overtook the compound. First, I heard the stridulation of the insects, and then the resonant calls of lovesick frogs. Then I felt large soft things falling on my head. I lit a candle and saw that it was raining large, fragile-winged termites. They popped out as if by magic, and were fluttering off on their one "big fling" in their mating flight before they crash and are destined from then on to be burrowing under ground. There must be a moral lesson, or at least an essay, in this metaphor of the high-flying life!

The recently-shed wings of these termites littered the floor. The now wingless termites were scurrying away, no longer quite so giddy after their "maidenhead flights" clipped their wings, bringing them to the crash-and-burn phase of their brief lives. I knew from my first exposure to these postdrought emergence phenomena when I had entered Nigeria and saw the coming of the rainy season, what follows the piling up of the insects under candlelight or lanterns. The toads and frogs who appear as if on cue following this same phenomenon lead to the slithering of snakes. The snakes can almost be heard in the dark in the next stage that reliably follows this froggy cornucopia.

A new weird phenomenon appeared to my inflamed imagination around 3:00 AM. I could see light on the ceiling! In the inky black night in the rainforest, the slightest glimmer seems remarkable. It turned out that this was no glimmer. Somehow, immediately following the rains, electricity returned to the CME, and I was seeing the reflections of lights left on when the power failed, weeks before! This is too precious to be wasted! I jumped up and wrote two cards and a serial letter, and tried to find a plug that might charge the computer battery. I did, and felt like I had accomplished all the goals of my brief stay in Nyankunde, and could go back to bed.

Unfortunately, just as I started to drift off again, there was a tumbling rush of sound from the birds, indicating dawn. I was supposed to be at the hangar before 7:00 AM. Great! I have nearly three hours to enjoy the birds and watch the arrival of another day.

In one way it is good that I have this weather delay. When I had stuffed the computer into my bag to hide it on approaching Bunia, I heard a "bleep" and looked to see that there were no indicator lights on. When I got it here, I discovered that the computer had been accidentally activated. The computer was dead as a mackerel in the Sahara, dead as any possum trying to cross any road. Its crucial battery was drained to zero. So, this quick charge delay gives me a brief power reprieve until I have to face this whole sequence again.

7 DRAMATIS PERSONAE

IN FLIGHT FROM NYANKUNDE, REFUELING AT NEBOBONGO, AND ON TO ASSA

July 7, 1998

I loitered over the generator in the MAF hangar to charge the batteries for the computer. The AC line was rigged to power a tape player. The tapes lay all around on the workbench in the disarray of tools, metal shavings, oily rags and spare parts for the aircraft being worked on by a couple of the MAF pilot/mechanics. This would be like almost any garage, with the pile of audiotapes, and faded posters on the walls, but for a qualitative difference apparent on a double take. The posters were not pinups but scripture verses. The tapes were hymns rather than honky-tonk music. There was no swearing at the obstinate, frozen, rusty bolt. As in all other duties, these dedicated folk have undertaken, avionics is the Lord's work. I felt like a bit of an infidel in unplugging the hymns for recharging secular batteries, when the music had so obviously been elevating the atmosphere of the workplace. While the charger trickled, I supervised loading the plane with the supplies for Assa while André and Sonny and their wives watched.

PROTÉGÉS OF THE LATE PAPA DIX

André ("the *dentiste*") and I had made the last excursion together in 1996 into Zandeland to Assa, Banda and Nebobongo. His is a remarkable story. It links the earliest history of the Zande "mission field" with the present indigenous principle players. A Butte, Nebraska farmboy named Earl Dix (called "Papa Dix" by the natives) had experienced a "call to missions" in the early part of this century, and advertised for a stout wife to accompany him. Within a week, he had packed up his worldly goods, including his trusted varmint rifle from the farm. He also carried a wealth of practical mechanical sense, learned the hard way by repairing farm equipment critical for harvest; and, lest we forget, yes, the wife, who had answered his ad as his "helpmate" in the fields. With all in tow, he sailed off to Africa. They set up a mission outpost on a hill in Banda, a remote Congolese village, and built a church, a school and a hospital, in that order.

Papa Dix befriended the local chief Sasa, whose grandson, Emmanuel, was recently elevated to that position and most recently was ordered to dig his own grave. Papa Dix impressed the natives. His hunting prowess became legendary. Once, using his small caliber varmint rifle, he dropped an elephant with one shot. While hunting at dusk for guinea-fowl for dinner, Earl felt a "presence" and turned to face a bull elephant. The giant raised his trunk with mouth gaping and trumpeted. Earl paused to say a prayer, aimed, and fired a single bullet through the roof of the elephant's mouth, into his brain, killing the huge beast instantly. His prayer, incredible aim, or dumb luck established him as a legendary hunter in Zandeland. He introduced motorized vehicles and kept them running. His devout piety, and his capacity to feed and organize a large mission community, also earned the respect of all those with whom he worked. His biography, part piety mixed with the brash bravado of anyone with the temerity to take on Africa for over half a century, is entitled *Earl Dix: Adventurer for God.*

Mrs. Dix survived Earl and the Simba Revolt that lead to Patrice Lumumba's rise to power and Congolese independence from Belgium in 1960. Many missionaries were killed during this period, among them GWU medical graduate Dr. Paul Carlson, shot as he tried to help other missionaries escape the rampaging, looting army that is a standard feature of African revolutions. Mrs. Dix had continued to work in Zandeland, having produced a prolific family of "MK's" (missionary kids), such that the name Dix is a common one in the mission community in the Congo.

Papa Dix identified young boys with high potential. He promised them that he would help them to improve their lives if they did their schoolwork, practiced religious devotion, and worked hard at the more practical side of supporting themselves and their community. He didn't let the boys know the entire truth about how they might benefit from some of the various projects he organized. For example, he set them to the lucrative task of scouring the bush for a plant called *Rauwolfia*. The bark from the root of this bush is the source of a drug reserpine, used to treat high blood pressure. Papa Dix started by feeding people with game meat, largely elephant meat, through his bravery and the accuracy of his varmint rifle. Soon he became a large exporter of ivory, and then the single largest supplier of *Rauwolfia* to the Swiss pharmaceutical giant Ciba-Geigy, a firm with a lock on the reserpine market at that time. When his industrious and studious protégés asked why they must produce still more, he told them it was because their school fees had yet to be paid. Without telling them, he had already paid their school fees for several years, and what they were working for would support their years subsequent to graduation. This constituted the African equivalent of an insurance policy, trust fund, and savings account. Two of these Azande boys, André and Inikpio, grew up under his scheme into his prize students.

ANDRÉ THE *DENTISTE* OF THE ZANDELAND BUSH

André is his chosen French name, and far easier to attempt than his Pazande name. His Pazande name happens to be, hold on, *Ngbamboligbe Kunangbangate*. This light-hearted, grandparent-inflicted name means "God is so much good, but man is bad." Would you not be glad to be so edified at every calling of your name? As I said, he is called André.

Both André and Inikpio graduated from Papa Dix's school in Banda, and were selected for community medical work. They were sent on for further training at the CME in Nyankunde. André was trained further to be the specialist for problems in the mouth, head and neck (which is how he had been selected to accompany me on the prior goiter project). He was sent away to Senegal for a special training program as "bush *dentiste*," or independently practicing African dental technician.

André was born in Banda with much family around Assa. His father was selected by Papa Dix to be one of the teachers in Banda. His father later developed a malignant African melanoma (cancer arising in the pigmented cells of the skin). In Africans, this usually arises where there is *less* skin pigment, in this case, under a toenail. On the last visit to Banda in 1996, André's younger brother brought their father to me on a bicycle without tires. I evaluated him and found that he had extensive, life-threatening spread of the cancer. He was taking an antimetabolite drug with limited effectiveness to control this disease. Just as we were examining him, a young girl was brought in with an obvious Burkitt's lymphoma. This is a horrendous cancer of the immune system that presents with enormous swelling of the lower face. As it happens, this tumor *does* have a curative sensitivity to the drug André's father was taking. Without hesitation, he turned his supply of the drug over to his son, in effect, passing life along, saying "It is all for the best." André's father died a short time later. We will learn in Chapter 15 about the effect of the drug on the young girl with Burkitt's lymphoma.

DR. SONNY MWEMBO

Sonny had come up to Bunia to meet me for the first time. He presented me with a hand-written note from Ahuka, introducing him to me as Ahuka's surgical substitute. Ahuka accompanied me on the first six trips in to Assa. Ahuka had gone from being a postgraduate doctor trainee learning thyroidectomy with me to being the CME chief. He had been called away as the Congolese representative of the new Pan-African Association of Christian Surgeons meeting in South Africa. This group is attempting to institute training periods that are similar to postgraduate surgical training. African physicians are selected for further training that is an African-appropriate, "surgical residency," using locally available techniques. I have edited a book on "appropriate technology" to be used in teaching surgical techniques in the developing world (*Surgery and Healing in the Developing World*, Landes Bioscience, 2000). Sonny Mwembo would be one of those chosen, and for that reason he would be accompanying me as the "local surgeon." He is Congolese from Kisangani, so he spoke Lingala, Kiswahili, and French, but not Pazande. As most other young professionals of his era, he had part of his training abroad, in Romania in his case.

ÉMILE ZOLA

Émile Zola (his Pazande name is *Zefuyu Bakarawa*) was born in Assa. He would be making his first trip home since leaving for training as a scrub nurse (surgical assistant) at CME over eight years earlier. He was being groomed to run a mission hospital in the remote reaches of Zandeland, most likely at Banda, where I had operated for two days on my last trip. In moving from Pazande-speaking Assa to the more cosmopolitan Nyankunde (after all, it has a road and intermittent electricity), he had retired his Pazande name. While at school, studying French, he spotted the name of an author, Émile Zola. "That's it!" he said, so I was being accompanied by Émile Zola on his first return trip to his familial home in Assa, where he might, once again, be called by his boyhood name.

A runner alerted his large family that he would returning to Assa, accompanying "the *Bwana*." He was wearing his best for the occasion of the reunion. He is a local boy who had gone away and made good. He was wearing a watch and carrying a transistor radio—a success story by any African definition. It did not really matter that time is of little relevance in Assa, or that there are no radio broadcasts that reach this remote region: he was equipped for

35

life in a city. He would be our scrub nurse in what would be called the operating room (OR) in America, but is called theatre as the Briticism goes across Africa.

"ENDLESS BROCCOLI" OVER THE GREAT ITURI RAINFOREST TO NEBOBONGO

We sorted out the stuff to be left behind, such as processed food, salt by the kilogram, soap, matches, batteries and clothes. Then we packed in the essential medicines, surgical instruments, and a large storage battery. This was needed to power OR lights and the "phonie" (the short wave radio) if it could be repaired. The phonie might allow rapid communication with the outside world and also has the life-saving function of warning the villagers of soldiers plundering the bush of people, food, or *matériel*. It was used this way during the Simba revolt and unfortunately has been continuously needed for this utility in various subsequent civil wars and raids.

We would fly direct with "Four Plus One" as the radio call to base would have it, the pilot Lary, passengers André, Sonny, Émile and me, and enough fuel to get us to Nebobongo. Nebobongo is the last outpost supplied by road, and therefore the one most likely to have fuel brought during the dry season over passable roads before the rains mired them in mud. We will stop to refuel and then regroup for the flight to Assa.

OVER THE CANOPY

The Ituri Forest is large, second in rainforest area only to the Amazon basin. It looks like a sea of endless broccoli from the air. It is magnificent! I am staring down from my copilot's seat, with the helmet headphones monitoring the calls in several languages until they fade away. I am bird watching from above the unbroken sea of vegetation reaching toward us. I see the shadow of the little Cessna on the canopy dancing like the colonies of egrets flushed from their rookeries by the roar from our plane. I recalled being on board the HMS Danmark, the "tall ship" training vessel of the Danish navy that sailed into Washington in 1976 to help celebrate the Bicentennial. As I stood at the wheel of this frigate, I looked down to see a brass plate on which was engraved the inscription: "Oh, God! My ship is so small, and thy sea is so vast!" I am looking down at the trackless rainforest from a Cessna with a tare weight of 740 kg cruising at 130 knots at 11,000 feet. There is a 360° horizon of sameness. I thought about the plane going down here. The lucky ones would be killed on impact in the canopy. I reached again for the security of my GPS.

The trees below, when one can pick out a tree from the forest, are complex systems of their own, hosting the birds flaring from them and the primates scampering away from the unnatural aircraft noise. I see some trees in which only half the crown is in magnificent bloom against a darker green, flowerless opposite side. These trees are probably monoecious, i.e., they have separate male and female flowers on one plant. There must be some ingenious means, not immediately apparent or recollected by me just now, to avoid continuous self-fertilization. Perhaps there is staggered flowering or controlled production of scents to attract pollinating animals. Perhaps the individual trees are self-sterile, like corn.

I can see the occasional glint of sunlight off water beneath the foliage. There may be whole river systems obscured to me from this height. The forest canopy is so dense that it is confluent, overarching the rivers beneath. Closer to the Ituri River, named on our aviation map with the nearest airstrips (and sometimes segments of roads) flagged for emergencies, I can see the ribbon of river as it snakes through rocky gorges. These stony hard places that show white water rapids throughout the constricting confines of the gorges are the cooled residue from the nearby Ruwenzori Mountains—the "Mountains of the Moon," which have been beckoning to me from my first over flight a dozen years ago. They are as magnetic to me as they were to Richard Burton who was one of the earliest Europeans to be pulled over by them. During each visit, I had made plans to climb them, but I was repelled by new wars from new factions who kept using them as sanctuaries from which they cannot be routed. There is said to be an army of over 180,000 well-equipped troops spilled over from Uganda in the Ruwenzori just now. Yet beneath the wings of the Cessna, I see only the endless broccoli and the few visible creatures that come up to the crown or over the canopy.

If I were looking down at a temperate forest, it would be much more homogeneous; all Sitka spruce in Alaska, or lodge pole pines in Wyoming. Here the overwhelming superficial sameness is an illusion. At ground level, you would find that almost every tree is different from its neighbor, in an explosion of speciation. This cradle of life must be the mother of all biodiversity!

I talk with Lary through the headsets. I take the controls for a while and experience, as always, the twin sensations of flying. First, there is the liberating sense of the ease of slipping through this thin medium with the tension of realizing how abruptly things can change. Then there is the obligation to pay attention to a deadening series of iterated details while being deluded into the feeling that "nothing is happening" during this droning plunge, both laterally and vertically. I fly only in uncontrolled airspace by direct sight, weaving around

37

clouds, keeping course and altitude until I am nearly relieved by Lary's casual resumption of the yoke.

We have been talking not about flying, nor about Africa, and only briefly about my medical, anthropologic or writer's mission. We talk longingly about hunting, an avocation that may well be a prime candidate for "first love" for each of us. Lary was born in Wisconsin in a large family supported by his dentist father, but they still hunted for meat. This year he and his brothers had a sentimental family reunion and had all gone hunting, this time reversing their previous hunting history. The sons had taken their elderly father to hunt elk, perhaps their last hunt together. I understand not only the elk-hunting part of this story, but even more the importance of the occasion. With sparse transmissions to monitor from the few aircraft anywhere near us, we got to tell a lot of hunting stories. Lary has never been to Assa, but had been eager to get to this remote spot on his map. "Just wait until we get there and let me introduce you to some *real hunters*!" I promise.

"From what I hear, there will not be any hunting this trip, and the folk left at Assa are just lucky enough to have survived being hunted," replied Lary.

"And if any could, they would," I answered. "My bets would be on the prey over the predators in this chase." I am thinking of my fellow-hunter/guide Jean Marco, and hoping he is all right, but have heard no word about his well-being.

With Lary at the controls again, and me in my reveries staring down into the rainforest, we approach the glide slope over Nebobongo. We circle once to scare off any wart hogs, goats, children or vultures that might be on the strip, and settle in for the heads-up final approach, slipping through the canopy layer cut away on either side of the strip. "Touchdown, Nebobongo!" Lary calls through the radio.

"We are praying for you," comes back the response.

"Thank you!" Lary calls back, with a smile, then explains, "That is my wife!"

8 DESTINATION ASSA, THE PLACE AND ITS PEOPLE

REFUELING IN NEBOBONGO AND ON TOWARD ASSA

At Nebobongo (I love this name), hundreds of people lined the taxiway, getting eye-filling loads of grit from the prop wash, while their tattered clothes and their jaunty, home-made hats of palm fronds were whipped and scattered at our turn. We rolled the barrel of aviation gasoline toward the plane and poured buckets of fuel into the wing tanks through a filter made from a coffee can and a muslin screen.

Mary Jane Robertson, the Canadian nurse/midwife turned community developer, came to the plane to greet us. She introduced a young German doctor newly arrived for a short term of service. He wanted to talk about goiter (enlarged thyroid gland). He said, "I never ever see so many and so gross!" I told him about the higher incidence farther from Nebobongo and promised materials on treatment and prevention. I shared some of my experience with him, warning him about preoperative treatment that patients would require before surgical removal of the goiter. The rich blood supply of the goiter dictates medical intervention before surgery. One encounter with an unprepped, profoundly hypothyroid patient in the operating room would put him off the surgical approach to the thyroid forever! The hypervascularity of the goiter in a patient who has not been pretreated would be a memorable bloody mess that no surgeon should ever experience more than once.

I really should spend some time in Nebobongo, which is a nearly ideal mission hospital setting for a medical student elective of the kind I had first experienced in Nigeria. The facilities are nearly adequate. There are supplies that can be ordered and anticipated because of intermittent access by road. Finally, there are experienced personnel like Mary Jane who would be very helpful and could supervise the student's experience. Ironically, this relative development is the reason I have passed through Nebobongo. Knowing the destitution of the more remote Assa station, I considered Nebobongo "developed."

We picked up the letters to be carried on to Assa, some of them dated back to my last pass through, now nearly two years old. There is a special compartment in our unofficial mailbag called "hot mail." In this group are letters that require an immediate response. The recipient is required to stand by the plane, open the letter, and respond on the same letter. Despite all the turmoil and emotion of the arrivals and the departures, like the telephone, it is a preemptory demand, as if your local postman rang your doorbell and insisted that you open your mail and respond to it immediately. But, if the interval until the next mail is months to years, it is one of the few ways to get anything done within brief lifetimes.

Bidding farewell to our friends at Nebobongo, we strapped into the refueled plane (no fuel need be expected at Assa) and Lary called out the mandatory "*Attention!*" to clear the prop area and started our single engine. I realized then that I was the only veteran returning to Assa. These passengers and the pilot were making their first trip there; whereas, André had only been there once before—last time, with me!

In a roar that scattered tree fronds, sticks and stones as well as chickens and kids through the waiting crowds who can never quite get used to the downside of any mechanical advantage until after the fact, we bounced off the grass strip of Nebobongo.

This is my last leg, toward what travel agents might call "Destination Travel." By the ultimate definition of that term, you surely do not get to Assa en route to anywhere else! To borrow a phrase I had first learned in Nigeria, this is an "arrival."

ASSA DRAMATIS PERSONAE

BULE

Jean Marco is the second-born son of Pastor Bule. He is easily the most capable man in the village, holding Assa together, following in his father's footsteps. The first Christian missionary to reach this region was an American named Pierson, who wore a pith helmet and was borne in a sedan chair. The indigenous people could never quite master his name, so he was, and remains known today, as "Pastor Piesey." He managed to bring in a Model A Ford into this roadless district. Its rusted frame is resting in state at Assa station as a monument to the first—and the fifth to the last—vehicle to be used here. He had a green thumb, and cleverly rearranged native plants to decorate the village. He even imported a few South American exotics such as palm trees and mangos, now in bloom at Assa. Along the "road" to Assa, a bicycle track in reality, the trees sport bromeliads. These are native epiphytic species with waxy green leaves and flamboyant spikes of colorful flowers at their center. Pierson neatly arrayed them at head height, a nice decorative touch.

Pierson wanted to establish some form of communication before the introduction of the "phonie," a short wave radio. Fortunately, he brought a young man to the village who made a name for himself working in the Congolese gold fields where he learned Kiswahili. Bule was especially well known for being a master drum carver, but he was also a blacksmith, an herbalist and a practical jack-of-all-trades. He was the one indispensable man in this outpost, which needed to be self-sufficient. His gold field name was particularly ironic, since "Bule" in Kiswahili means "useless!"

What a bargain Pierson got for bringing Bule to the Assa station. Bule carved the master drum! The "talking drum" of Zandeland was established with this central "node" in a 35-km relay of messenger drums (**Figure 13**). A skilled operator could beat out messages announcing events such as deaths, forecasts, chief's orders, and warnings. Bule carved a large cylindrical drum from a hollowed-out log. It was carved thicker on one side of the slit (the "parent") than the other (the "child"). With natural latex coating short drumsticks, he can beat out a rhythmic, two-toned, low-pitched, long-carrying message in a code he and the other drummers and most of the senior citizens of Zandeland understand.

The other village drums pick up and relay this message in a sequential ripple that can be transmitted like a game of "telephone" all the way to cities as far away as Kinshasa or Kisangani. Ironically, by the time the message reaches any urban center, the message is not likely to be understood, not because it was garbled in relay but because in an urban setting of transistor radios and boom boxes, the citizens no longer "hear" the drum. There is a radio vacuum in Assa. Émile's transistor radio is a useless bauble to show off proudly but it receives nothing. Here, people still need to rely upon the drum for important "local news."

How important that news can be was dramatically illustrated during the Simba Revolt. This turmoil brought death to many Europeans, and to many more opposing Congolese. Patrice Lumumba came to power, temporarily aligning the new government with the communist Eastern Bloc. As a reign of terror spread through the distant bush, the "talking drum" always forewarned of the whereabouts and approach of the marauding Simbas, and allowed the hiding of persons and precious things (like the "phonies") before their arrival. During the Simba Revolt, Bule, the drummer, was the most severely beaten person who still survived in Assa. With him at the time was one other survivor, Metasela, the cook at Pierson's Assa station. Timoteo, a friend of Metasela, was the father of Yuni, my housemaid on previous visits. Yuni is a hard-working helper who was

41

a heroine during the most recent Assa sacking by Hutu soldiers and their temporary allies in President-for-Life Sesse Mobutu's army.

The master drum has two lateral extensions that would be handles if the drum were small enough to pick up and carry. The handles are largely decorative in this nearly immovable master drum. It rests on a fixed base in its own special central village location, adjacent to the site where the new church has been in the stages of completion for the last several visits. So, what kinds of decoration did Bule carve on the decorative handles of the master drum? He used two important influences on his life that moved him to select the surprising images.

On one end is the carved head of a Cape buffalo, the most fearsome of the big game around Assa. It is the biggest source of coveted but rarely enjoyed meat. This animal also accounts for the most human deaths from animal attacks in Assa. The Cape buffalo bears a cantankerous grudge and seems to have a vindictive streak, turning the tables on the hunter. I can confirm this from my extended circle of late hunter friends. Bule's first close encounter with a wounded Cape buffalo is commemorated on the left side of the drum.

On the other side there is a carved miniature Cessna! "The audaciousness of man, that he should presume to fly like the birds! How do you pull it off?" I must confess a sense of wonderment each time it happens to me again. I hope to take Bule on an airplane ride to experience what the birds must take for granted but I doubt I ever will.

The drum, carved by Bule one generation ago on his first encounter with white men and a ferocious Cape buffalo and the airplane, really represents *Africa*. *Ancient* Africa with all its primeval fears and natural terrors in the bush on which we still depend; and *modern* Africa, and just how do we cope with and use these special tools to help us in adapting for our survival? *Communication* between these two different worlds may still be possible, more by resonance than direct understanding.

A DRUM OF MY OWN

Following my third and fourth visits to Assa, the group had got together and thought of gifts they could present the *Bwana* that they thought I would appreciate. *Bwana* is their name for me. It is applied to all outside white men and is a name with which I have never been comfortable. It simply means "Sir" or "Mister," but is used in prayers to mean "Lord." It conjures up images of colonials in pith helmets, hardly the way I look or feel—but, then, I am white. Bule was commissioned to prepare one of these gifts. He formally presented me with a drum, a miniature carving of the master drum, with a pair of sticks to beat upon it (**Figure 15**). I thanked him for it, and thought it would make a good decoration or a toy.

Bule, however tugged me over to the master drum, while I was still carrying the smaller version. He then stepped up to the podium at the side of the drum under its open-sided, thatch-roofed shelter. He stretched and then paused, almost identical to the ritual of the concert maestro before waving the baton and bringing art to life. This is a process Bule has never seen to mimic. Perhaps it is the other way around, with most other maestros mimicking the African performers. With his eyes closed, he began beating a rhythmic message on the master drum. He stopped abruptly, muffling the master drum with both of his hands. The melody lingered on. There was an after tone that I thought might be the distant response of one of the relay drums. Bule came over and muffled my drum. There was silence. He repeated the process with the same result. The profound meaning of his gift moved me. Wherever I may be, there will always be a resonance between me and the people of Assa. Count on it!

JEAN MARCO

Bule's son is called Jean Marco. But first, it helps to know his real name, *Pung Balate*. Jean Marco, his French name (usually abbreviated by those who speak to him in other than Pazande as "JM") is his own choosing. His grandparents bestowed his Pazande name upon him. This sometimes leads to results that vary from unfortunate to hilarious: I have kept records of several such names as examples, such as "Looks like he is going to die!" Bule's parents lived a long way from Assa as you might conclude from the story of how he was brought here by Pastor Piesey. During a prolonged absence from the distant parents, Bule's wife, already well along in years, was giving birth, when Bule traveled to follow up the drum message of the good news, even before the outcome was fully known. When Bule delivered the unlikely message in person, that one of Assa's eldest and least fertile wives had just delivered a healthy son, Bule's father blurted out his grandson's name: "*Pung Balete!*" The literal meaning of this is "There is nothing in my mouth," or, in liberal translation, "I am speechless!"

JM is my closest companion in the bush and on the hunt. I have had whole days of close communication with him with never more than the passage of a few words in one of six languages he uses and only one of a couple, at best, that I can use here. He is *Pung Balete* to me, but JM in all other third person references.

JM has surpassed his father's ingenuity. He is a strong, good-hearted, clever entrepreneur and a loyal, community-spirited fellow. He has taught me more about how to live in Assa than any other person has. He is my number one hunter. He quickly points out that if he worked very hard at it, he could get to be only one-tenth the hunter that a couple of the elderly "retired hunters" in the village once were. These hunters were armed more with their tracking skills and knowledge of animal behavior than with the spears they carried. The men of Assa respect hunting skill and sharply attuned awareness of bush craft. They were at first amazed that a white man might know which way the wind was blowing and what significance that might hold.

Bwana is not here in Assa to "teach the natives all about everything." I am a highly skilled hunter by North American standards, and if I continue to hunt every year with JM in the bush, I may some day get to be one-tenth the hunter he is. The hunt is an opportunity for a turnabout in our relationship. They get to reciprocate with *Bwana* after he has been operating all day in theatre. They can take him out and show him things that both parties thoroughly appreciate as hard-won skills. I have gotten the better of the deal in this exchange over the years. Unfortunately, things look gloomy for the hunt in the oppressive militarized circumstances surrounding this visit to Assa.

INIKPIO

Inikpio is the second of the protégés I named earlier (along with André) of Papa Dix. Inikpio came from Assa originally, and went through school at Banda. Through his own native intelligence and diligence, he worked his way through nursing school at CME Nyankunde. More recently, he graduated from CME as an anesthetist and returned to Assa with his wife, Tasamu, and his extensive family, to head up the Assa health work. "Inikpio" is another Pazande name that should be translated to recognize what long-dead grandparents can do to baptize a newborn ironically with a heritage that may be a bit of baggage to carry as the head nurse of the entire district's health care: "Inikpio" means "He who has seen death!"

Tasamu is an accomplished nurse midwife. She is a graduate of the CME nursing school. She was born in a village along the eastern border of the Congo in the area influenced by the genes and trade of the Arabic slave-trading camel caravans. She has strikingly handsome and different facial features from those conveyed by the more Bantu genes apparent in the Azande/Mbisile hybrid tribes around Assa. Tasamu bears a striking resemblance to a female version of NBA star Scotty Pippin. I helped Tasamu do several operations at Assa early on, although she defers during our surgical marathons with guest surgeons operating and acts as our circulating nurse or anesthetist. I would say, impartially as I can make such a judgement, that she has the more gifted set of hands than those of any others' she is assisting during our visits, including mine.

When Inikpio married such a high-value woman, the *lobola* (dowry) demanded by her family was a heavy burden, in the thousands of US dollars, which the mission had to absorb. In comparison, the whole district's current monthly budget for health care, including salaries, drugs, operations, and supplies is $130.00 US. Tasamu has been a rather good return on that investment. Their marriage was jeopardized during the separation of Tasamu and Inikpio when he was living at CME, on clinical rotation at Bunia, completing his nursing studies, but not alone. That this transient indiscretion has been accommodated, and that the husband/wife team is together at the heart of the Assa medical mission is personified in the flesh of the child born after his return. The child's Pazande name means "Forgiven."

I have walked around in the bush near the hospital with Inikpio. He is not a hunter but he made a living with and for Papa Dix in the bush finding *Rauwolfia*. He is a superb ethnobotanist, and can identify various bush medicines on a casual "walkabout." His knowledge would keep a drug company busy in clinical trials for years. He wrote a proposal for the continued application of the Iodine Repletion Project in literate French. I forwarded this document on to the International Council on the Control of Iodine Deficiency without so much as an explanatory or introductory cover letter. He carefully recorded for me each of the operations he had done in the interval between my last visit. One of these was a difficult bowel resection on a man who had come in with an obstructed bowel from a strangulated hernia. The man had happened to be the chief of Ebale, a village that had participated in our goiter study, many days from Assa. The chief ordered his villagers to tie him to his chair, and to tie the chair to a bicycle. That the bicycle had no tires was not important. That he was in stoic agony was also not to deter them. He ordered the villagers to push him on the bicycle until they reached Assa, since that is where the doctor is.

When this sorry looking dispatch arrived following the runner who announced their coming a day behind him, the chief of Ebale was dehydrated and nearly dead. Inikpio ran in intravenous fluids, and set about the several methodical steps in sequence to relieve him. "First, put in a spinal anesthetic to see if the abdominal wall relaxes enough to reduce the bowel into the abdomen." No luck. "Then make an inguinal incision and check the bowel within the sack. If it is black, just bring it out of the abdomen and exteriorize the dead bowel loop. When we return we will put the two exteriorized viable ends back together. This is how we would do it when we return." I used his two sleeves of the long-sleeved shirt that had once been mine, showing him how the inside layer of the bowel could be stitched with a running absorbable suture and the outside stitched

45

together with an interrupted layer of silk. "Then check for patency of the anastomosis, thus, and then close up the abdomen." Just so. For someone as astute as Inikpio, there is no need for the usual "See one, do one, teach one" sequence typical for surgeons in training. The first one he saw was on his shirt sleeves as mock loops of bowel. The next one was on the bowel of the chief of Ebale. No only did the chief do well, going home in triumph 10 days later, but he had a feast thrown to commemorate the event upon my visit to Ebale six years ago. "But," I protested, "I did not do anything; I wasn't even here!"

The chief knows that rank hath its privileges and knows protocol in these matters. "But," he said, "You taught Inikpio!"

I am proud to be identified by my protégés. I have a small flash of "out of body experience" whenever I see either JM or Inikpio walking through the bush coming at me. I could think of them as "alter egos"; but, then, I realize it is a visual recognition. They often wear clothes that were my favorite standbys about a decade earlier! I tried to explain this feeling to good friends in the University of Colorade, Dr. Alden Harkin, Chairman of Surgery and fellow resident at Harvard's Peter Bent Brigham Hospital and his wife Laurie, another fellow resident in Boston. Laurie joked that some might consider this recognition more like an "out of mind" experience!

LAZUNGA

Lazunga is the hard working school superintendent of the only education going on anywhere that I can detect in this part of the Congo at this time. He had hunted with me in the bush. We also shared ideas on how to start community development in Assa to lift people out of the grinding poverty that has entrapped them here. To encourage any kind of economic development involved some idea, then risk, and concerted effort to bring it to fruition. JM understands that and so does Lazunga. Most of the others, alas, have the ambition to become full-time dependents on the largesse of a handout from someone somewhere and will wait for any promising lead. I often happen to fall out of the sky at the time some of the younger mendicants are practicing their finest speeches, some in English, about how worthy they are to be adopted by me. Lazunga understands the role of education as one of the ladders to climb out of despair. Many people in Assa are mired in the endless waiting for conditions to somehow improve, as they continue their entropic slide into total collapse.

Lazunga understands self-improvement in the abstract, but his son is something more concrete. Lazunga has come to me regularly with desperation, seeking funds to get his son to Bunia for school. He needs school fees. Oh, yes, and his living expenses. Well, all right. Be sure to add in his transportation to

Bunia. Well, now, remember that total is already much more than the monthly support of all of the Assa medical projects. Oh, and also for his wife, and, did I mention his family, and the sister who goes with them to care for the kids.

I usually cannot stay long enough in any of these recitals to ever hear the end of the list. Inevitably upon my arrival I will have a list of petitioners who need to see me urgently and alone, for just a few minutes, and no one else should know the subject of this conversation. I often telegraph ahead, that I understand their generosity, and their humility at not wanting everyone to know what they are planning to donate to the community, but they might make these charitable contributions more directly than through me! That still does not discourage a number of the more advanced mendicants who come to my door with what is now rehearsed to the point of an absolutely compelling sales pitch. It comes down to this: You have it; I don't; I need it; you, therefore, good brother, whom I love dearly, will give it to me. It is all so simple!

Besides, they are quite generous to me. One quaint gift that showed appreciation for me came from a "committee," one of whose members was Lazunga, and another a former pastor here named Pastor Tanda. They once presented me with a pullet upon my departure, since I was making a trip a long way to America, and I would surely be hungry along the way. I was not sure that the flight attendants on a transatlantic 747 would appreciate the squawking of a trussed chicken in the overhead bin. The gift accomplished its purpose of letting me know that they were concerned enough about me that they gave me a family's protein reserves for the month.

The committee got together and puzzled over the bizarre finding that "*Bwana* likes *old* things." Now, I should quickly add, for the correction of many of my friends or close sartorial advisors, such as my sons, that this conclusion was not reached after a review of my wardrobe. They had noted that I showed interest in the original Azande artifacts from the time of earliest pre-European conquests of the area. I was particularly interested in the Azande blades, a stylized characteristic piece of early Azande technology in the smelting of what could be called a "late Bronze Age." I had once admired an Azande war knife, and they remembered that in my absence.

They had gathered around a fire and retold a traditional tale of a local Mbisili hero. He resisted the conquest of the Azande warriors who had over-run this area of peaceful Mbisili Bantu around four centuries ago, before any Europeans knew of this area or its population dynamics. The local Mbisili seized his opportunity when he caught his captor off guard, and killed him with his own Azande blade. He was then so frightened of the consequences of this bold act, that he buried the blade in the banks of a stream and fled. His act of bravery was told for generations without any doubt that he had been the last of the Mbisili to stand up for independence, before they were absorbed into the ruling culture of the Azande people. As in any mythic tale of this sort, there was some suspicion that the story may actually have been based in historic fact that had been embellished and canonized over time. The committee commissioned some of the local young men to help them search around for evidence. They checked the beds of streams that were known as likely spots and dug up a good deal of the countryside around what might have been a hiding place. No discoveries were made of any interest to the committee, who then consulted JM. He pointed out that the course of the streams varied from one rainy season to the next, and that they should check the bends in previous rivers, where only little valleys suggested that a river had once run through the area. They tore up a good deal more geography, until one day they found an artifact and carried it to Pastor Tanda, who had been a repository of local lore. He looked over the site and agreed that it was compatible with the story, and then checked out the Azande blade. It was classic, in style and forging and looked exactly like the "treaty" blades that were fashioned to last a long time. They were used to seal a deal such as a marriage contract, or a peace negotiation, or could even be used as currency reserve, like a "federal reserve note" against which future obligations could be withdrawn. But, Pastor Tanda observed, the blade is hafted to this very old rotten wooden handle. "We surely cannot give this gift to *Bwana* like this, even if he does like old things." So, they chipped away the crumbled fragments of the ancient wooden handle, and applied a freshly cut limb which they carved carefully and then blackened with shoe polish to make it far more presentable. When I was leaving Assa after a trip to work on the goiter project in 1990, the "committee" triumphantly presented me with the newly hafted spear, along with the retelling of the story I had heard many times before. I now had to carry back in my luggage, somehow, a genuine antique weapon, smuggling on board a freshly hafted spear. With tolerance for on-board weaponry limited in most airlines, I had to make some modifications. When I got to Nairobi, I had unhafted the spear, carefully wrapped the blade, and put it in my checked luggage. At home, I gleefully trekked down to the Smithsonian Museum of African Art and had the curators there appraise it and evaluate it. The evaluation read, "Early Azande blade, perhaps four centuries old, used in treaties and to secure contracts. Every bit as good and probably older than the one we have on display, and we would love to have it as a gift or loan for our collection, but what were you doing trying to paint it with what looks like shoe polish?"

THE TALL POPPY IN ASSA AND IN AFRICA

I was told on my first visit to Assa that there was an over-achiever who was born and raised in Assa, showed great promise, and with extraordinary support, achieved a realization of much of this promise. His name was Finasa Babili. He was identified by "Papa Piesey" (Pastor Pierson, the original American missionary who was the founder of this remote mission station) as a young man who showed high intelligence and potential for community leadership. He was picked out by Pierson for extra tutelage, in language and science, and sponsored for secondary education, being sent out of Assa, first to Nyankunde and then to the National University in then-Zaïre, when it was (briefly) still open. He was being groomed for a leadership role among the Azande. He returned to Assa and married a local woman, Bibiana. When Bibiana was born, Finasa's father marked her front door, securing her for a later marriage to his son. They had a daughter, Julie, and then later, when abroad, a son Artemas. But, others in Assa also noted his rapid rise to prominence from his humble beginnings, and he narrowly escaped several "accidents" that seemed to cluster about him during any return visits to Zandeland.

When he was spirited away to Nyankunde after an attempt on his life by poisoning, a decision was reached there that he should be the first known Assa resident to get the big chance to study in America. He eventually received the first graduate degree known to Assa, a M.S. in Chemistry from the University of Colorado. With substantial help from the mission and his considerable competence in bootstrapping himself up to this advanced educational achievement, he returned, well-equipped to help his Azande people in further educational and developmental progress. Having narrowly escaped several attempts on his life nearer to his birthplace, Assa, he was sent to Isiro, the closest thing to a town in northeast Zaïre. He taught science in a secondary school there.

I recalled that I had hand-carried a letter from Babili's family on one of my earlier visits, and enclosed was a J.C. Penny portrait photo of his son Artemas and his wife Bibiana, taken while they were living in Atlanta. This created quite a stir, which I did not understand. The crowd of Assa people passed the professional portraits around, showing what appeared to be a young African-American man dressed in a suit, posing in a studio. "That cannot be an Assa boy," was the consensus. It appeared that a family had escaped into a different and immeasurably better world. Not everyone was rejoicing with them in their good fortune.

When Finasa Babili was teaching in Isiro, an uncle visited him from Assa, a long trip away on footpaths, and, just like old times, they went out in a dugout canoe for a fishing trip. What happened next was never made clear, but

49

Finasa was almost drowned and made a hasty escape to the Pazande-speaking part of the Sudan. He had just begun a new teaching post in the Sudan when his wife left to visit Assa. While there, a cryptic and terrifying message was received: her young and previously healthy husband had suddenly and mysteriously died in the Sudan. The suspicious circumstances, having followed several attempts by poisoning and drowning, were never resolved. The widow now lives as an American with her own grown children in Georgia. Fully one third of the letters I would later hand-carry out of Assa were addressed to Bibiana, the Assa escapee.

The meteoric rise of her late husband, and its consequences, are lost on no one in Assa. I have seen similar object lessons in Africa in tall poppies that have outgrown their roots in the estimation of the communities from which they had arisen. The one person that Assa folk might really envy would be Bibiana, with her American kids. The tragic circumstances that formed the bridge to her new life might even have been worth it. She now has the benefits of no more risk to herself or family and comfortable circumstances in American security. Africa had extracted its due. The remains of this Assa family are now immune from Azande sorcery.

ASSA: DEAD AHEAD

While closing in on Assa on the flight from Nebobongo, I thought of all the conflicts my friends in Assa must find a way to live through. As though it is not enough to have malaria-infested *Anopheles* mosquitoes, contaminated drinking water, Green Mambas, Cape buffalo, and prowling leopards, they also have to deal with poverty, hunger, and disease. If they can survive that, and the envy of those who are not doing as well, the crushing blow of war has overrun them again, with the ragtag remnants of the last war still marauding as a new civil war is rekindled. As we slip down lower over the tall elephant grass, I keep looking for buffalo and elephant, but am aware that far more sinister forces are now loose in the bush.

And, now, here comes the Assa area, as we slide over the deep green of the *mungas* in the fresh verdure of rainy season. What new and unexpected things will pop up out of this fertile, myth-growing area this time?

PART II

OUT OF ASSA

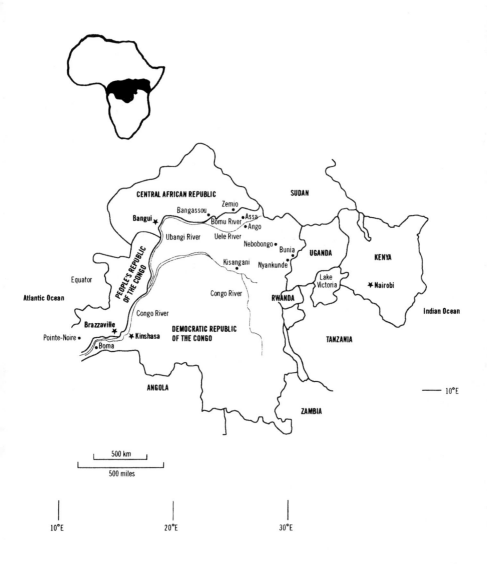

**THE PEOPLE OF ASSA, SUFFERING CONTINUING INFLICTION
FROM THE CIVIL WAR THAT OVERRAN THEM SINCE MY LAST
VISIT, AND AS RECENTLY AS JUST LAST WEEK**

July 7, 1998

POWER UP!

I am in position in the previously equipped theatre (operating room, OR) for which André should have full credit! I am sitting with the computer on my lap and the charger between my knees after he has hot-wired the connection between the solar battery from the theatre's solar panel overhead on the roof to the new battery that we transported to Assa on our flight. That is the good news—he did something I could never have done to get power trickling into my battery so that I might continue my narrative of this experience.

Now, for the bad news: Someone came in the night and stole the solar panel off the roof.

For now, you will be able to read what I have learned in Assa, and we may be able to get a few operations done under the previously solar powered OR lamp, now illuminated by the new battery. These expedients are not sustainable indefinitely, however, as grateful as we may be that it is a new battery that is hooked up to this jury-rig, since it is not getting any newer, as it might have been self-renewing with the solar panel overhead rejuvenating it daily. Once again, when it is dark as the sun goes down, it will get dark, not only inside the houses, but possibly in this machine as well.

**RETURN TO THE EVENTS OF THE ASSA ARRIVAL
WHEN WE CAME IN TO A DESERTED AIRSTRIP,
BUT SHORTLY WERE TREATED TO A MUTED
BUT JOYFUL RECEPTION**

When we circled familiar areas beneath the wings of the low-level flight, I recognized *Zala*, the marsh that becomes a water hole in the dry season. It is one of the most frequent hunting venues we have. There is a platform in the canopy from which we might be able to spend the night as we once did. We flew over the hill and could see the airstrip where the grass was freshly chopped down by hand. This is the rainy season, although I am told that the rains have not been as strong as usual either in Nyankunde or here, despite the heavy soaking on the night of my arrival in CME. That storm was a demonstration of a more usual phenomenon at this time of year and why I was treated to the termite hatch on their ephemeral wings. Despite the sparse rains, the countryside is very green, especially over the mosaic of the "*mungas*," the bare volcanic rock mounds that are sometimes hollow and often broken through at points where caves are formed. Bats by the thousands congregate in these caves, depositing millennia of guano, the only real soil enrichment found around here. It is mined and transported as fertilizer for kitchen garden plots around shambas.

I have hunted these parts often, so often in fact, that I was almost getting to know them, a fact of life to those here, and always a surprise when I revealed that I did not know exactly where I was. After talking to pilot Lary about elk hunting and other stories, I grew eager to be tramping the bush again and hunting big game in Assa. If not big game hunting, I was anxious just to be tramping the bush, even if it meant going among these big brutes unarmed!

Nevertheless, let there be no romanticizing about the danger down there. We were flying at several hundred feet altitude for the express purpose of spotting game, since Lary was making his first approach to Assa, having flown over and identified the last mark on the map as Amadi, a tiny village on the Uele River. What looked like a well-clipped putting green was actually 15 feet of elephant grass and would take a very large creature to be seen even if they were bolting away in full flight from the sound of the low-flying aircraft. On past approaches during the dry season, I have typically seen small groups of elephants and Cape buffalo milling about, and the darting retreat of bushbuck (*Tragelaphus scriptus*) or waterbuck (*Kobus ellipsiprymnus*). So, I now know that in the rainy season it is not easy to see big game from above, or below, until it is often too late. We did see several *Zigba*, giant forest hogs (*Hylochoerus meinertzhageni*), of the kind that furnished the last *fête du chasseurs* when Jean Marco had been gored by one that he killed with his muzzle-loader. The giant tusks of this creature, which I had photographed next to Jean Marco's leg wounds, are now in circulation with the renegade soldiers who were here only last week. This soldier's visit is a story to be delayed in its telling, lest it dampen the joy of this reunion. Our reunion is one of the two events that has broken up the enervating sameness of the destitute lives of the people of Assa, and the only one recently that has been a happy one.

ASSA, AT LAST, THANK GOD! —
FROM BOTH THE GROUP IN THE AIR
AND A MUCH BIGGER GROUP ON THE GROUND

Where is everybody? By now there should be a dozen folk on the airstrip, with Kati or one of the others driving the gasping and coughing old Bronco down to pick up our gear! I told Lary that I wanted to introduce him to the *real* hunter behind one of my stories. I wanted to have him and Jean Marco shake hands in the event that it was possible to hunt if he could come to retrieve us a day or two early—that is, if there were any weapons of any kind not already purloined. Lary was in a hurry to get away to make it back in time to Nyankunde under VFR before getting caught up by the sunset. He wanted to avoid being trapped by any official wanting to come from Ango to go over again all the *matériel* I had imported into this zone from within the Congo itself. Lary wanted to get into fewer official hassles by being gone, if and when Ango officials were to arrive, unceremoniously clutching onto the back of Inikpio's "*Piki*," the Kiswahili name for a motorbike, possibly the only transport system left at Assa.

We off-loaded and then sighted a very eager fellow coming full speed through the tall grass on his bicycle. From a distance, I could see it was Jean Marco—*Pung Balete!* He came over for a greeting around to the others as well as an introduction to Lary. I did not stand on the usual greeting formalities which would require that I banter around for a long time to ask about all family members present and gone beyond. Lary was seated and strapped in ready to roll, so I asked Jean Marco if we could hunt with Lary if he returned sooner, with which Lary enthusiastically concurred. Jean Marco looked shocked, as if I had fallen off the moon, instead of having come around the globe a bit less far than that. Did I not know what has been going on? It is quite hot right now, was the translated response, besides there being no weapons of any kind and we are not wanted out in the bush from which people are just now returning.

So we worked out the possibility that later André could get a permit to go up to his forest hideaway 20 km by road from Nyankunde, and 12 km by over-mountain fast retreat on foot. This fast retreat method had been used rather regularly during the fierce civil war that he would be telling me more about later. Perhaps we would get back to Nyankunde and seek a hunting site near there as a possible consolation prize. By now, Lary attempted once again to get rolling, and he took off as the group began to gather. They certainly *did* know I was coming, and there were four of us arriving. They knew of André's return. He had been here with me one time previously. He was a Zande whose native son homecoming I had witnessed at Banda last year when I took the final photos of father and son. They knew of the arrival of Émile Zola, a returning native son who is being groomed to be the local health care worker for Banda, but who is taking advantage of this flight on me to make his first return trip to his family in the eight years since he has been in Nyankunde. They did not know of Sonny Mwembo, who has not been this far from CME, a surgeon classmate of Ahuka's from Kisangani, whom I will help operate in the clinics we visit. As, the crowd gathered, I had a sudden thought as Lary took off—I am the only white face in all of Assa—when André laughed and pointed out, very respectfully but not entirely accurately, "...within a 300 kilometer radius, you mean!"

FACES FROM THE CROWD OF ONRUSHING WELL-WISHERS

The next person I recognized was Lazunga careening forward on a bicycle. He is the tireless School Superintendent and the master of impossible tasks in this very poor region. It was his son that he came to see me about last time tearfully, with a letter asking to have him supported for schooling at Bunia. I said I would help, and I then learned that the "Geelhoed Foundation" would be supporting him, along with his wife and children in Bunia until graduation. Now he is in Ango. Lazunga was trying to put together a small ceremony of welcome at the airstrip. I knew that a much bigger one would hit us when we walked up to Assa. At the moment when Lazunga was assembling the group for a prayer of gratitude, we heard a whoop of greeting. Flying toward us were a woman and two nearly naked girls, nubile teenagers falling out of their very tattered rags, a picture of African desperation caught in the one happy moment of their recent lives. They were the mother and sisters of my fellow traveler Émile Zola who had left Assa for Nyankunde and study eight years ago. Seeing him for the first time in years, recognizing at a distance the boy who made good, they ran until they were breathless, tearful and sweaty. Excited as they were, they had to restrain themselves, however, while a prayer was being offered with some greater formality than their impulsive joyful greeting warranted.

There was no Bronco. I saw its hulk later when I was on my search for a cigarette lighter plug-in. Eventually the garden tractor putt-putted down the hill with the rusty trailer that would haul our gear and the precious medicines up the hill. With an apology to me, André interpreted "We will have to walk!" That is exactly what I had hoped to do, saying, as I slapped my arm around his back "Jean Marco and I have never walked these bush treks before, and I am usually carried in a sedan chair!" This is an old joke relating to the first missionary fellow who reached this place, a man named Pierson whom they called "Papa

Piesey." He was a portly fellow wearing a pith helmet and made his august rounds carried in a sedan chair, something they had half-expected to have to do for the doctor on my first visit. I told them they could do it for me only if I had a dripping Cape buffalo hindquarter on my head at the time.

So, I walked up the hill at the head of the procession (protocol must be served) through the dense grass and the forest toward Assa. The procession grew and others came to shriek when they recognized the boy from Assa who had been to the big city of Nyankunde to return to visit his origins, proudly carrying a transistor radio. When I would stop to wait while greetings were exchanged, I took a few photos of homecomings, and saw that no one would move along until I got started again, since no one was allowed to process before me. I watched the social order during the day's greeting rituals, while smiling through a lot of language I did not recognize and some that I did. The old social amenities came back to me quickly and were said in all directions. We arrived at the house, after I had stopped to admire the now completed church. There was Bule, and Inikpio came riding in on his *pikipiki* (motorbike). I saw many familiar faces and a few that I did not see from among my old hunting partners. On several occasions when I mentioned their names, there was silence. I was told that Pastor Tanda had died on March 31, 1998, and later we visited his grave.

Four chairs had been placed in the shade at the house next to the cistern of the adjoining house (formerly nurse Ruth Powell's house, and now Inikpio's and Tasamu's). The cistern is at a site significant for an event during my last visit that André reminded me and the rest about later. I sat here in the bushes that were stained with blood from the bushbuck I had shot on the last trip, at the site where it had been dressed out and all the meat distributed. The next morning I was waiting in the camouflage outfit, now impounded in Bunia. The quiet wait at dawn was interrupted by a big wild cat that walked through the bushbuck's scent only two meters from me. I gave chase to see and photograph it, since I had not seen a cat in Assa before. When Jean Marco arrived, he saw the tracks. He told me in answer to my story "*Seulement un chat in Assa: c'est chui!*" (the leopard).

Ruth Powell, according to Kati, her driver, had been transferred to the Comoro Islands. The chief pastor of the local church stood forward first as the arc closed around and we all looked at each other. The men were all to my right in one large group around Bule and the women were all in a ring around the shade of the tree at the side of the house where a chimp had been chained up during my earlier visits.

With a fore singer, they all clapped and chanted a song thanking and praising God for the visitors and for the return to give them hope. They were genuinely happy, and it was also apparent that this was not the usual state of affairs recently. Several prominent people gave small opening speeches in a strict social order. I replied in a briefer note with the six or eight Bangala greetings and Pazande salutations I could come up with at that moment, electing not to try to stumble around in much French. Then after repetitive thanks, a receiving line was set up. I shook the hands of the senior males, then all the women with their babies clutched at their breasts, and then all the toddlers with their scabies-covered extremities, solemnly offering their paws to me with round-eyed wonder. I am home.

Now the bad news. There is not much to home. The first thing I noticed is the copy of Rembrandt's *The Man with the Golden Helmet*, prominent on each of my earlier visits, is gone. My surname means "golden helmet" in Dutch and this picture has mysteriously appeared here in the Congo and in the Bronte Hotel in Harare and elsewhere along the way in my travels, a coincidence that keeps preceding me. Fortunately, *The Man with the Golden Helmet* is not lonely. The bathroom fixtures, every mirror in the house, and everything screwed in or with plugs were keeping him company. The whole of Assa was swept clean for the processional and my arrival. This task was easier than it might have been because before being cleaned, the house had been cleaned out by soldiers. Chairs had been carried in from the bush where they had been sequestered in the raid, but very little escaped here.

The hero from the time of civil war that should get high marks was Mawa, the nurse from theatre who was here when Inikpio was at Nyankunde. He is not here now. He carried most of the medicines and OR equipment he could into the bush, and almost everything he squirreled away has returned. Nothing that the recent raiders took has been recovered, and that was almost everything that was in the house, and little they had wanted or could use from the hospital.

I was ushered into the house and sat drowsily as we all looked at each other grateful to be here together without a lot of extra words spoken. But when I asked questions about recent events or about people I did not see—like the cook, who had been among the most severely beaten men along with Bule who did not die during the Simba revolt that created Zaïre nearly 40 years ago—I got a translated response from Jean Marco via André:

"This day is one of great joy. We are so happy to see you again and to know that you have returned from so far away letting us know that you and others are still thinking of us, our hearts are overflowing despite many troubles. We want to enjoy this happiness together. To answer the questions of what has been happening recently would lessen that joy and bring most of us much more pain. So, let us not speak of these things you ask. It is true what you heard, that we were attacked again, and that what little we had was taken away, and that several of us were killed. But to repeat their names and these stories so soon would be to relive the awful events of the last weeks again, and we are here instead to rejoice with you and with God who has spared us to see you again."

"*Welcome to Assa, therefore, and may we all be so grateful to be alive, that we can hold back the telling of our troubles and glory instead that we are here and alive together to start over again.*"

10 THREE OBJECTIVES

THE THREE OBJECTIVES FOR THE WORK IN ASSA ON THIS TRIP INTO THE BELEAGUERED AND DISCOURAGED VILLAGE

In this fulfillment of an earlier promise to return this year, notwithstanding the disruption of a continuing civil war, I had a continuing agenda. This plan was tripartite: 1) the *medical/surgical* work and its resupply and training mission; 2) the *linguistic anthropology* study of the population begun last visit; 3) the *writing* of this experience as a *book* describing the situation of the people of Assa as an appeal for further support.

The primary purpose of my mission to Assa is medical. A large part is teaching the personnel in this isolated outpost and encouraging them to carry out the medical and surgical work during the long intervals when they are without outside help.

My presence in Assa, if it represents nothing else, is a promise fulfilled: it assures the people here that they have not been forgotten. They are justified in feeling abandoned, by the European and American missionary withdrawal, and the absence of any other multilateral, nongovernmental aid agencies. They have certainly been tortured, plundered and devastated by their own government. They most fear their own "national" army, which travels without a supply line, living "off the land," or to borrow a phrase from the American legal profession, they "eat what they kill." Whoever could claim to have a chicken or a wife before the army (of whatever stripe) comes through cannot find either after the armed marauders have passed.

The inhabitants of Assa desperately seek any form of outside "connection" for help or guidance; or even so little as an open-handed friend who is not rapaciously coming after what little they have. They are eager to show what they are justly proud of, at present, their simple survival. They have so far adapted to the loss of the few possessions they had. And, after all, they are adapted, by definition, since they still exist.

THE MEDICAL MISSION

The primary medical mission was the same as it was from the start and from my first trip here. At the founding of the Assa mission station the attempt was made to address the unmet needs of this population. Before the establishment of this mission station, the people had no modern medical, surgical, obstetric, pediatric and public health services. Many required urgent surgical care. The original missionaries did a survey and found that almost all men and most women had unrepaired hernias, a common cause of emergency bowel obstruction and a frequent cause of death in preventable misery. Obstetric disasters were frequent. In the absence of any regular form of perinatal care, both maternal and infant mortality rates had been high before the institution of a program of midwifery. Endemic hypothyroidism, however, is the most serious problem of this population. Its incidence is by far disproportionally greater than that seen in other areas of undeveloped Africa in the 23 nations of my experience in this continent.

Hypothyroidism means that there is insufficient thyroid hormone made by the thyroid gland for normal metabolic function in the adult. Hypothyroidism also has profound effects on normal development in the fetus and child. This may be due to a number of factors, most common of which is insufficient iodine intake in the diet, or factors called goitrogens that render the thyroid incapable of using what little iodine might be available to make into usable thyroid hormone. Iodine is often found in the diet of people living in salt-water coastal areas of the world, as it is concentrated in the oceanic food chain. Iodine is frequently deficient in areas that are remote from the sea, have volcanic rock as the ground base (since magma from the earth's interior has almost no iodine), or areas that were glaciated or subject to alternating seasons of inundation and desiccation.

Except for the glacial history, these features describe the central equatorial African rainforest around Assa. To add further compromise to the lack of dietary iodine, Assa's only staple starch is a goitrogen. Cassava is a root crop imported with European explorers from the New World. It requires very little care in its cultivation. Few pests ever attack it because of its high cyanide content. The root is harvested and dried like a log. After this dried log is soaked to remove the cyanide and pounded in a mortar and pestle into a floury paste, it is cooked and eaten as every meal's staple ingredient. A cyanide metabolite from cassava ingestion blocks utilization of what little iodine the diet can provide. Suffering both iodine deficiency and a dietary blockade to iodine utilization, this Central African area has world record profundity of iodine deficiency. The other parts of the world with iodine deficiency such as the Great Lakes area of glaciated America or the alpine areas of Central Europe, add iodine to salt, a ubiquitously required mineral. In Central Africa, salt itself is a precious commodity, difficult to transport and preserve, particularly in the rainy season. It is so precious that it would never get to women and children, the population most harmed by iodine deficiency.

The iodine deficiency is reflected in the adult by goiter, an enlargement, under the influence of thyroid-stimulating hormone, of the thyroid gland. Sometimes the thyroid gland becomes swollen over a hundred fold to grotesque proportions, sometimes even compromising breathing (**Figure 6**). The real tragedy of iodine deficiency comes with congenital hypothyroidism in a condition called *cretinism,* in which normal prenatal and childhood development fails (**front cover, Figure 30**). The infant never gains full stature, neuromuscular development or normal intelligence. In severe cases, the cretin may be deaf-mute and imbecile. In Assa and the surrounding villages, the goiter rate was nearly 100% in adults and children, and the cretinism rate was 11% before any intervention was undertaken.

During my earlier visits to Assa, I joined a study of hypothyroidism in this endemia, and tried several methods of management and prevention. Iodine repletion was attempted by the use of Lipiodal, a "depot" injection of slowly released iodine in poppy seed oil. This simple public health measure dramatically reduced the cretinism rate when given to women of childbearing age. It also shrunk the goiters in many adults, some of whom sustained breathing compromise from the goiter pressing on their airways. Those patients with life-threatening breathing problems were selected for thyroidectomy. We operated in the bush clinic set up to care for these patients (**Figure 7**).

Medical and surgical treatment and wider application of methods of prevention quite remarkably changed the individuals treated by normalizing their measurable thyroid hormone and thyroid-stimulating hormone values and their metabolic rates. The changes in these numbers, intuitively a good thing, was met by skepticism by some who asked if there was any measurable improvement in quality of life along with the demonstrated correction of endocrinologic numbers?

One of the inadvertent consequences of normalizing thyroid function is that the patients increase their appetites and consume more calories if they are available. Note that this *medical* program was designed to address *hypothyroidism,* and by these measures it was a success. If a broader view is taken of the consequences for the society of which these improved, treated individuals are a part, some startlingly counterintuitive consequences may be uncovered if a broader, societal view of the treatment of endemic hypothyroidism is taken. We restored a micronutrient that resulted in an increased demand for food without concomitantly increasing food supply in this resource-deficient environment. This created hunger. Furthermore, hypothyroidism causes a dramatic impairment of fertility. An immediate consequence of normalization of thyroid function was a population explosion, especially when accompanied by the improved perinatal and obstetric services developed with increased survival of newborns. This meant that the hypothyroidism program, addressed successfully as a focused medical program, had resulted in an increasing number of hungrier consumers.

Increased food demand thus created adverse social and environmental consequences. Assa is in a region of marginal food resources, mainly based in hunter-gatherer activities, and limited agriculture, made more difficult by thin soils on rocky volcanic ground in a rainforest environment. The problem addressed as medical was embedded in a complex system of adaptation to this environment, and addressing one vertical focus may have disturbed that system in which hypothyroidism had been conserved. Over a period of observation following intervention in hypothyroidism, a plausible interpretation presented itself. Hypothyroidism may be an adaptive population response to the constraints of the environment that limited the population and individual demands and impact upon the marginal carrying capacity to generate sufficient calories to be sustainable. Medical intervention in a vertical program may even be maladaptive. What measures of individual and community change could reflect on the quality of life benefits that were the humanitarian aim of the mission?

LINGUISTIC ANTHROPOLOGY

Critics challenged me to measure changes in quality of life using a methodology not mired in a cultural prejudice. I turned for help to a unique field of linguistic anthropology. "Color linguistics" studies the ability of an individual to differentiate and name as many different colors as can be recognized in an array of 330 different "Munsell" color chips (**Figure 16**) that cover the color spectrum visible to humans. The more colors that can be reproducibly recognized and named, the greater the degree of color discrimination. This may take different patterns in color criticality for individuals or population groups. For example, some males have red/green color blindness. For some equatorial jungle populations, critical subdifferentiation of the greens may be important. This would be a useless differentiation system for Eskimos. Eskimos might have several hundred words for snow, for example, since differentiating different types may be important to them. This Central African population lacked even one word for, or concept of, snow. Increases in criticality of color discrimination could have implications for adaptation, and, if demonstrable, a nonculture-bound test could be applied to show a qualitative difference that could be correlated with the endocrinologic data.

A standard color kit was developed with a method for administering this series of "color interviews" through the naming of colors and the foci of all colors subsumed under the name. The kit had been tested in a worldwide color survey; and, I carried this methodology with me to the Congo during my last visit to field test it in Assa. After doing the day's cases in the operating theatre, I would scurry to round up informants for the labor-intensive and time-consuming color interviews in Pazande (the home language) or Bangala (the market tongue). In a few instances we did color interviews in each language on different days for the same bilingual informants. It was very hard work, both for the interviewer and the informants. Each interview and the recording of the data took more than four hours in each language. It had to be completed while there was light to see, recognize and name the color chips. There is little "twilight" on the equator. Equatorial equinox means that with little warning, darkness falls, ending the color linguistics testing in whatever stage it was at the time the light faded quickly away at jungle sunset. After much effort, the data were packed up and carried out of Africa for analysis with a former linguistic anthropology instructor, named Rob MacLaury, now resident in Philadelphia.

He had enthusiastically noted the much higher discrimination of colors in the home language Pazande than in the market tongue Bangala, and proposed a further testing of the hypothesis that objects of the same colors would be identified differently in spatial configuration according to their similarities or differences. On this trip, we increased four-fold the number of informants to give us complete color interviews in each language on subsequent days. We were also able to configure both colors and objects in triad patterns of similarity or dissimilarity when the informants were given instructions in the home language on one day and the market language on another day. This experiment would suggest the pattern of influence of language on thought, the so-called "Sapir-Whorf Hypothesis."

Now, it may not be readily apparent to the reader just what I am studying in the hypothyroidism survey, and what my motive and methods might be in treating this condition and trying methods to prevent it. "Doing science" in what might be euphemistically called "field conditions" is often more complicated than within a controlled laboratory setting. The field study can't eliminate noisy distractions and unwanted variables outside the controls of a laboratory setting. Assa is "far afield." *Especially* in the settings of a less complex society as is present in Assa, the doctor would be given some benefit of the doubt as to what he or she is trying to do. The individual patient emerges from the operation or requested treatment with obvious and quick improvement. Mission accomplished.

Try that with the convoluted, laborious, even if superficially quite simple, scientific methods of linguistic anthropology! I have just attempted a brief explanation of one set of methods to you. You are literate and reading it in English, a language into which you were born. You have been acculturated to appreciate the scientific method. It has brought benefits individually and collectively to the society represented by those in which the author and reader are resident. How easy is that to explain in Assa?

We have a method that will study the cognitive "hard-wiring" across a wide spectrum of cultures, languages, and environments. Try to explain this subtlety to a group of informants one must interview one at a time for long periods across great gulfs of culture, linguistic skills and impatient skepticism on what the return benefit might be to anyone at all! If I had not previously earned their trust and this important entrée to do this study through the credibility of the medical outcomes they had witnessed, they would wander off even earlier to their garden shambas to do the real work of staying alive rather than this arcane ritual to humor the *Bwana*. It was very difficult to hold the informants in one place, let alone obtain their interest, in this extended data-gathering stage of the linguistic anthropology study.

Captivating attention is what I had deliberately sought *not to do*, when carrying the color kit through the Bunia border. "What is this?" the "customs officer" *sans* uniform asked of me, holding up the black plastic recipe box that had the color chips stuffed inside in sequence for the study. If I had explained that this device was a scientific instrument for critical use in a linguistic anthropology study, he might have sliced it open, or confiscated it to see if this could be value-added in ransoming it back. But the black plastic cover of the recipe box has a special stick-on cartoon. It is "Spiderman" spreading his net. After the official looked at this absurd cartoon for kids, and spilled the Munsell color chips from the box, he just shrugged when I said, "It's a toy!"

The customs officials were probably thinking, "What weird and wonderful stuff these Americans seem to travel around with. Just exactly at what age do these zany Americans put away such childish things?" As effective as this disguise into triviality makes the color kit, the same box has to be used with the informants looking quizzically to see what manner of odd fetishes this odd American stencils onto his tools and toys!

Let me describe what this study *could not* do. I could not do color interviews on cretins before and after treatment to see how much their cognition and communication was enhanced. A severely effected cretin is deaf-mute and profoundly retarded, so that a complex interview in subtle linguistic discrimination in color and spatial relations is a nonstarter. To reduce the variables, the informants were limited to bilingual males 20 to 60 years of age resident lifelong in Assa who had obviously improved under the hypothyroidism program. Many untreated informants could not pull themselves together long enough to complete interviews. After treatment, they were able to complete the interviews with interesting results. Some were still naïve about the scientific intent and method. An informant would ask, in all innocence after the successful completion of a long interview series over several days, "When will I hear whether I have passed the test?"

"Doing science" with makeshift materials and methods, while sitting on a log in a thatched-roof hut as the sky is darkening with dusk or storm clouds, and still maintaining standardization for reliable statistical tests only *sounds* romantic. In repetitive fact, it is not! To respond to skepticism in peer review that comparative cognitive data must be forthcoming to confirm a real human benefit following the hypothyroidism management program, I must carry back scientifically rigorous studies. For the population under study, the improvement is self-evident. Participation in these taxing interviews requiring concentration on iterative tasks is not necessary.

Ironically, if only the informants could have responded to a similar test when obtunded in profound hypothyroidism, their ability to sit still for prolonged periods and carry out low-level cognitive tests repeatedly with a low energy expenditure would have been optimal for study purposes, even if their response times would have been much slower. Now that they have become euthyroid, they are restless, and can think of many things to which they might apply their new energy instead of sitting through a prolonged test which, somehow, must humor *Bwana*. In spite of these difficulties, the scientist in me felt compelled to pursue the study, even as the physician in me knew that the study was an unnecessary procedure with little benefit and some potential harm for the informants. As in many other medical settings, the physician must balance these competing instincts and make decisions for the greater good of the patient and community.

WRITER IN RESIDENCE

On each occasion when I return from one of my "surgical adventures in the African bush" I am told: "Oh, you *must* write a book about these experiences!"

"Oh, but I have!" I respond. "I travel like an excited squid, leaving a cloud of black ink in my wake." On every occasion of my ventures into the unknown, I have carried a reporter's notepad, a portable tape recorder, a camera, and write about each of the experiences in a serialized journal, letters, and even serial postcards! Many of these book-length written records have been passed from hand to hand in fifth generation xerography, and I am always about to put the completed text into book form when the next trip interrupts me. I also identify myself as a *writer*. How can I continue to be called a writer without having these books published? I have written hundreds of medical papers and several medical books. These efforts were part of my profession as academic surgeon. A real writer writes because he or she must. Joseph Conrad was a writer. Publishing my work also makes it possible to extend the reach of my journals beyond those to whom it is sent or those to whom they pass it along.

Using a policy that NASA refers to as "redundancy in depth," I will continue to write my summary serial letters, daily or at least weekly, and have always used the "down time" around theatre and whenever there is light to write longhand what I am doing here. At least these manuscripts should be able to be collected upon my return if the electronic media fail for any reason, man-made or otherwise, by accident or intent.

But, I have entered a new age as a writer. I am now here in Central Africa, without a reliable source of electricity but with my untrustworthy smuggled laptop computer. I can now generate my observations from the field, and some time through some means actually transmit it back to individuals following the events as they happen and perhaps even rendering support for the missions. The telemetry on this trip will take principally two forms: E-mailing the messages back as attachments if I can find a functioning phone somewhere from Nyankunde to Nairobi, and surely when I arrive in South Africa, and posting back the written journals and downloaded floppy discs.

The computer is a very desirable asset. Its capability, when powered, enables the creation of the record of another still-more-stimulating experience than each of the others that preceded it in this Central African series. So desirable is it, in fact, that its nearly sure fate will be to be stolen, most likely by Congolese government "officials" whose "benefits packages" consist mainly of predation of items such as this from sources such as I. As a consequence, I am making sure that I copy the material I type into both the hard disc, and on a formatted disc stored separately, so that all the information the computer contains does not disappear when (not if) it does.

I speak with experience on this subject. My first month in Mozambique in 1996 was recorded by a hand-written series of journal entries in a student's exercise book. I was relieved of my tape recorder, camera, and prior portable computer equipment by two bayonet-wielding bandits who fell from trees overhanging a secluded park-like Maputo road. I will try to post this disc from a safe place, most likely upon an exit visit to the US Embassy in Nairobi. If it is not possible to e-mail it directly from the embassy, I will put the disc into the diplomatic mail pouch (as I did during my term as Senior Fulbright Scholar) or mail it from Kenya's more secure postal service.

I have never, ever, mailed *anything* using the Congolese post. They sell stamps, and collect fines if one is caught using a foreign postal address, but these are the only two aboveground functions I can determine that the Congolese post has. Others have told me that if a letter, with nothing of any value, is given over to the Congolese Postal Service, it has about a 5% chance of arrival at its destination address outside the Congo. If there is something of value in a package being sent out, it has no chance to make it to its destination, since it will be stripped out of the "flow" of items, all going nowhere, and pillaged with the same certainty that unaccompanied luggage will "go missing." A letter coming from somewhere else into the Congo is already assumed to be more valuable than anything that is going out, so these are doomed by their stamps or return addresses. I hope to be generating and carrying a manuscript and disc that will make its way around these internal diversions to a reliable postal service or electronic relay station.

Mary Jane Robertson at Nebobongo tells a story that illustrates the nonexistence of the Congolese Postal Service. A government official (this one even had a uniform) tried to levy a fine upon her, since she was using Kenyan stamps and passing letters to whomever had come through to drop in the Nairobi post in transit. The man wanted a fine of $500.00 US. So confident was she in the inept and corrupt civil service that she challenged them: "Here is the check for $500.00 US (the 'official,' of course, wanted only US currency for the 'fine'). Here is also a letter addressed to my mother in England covered with legitimate stamps of Zaïre. When the response from this letter returns here to me through the Congolese post, I will turn over to you this check for what you say is my fine." Of course, no letter or "official" ever returned, and all of Nebobongo still uses traveler-carried mail.

The terms applied to some of these agencies have the ring of a Zen koan. "Consider the Congolese Postal Service." Or, "Consider the Maputo Sewage Treatment System." Or, "Consider the Nigerian Zoning Commission." A civil servant in Nigeria illustrated the point with the following exchange: "See that eight story building over there?"

"No, I do not, but there is a smaller four story building in front of us," I replied.

"Ahah!" the Nigerian poked his hand in his pocket. "Fifty percent in pocket!" He went on to ask, "Do you see that bridge over there?"

"No, I see no bridge over there," I responded.

"So, you see! 100% in pocket!"

If the problem of how to get my Assa story posted *out* of the computer and back to my US base can be resolved, the bigger more immediate problem is how to get the story *into* the computer. First, I have to find enough time and light to type it in. I am a relatively recent convert to word processing. There is often a tension for the use of time in either *having* certain or further experiences or *recording* them, with one of these uses possibly excluding the other given a finite amount of time and light each working day.

Second, how will I feed the ThinkPad? I had brought my A/C and D/C adapter chargers and a second new battery. The A/C adapter is a nonstarter here where there is no generator, no current, few wires, and no electrical outlets. All have gone away with the last pass of the marauding army. Many of the wires are now being used as snares to catch bush meat. The computer battery can be used for about three hours before it is discharged. I had also purchased a D/C adapter for use in aircraft or the cigarette lighter power source of a vehicle, should either be available. The hulk of the stripped Bronco is parked behind huts here at the compound, another bit of spoor in the wake of the passing troops, with nothing useful anywhere near it.

The new storage battery we had flown in with from Nyankunde should be useful, and was intended to power the vaccine refrigerator, the free end of the "cold chain" for vaccine here designated for the end users. This storage battery also powers the operating room (OR) light, a jury-rigged contraption of copper wires running from battery terminals to a Toyota headlamp taped on a frame of pipes. This energy source was renewable, as it could be recharged from the solar panel on the roof of our OR. Renewability only lasted one day. The solar panel was stolen off the roof on the moonless night of my arrival here. We will continue our operating and refrigerating vaccines now powered by whatever charge we carried with us in the Cessna, but after this battery becomes flat, the OR light will dim and the vaccines spoil. I worried about using precious electricity for my computer but decided to go ahead, thinking that the people of Assa would receive some benefit from my book. How often do you need to think about the morality of allocation of electrical energy?

I was amazed when my companions considered this electrical doomsday following the discovery of the theft of the solar panel an inconvenience, but turned quickly to other things that were more important issues. "We will do as much as long as we can, and nothing lasts forever, including the battery's electricity and us and our time here together. It is important to you and to us that you can use that machine to write about Assa, so we will see what we can do." And they did. Between André and Inikpio, the new D/C charger was examined at the plug-in end. A length of torn bandage was wrapped around the plug and used to spring the contact end forward, while a piece of heavy copper wire was twisted into a loop. The loop was taped to the outside contacts of the D/C adapter plug and the central contact at the end was tightly bandaged to a copper wire going to the other end of the battery terminal where it was threaded through to just barely make contact. Sparks would fly when contact was lost, as when anyone walked by, or when the light was adjusted to illuminate the patient on the table. Somehow, this fragile jury-rig was able to make contact long enough to recharge the computer battery for up to an hour's running when it was not connected. I would type in OR between cases, or when I was supervising a case they were doing, and then carry the ThinkPad back to the house at the close of the day. After all other chores were done, medical or linguistic, I can type for about an hour by the guttering flicker of a candle placed at the keyboard until the laptop bleeps (anywhere where British influence has permeated before American terms took root, machines "bleep," not "beep") to announce it is about to crash for lack of power as the battery runs flat. To the extent that you are still reading this, the fragile recharging system will have continued to revive the computer battery each new day in the OR.

　　　While life still continues to go on here, so will the story of Assa. Before battery life wanes, I will still continue to try to record it in bytes. What more, after all, can anyone or anything be expected to do in such circumstances but to just keep on trying?

11 REGROUPING IN ASSA

**SORTING OUT THE *MATERIA MEDICA*,
COMPARING NOTES ON RECENT HISTORY,
SETTING A PROGRAM FOR THIS VISIT,
AND ACCOMMODATING INCONVENIENCES OF MISSING
AMENITIES**

July 8, 1998

Thanks to the hot-wiring of the theatre storage battery to my D/C charger plug (**Figure 5**), I have borrowed enough of the energy from the battery in theatre to continue writing my story for yet another night. It is not easy doing things after 6:00 PM in blackness. I have a limited stock of candles furnishing the only light I have other than what comes from this screen or the tiny Mag-Lite that I have carried for a few years awaiting just such an emergency. Somehow, despite knowing more about this than most should, I had not figured on my day coming to an abrupt halt with sunset, especially since unlike a summer sunset, darkness comes early. We have to eat in the dark the standard Assa dinner (a feast by any standards of the devastated community) of a scrawny pullet chopped into palm fat and peanut oil as a condiment over a mound of rice. The rice makes a gravelly sound when chewed in the dark, for reasons that are obviously best left in the dark.

Then, somewhere out in the darkness, I believe in this instance it can legitimately be called the "Heart of that Darkness," I hear the strains of a hymn played upon the French horn I had scavenged in the US and sent here six years ago. The dark has not discouraged this fellow from doing his best with what little he has—the horn that came into his world from afar as a gift for which he is still grateful and expressing that gratitude tonight and every time it is played.

And, now, to complete the sound-picture, since the visibility is near zero, the "Talking Drum" of the Azande is coming through the cacophony of evening birdsong. The two-toned rhythmic message is meaningful to those who

69

can "hear" it—or simply setting a tone for those such as I who cannot. I am at home, in the dark and devastated Congo. I am among friends who can teach anyone a lot about life and how to live it gratefully, even joyfully. They live amid as many excuses to complain bitterly about their fate as any, yet they still shrug and say when asked about the details, "We must do only what we can and must."

FIGHTING OFF THE TROPICAL MALAISE
AND STILL NOT OPENING MYSELF
TO THE MORE DEADLY CEREBRAL MALARIA

So, I too, am trying to do only what I can and must. It is not easy. I have my own aching inflammatory reaction to re-entry into the tropics. I arrive with jet lag and the tropical lassitude that comes from irresistible eternal verities—like dawn and dusk, like no hot water and little enough water, let alone enough to shower. I am so lucky as to have a bed, how can anyone be so churlish as to now want sheets, or blanket or pillow as well? Part of my general malaise, I have only recently come to recognize, may be the central nervous system sequelae of starting up on mefloquine antimalarial prophylaxis. This is the way I felt during much of my time in Mozambique in the heart of its January rainy season with bad malaria cases and multiple deaths in women and children swarming almost as thick as the mosquitoes. I have not yet been too much troubled by mosquitoes, but I am now troubled by the mefloquine hangover. I am almost tempted to forego the prophylaxis, and would prefer the chloroguanidine hydrochloride, a less toxic but less effective drug not available in the US. I prefer this prophylactic antimalarial, except while crawling through swamps on the hunt with my friends in Assa in the heart of the highest malarial-risk rainy season.

ALL THE COMFORTS AND CONVENIENCES OF HOME
IF HOME WAS A RECENT TROGLODYTE EXPERIENCE!

So, I have the "*choo*," Kiswahili for "hole." I should not need the conveniences of flush toilets that have been around since Crete's Minoan civilization. So, in answer to the most frequently asked questions about what do I eat, and what do I —you know —do? The plumbing should be the first and easiest to dispose of. It isn't. There is a bathtub and a toilet that sits there in all its regal commode majesty, but is essentially the only chair in the house that is not portable, and is therefore still here. And as for water, it is available, in this rainy season, if I fetch it. I have just had the luxury of my first "cup and bucket" bath. This is clearly not a situation ideal for a running program, since getting hot and sweaty and smelly is not something one would want to do deliberately. Besides, why would anyone deliberately go out and waste calories that are precious and therefore to be conserved? So, for the last week and the foreseeable future, I was a highly attuned, and well-conditioned nonrunner.

I spoke too soon about the sameness of our regular feast, with boiled rice and a scrawny chicken. We have run out of the luxury of the chicken part and now have a gruel of greens for a topping. This is like the "*tua di mia*" of Nigeria, in which a gravy of some sort was put over pounded cassava, the staple here as well, with the exception that we have had the added luxury of rice for the carbohydrate staple, even if the rice is swept up with a bit of the gravel on which it is threshed. Dental crowns are unheard of here in Assa. The *fufu* or *tua di mia* of West Africa, depending on whether the language is Hausa, francophone, or the myriad of local languages, has a staple diet of some high-fiber, low-energy starch and saturated vegetable fat. It is palm fat or peanut oil here that makes the "gravy" over the staple base. With luck and industry, there is some condiment-style meat or greens added for protein. The condiments are used to make it look like a different entrée. This dish is often the single thing eaten daily. There aren't a lot of people with food allergies, bulimia, or lactose intolerance in Assa.

Because of my celebrity and their generosity, we eat three times a day, with the only variety being that the breakfast is lighter without the rice and gravy, but focused around the sliced pineapple and fried bananas. There is local coffee, and local peanuts, served either boiled or pounded into fresh peanut butter. This is not stored but made fresh daily. This is a good thing, because it is an excellent culture medium for *Aspergillus flavus*, a mold that secretes aflatoxin, a potent liver carcinogen. Since my initial arrival, I am an honored guest and thus am eating first and most of the best. That we should think of eating three times a day, not my usual habit even in my home base, is quite a luxury. The royal name for the Swazi rulers is "*Dlamini*" which means "Eater at midday." You have to be rather well-fixed to throw in a third meal, especially this frivolous one at midday.

Since I am writing an Odyssean travelogue here, I should describe local communication and transportation. This can be done succinctly. There is none, at least not until the plane arrives, whenever that will be. The "phonie" depends on the battery, and the battery has been out, which is why they had to guess when we would be arriving. They could neither call on the radio to tell us that things were very dicey over here with soldiers beating and shooting Assa residents, nor that the immediate, most severe threat had cleared. We have an idea that the plane will return for me and my team in less than three weeks when we hope to go on from here to Banda. There we will have to set up their looted OR with the one third of Assa's supplies we have sorted out as redundant. It could be plus or minus a few days of the July 22 planned date that we had hazarded as a guess.

So much for airline schedules. We will know that the plane is coming when we hear it.

Transportation, once again, comes back to that plane unless one is interested in a bicycle or *pikipiki* ride through the rainy season vegetation and "puddles and potholes." The rainy season "roads" here are nothing serious, mind you. It is just that they have swallowed whole lorries without a trace. The Assa station has at least three vehicles, all rusting in their final resting-place. A truck brought from Banda years ago has some major vegetation growing through its rusted hulk. It did not run even ten years ago when I was first watching it get transplanted with borrowed parts that were mainly jury-rigged. It is now just a carcass. The Bronco worked on my last visit but is now nonfunctional. It is under cover, but with a slashed right rear tire. The soldiers that came through last week stole the left front tire. There is no evidence of the cigarette lighter socket in the hole in the dash. Besides, the chances of there being a battery still present after the scavengers swept everything else are so slim that I did not even look. If it were not for the jury-rig on the OR battery no longer rejuvenated from the missing solar panel, I would not be able to communicate through this device either. Any communication would occur only if the messenger carried the message. My high-tech machinery looks less weather beaten and broken down than the other highly desirable items that have already vanished. I have to be wary of where it is displayed, used, or left unattended.

IT IS TIME NOW TO GET TO WORK

I have distributed the large stock of medicines and divided some of the instruments for relief of Banda's more devastated OR. I found a shipment of what is called the "first relief pack" of essential drugs and supplies. These are sent to the war-torn areas that have just had the most recent disasters, the civil war and a second hit in this case. They were sent by Med-Air, a Swiss NGO that uses the UNICEF "Essential Drugs List." I looked over what they had sent along, and it is good that it is here. I had promised the Swiss doctor I met at the CME Guest House that I would let her know that I had seen it and accounted for it. Not everything that is in the kit would I consider essential, and a lot is missing; but let's start with something. The MAP Travel Packs that I brought in were well-supplied with several items of high value that will be used well, particularly the antibiotics and other extremely valuable, time-sensitive (i.e., they expire) items such as antimalarials. I figured that my own cost for the mefloquine is about $7.00 per pill. With the addition of the surgical instruments, which should be semi-permanent additions, at least as long as they are in Inikpio's hands, Assa is restocked to go on. I didn't bring pontocaine for the spinal anesthesia because I thought it was already available in Assa. We will do our work under local anesthetic and morphine.

We have worked out the timing of our linguistic study so that we will not subtract too much daylight time from the time when the people will be out in the forest and fields trying to find food. But, we, too, need light to do our study, especially since it involves color vision. We have no lights, we will try to focus this in the afternoons after we get the string of cases we reviewed in consultations today, for operations tomorrow. Surprisingly, there were few goiters apparent. Hypothyroidism, here caused by dietary iodine deficiency, effects adults with goiter. When congenital, it causes cretinism. Cretins have stunting of both physical growth and intellectual development. Their stature, coordination, and productivity are usually profoundly retarded. We had treated the entire village with a depot iodine injection called Lipiodal. We did this toward the end of the missionary work of Diane Downing. White missionaries were withdrawn from the Assa station eight years ago. The blanketing of the area with Lipiodal reduced the incidence of hypothyroidism.

I was greeted, as always, by several very enthusiastic cretins, including Sasa, the old chief's half brother, and Bodo, the fellow who had incarcerated a hernia, one of the first "operations" undertaken in Assa early on. I saw a few of my goiter patients in follow-up and they had what looked like smaller, firmer goiters. By now, I have paid several calls for the sake of social amenities, and have gone to visit Pastor Tanda's grave. My last memory of him is carrying a big pot of stuff to the aircraft at my departure in 1996, holding it up and licking his finger with his lips, signaling that it was freshly produced peanut butter he had made for my journey. Despite the long trek back by way of South Africa and Mozambique, I did manage to get some of it back to the US for a sample of Assa to the Downings as Tanda's last tribute.

SO, NOW, TO WORK, AS BEFORE

I used to feel guilty about going out to go hunting in the predawn hours before operating, since I thought I might be holding up the team in the OR. Fat chance! When I said we would get an early start, it might be after ten before we had all the greetings, preliminaries and questions about family and how well each had fared and slept in the interval since last seen, 30 minutes before. So, our early start on "the list" was around 10:30 AM, an irreducible and obligatory stand-around time is required worldwide it seems. It quickly brings back to my mind what it is that I miss least about this operating business. As I have always said to my residents, "The only thing difficult about operating, is *getting to do it!*" Now, in Assa, this does not mean going through a politically charged and potentially hostile process of obtaining permits and reviews of credentials. In either Assa or the US, there is an entropic deliberative force that retards forward motion with the clear message that whatever we do not get to do today, will just be there available for us tomorrow, and will be that much less that we are required to exert today. The tempo of the ORs of the world I have frequented are sometimes set by the passive-aggressive temperaments of anesthetists. Now, fortunately, in Assa, we have no anesthetist, so only the local anesthesia, administered by the surgeons, is the rate-limiting step. We have already jumped one hurdle by the nonavailability of certain "inconveniences" of deprivation.

THEY ALSO SERVE WHO ONLY STAND AND WAIT

Who is our first patient, but Bule! He had an epigastric hernia that was bothering him, so that we fixed it under local anesthetic. It was an honor to take care of my good friend. I did not want to set a precedent as the white *Bwana* coming to do operations while everyone else watched. I made a point of prepping, draping, and then gowning Sonny Mwembo and his home-grown assistant, Émile Zola, the native son of Assa, being groomed to take over Banda when he finishes at CME Nyankunde. When Ahuka certifies him as surgically competent, he will complete his effort in training to become a local boy made good.

He affects the name "Émile Zola" which he prefers (as "Alberto" was the Portuguese name that Ahuka once preferred, that I now notice he is using less and less). After Émile's graduation at CME, he will be Banda's Inikpio. It is Émile Zola who had occasioned the grand flurry as he returned to Assa for the first visit after eight years at CME Nyankunde, and had the chance to come home with this team as we made the rounds in this series of surgical visits. I shook his father's hand and pointed out how proud I was to be here to support the team, especially his son's first chance to work in the village where he was born.

In confidence building, whether in US surgical residents, medical students, or paramedical personnel groomed to be the local health care resource in an environment such as Assa, I want it to be seen that *Bwana* is here to help them helping others. The more cautious they seem, with patient safety a high priority, the more independence they will get in decision-making. If they seem rambunctious and rough in cocky adventurism at the patient's risk, the trainees get much more closely supervised, or even interdicted from certain procedures, until that cautious confidence returns. I am pointing out to everyone who it is that did what, and show them by some distance from the OR table who is in charge. That takes about three times the amount of time to get anything done, since they are a bit hesitant, but appear safe.

Meanwhile, I am going to use this time, masked in OR, and sitting at the side as "consultant in residence" and available for help if needed, to plug my ThinkPad into the OR battery as they work. I will report what is happening here at Assa, even if this signal will take some time to get out along with me. This writing will also solve the problem of pacing in the theatre, while nothing much particularly seems to be happening. I should have had this jury-rig for the ThinkPad long ago!

Daylight is very precious to us, since we will need it to do the linguistic study. It is also the time that the other work of Assa needs to get done, their fieldwork as well as mine. So, if I can make things go a bit smoother and faster here in the surgical theatre, we can perhaps get one complete set of data done before dark this afternoon. They will have helped me toward my goal as I am helping them toward theirs here, a rather good trade in "foreign exchange."

12 SETTLING IN AT ASSA

LAUNCH MEDICAL AND LINGUISTIC WORK
WHILE TALKING ABOUT BUT NOT GOING HUNTING IN ASSA

July 9-10, 1998

IN THEATRE

I watched over some medical efforts and helped a full day in theatre (**Figure 4**), which including Bule's hernia repair, a hysterectomy (**Figure 10**), and amputation of a leg. André tells a story about a Zande from Banda who "learned surgery." His one operation, not unlike some US gynecologists, was hysterectomy. It was once said of a gynecologist in my Washington turf that he had almost single-handedly stamped out the dreaded disease called *uterus in situ*. Hysterectomy was his one operation and he plied it to something in excessive numbers for indications not always apparent to pathologists. Similarly, this Zande surgeon went to work at Aba, near the Sudan. A few years later André had come through this district and had heard a lot of complaints. The women of the area were remarkably infertile, and had lost some normal cyclic functions. They found out that the single common cause seemed to have been that the fellow from Banda operated on them all. So, the informant said to André, "Do not go near Aba as a Zande man, since the women there will kill you!"

There was no doubt about the indication for today's hysterectomy. The woman was genuinely relieved of the soccer-ball-sized fibroids pushing in on her bladder. The last case was a young man with a two-year-old open fracture of the ankle and bad osteomyelitis, resulting in draining abscesses and a large sequestrum in the bone. He is "butt-crawling" around and needs to get his other wasted limb in motion before contracture takes this relatively young man well beyond rehabilitation. He is being treated surgically with a below-the-knee amputation so that a home-made prosthesis can be fitted to salvage something of his life and get rid of this two-year-old ball and chain. He readily agreed to amputation, since he would have very little else left to him in life except to tend this dead and smelly limb and center his life around caring for it. It also shows the high cost of the neglected fracture care that is missing here. This fracture caused him not just a lot of morbidity, but changed his life to the degree it would have been impossible for him to do anything but waste away and die soon.

STORIES OF PAST HUNTS

We have told stories until into the night, and I filled one audiotape with André's halting rendition of tales of his early days as a renegade poacher. This earlier career nearly cost him his life. The obvious risks were from either the feet of angry elephants, or the fangs of the hungry lion. The interdiction of soldiers, who were also interested in the "white gold," was a more serious and inevitable danger. They were not above relieving him of the illicit ivory, the favorite currency of the local, well-armed kleptocracy.

A long story, taped in its entirety, described André's excursion from near Assa on July 18, 1983. He was going to CME Nyankunde to make a name for himself in the medical or dental profession if he could pass the examinations to get in. To get the funding to pay for this, he joined one of the "hunters" at Assa who took him on as an apprentice elephant hunter. They set off on a long hike with several porters, following the tracks of a band of elephants on a circuitous route ending up 60 km from Assa. Not one of these very astute "orienteers" had a clue where they were when they came upon the elephants at last, but suddenly it was pay-day. The hunter shot often, and was careful to have instructed André on his exit route so he did not find himself running into the elephants as they spooked. They might run randomly and trample the team of five hard-working fellows who were intent on getting meat and ivory. I probably was listening to the single biggest reason that elephants have become endangered in this area. Random distribution of high technology, "army surplus" rifles into the hands of a desperate band of bush folk, spells doom for elephants. Elephants represent a windfall of food and currency to them.

Five elephants fell. The hunters around Assa travel light, and continue trekking for days. They are often amazed at the extra equipment that I carry along in a backpack. They spent a full day chopping out ivory, and gathering up some meat. They had no other supplies and were lost.

The group gathered to listen to these stories had looked on with envy as I showed them the wonders of my GPS. I had once given Jean Marco my binoculars, the "twins"("*Bï*" in Pazande) as the Assa hunters call them. One hunter asked the naïve question, "How does the little animal get into them?"

I said, "Here!" handing them the reversed binoculars. "This is what the white man sees;" and flipping them around: "This is what Jean Marco sees without the glasses!" Now, I said about my GPS, "This will mean that I will only get lost one half as much which will now still be much more often than any of you do!"

André and the others had set out for home carrying ivory and some elephant meat, but nothing else. They had no food and no matches, so had nothing to eat until they tried eating the strips of elephant meat raw. They had only the water they drank from the streams they irregularly encountered and hiked all day until dark and collapsed, still unaware of where they were headed. After five days of this torture, when they were famished and exhausted, André came up with the suggestion that they follow any stream down, and he would find one of the two rivers he knew they were between. This suggestion of the "schoolboy" was met by derision, so the regular hunters split from him. They soon caught up when it was apparent that they had no better idea and were close to exhaustion. André made it out alive with barely enough time to escape the pursuit of the soldiers. It turned out that the most dangerous part of this formidable escapade was not the elephants or the overwhelming wilderness but the encounter with the soldiers. They had heard he was packing a 12 and a 10 kg tusk, and wanted to relieve him of this heavy burden, and also throw his body into the same river he had been following. But, he escaped Assa, ahead of the "poachers poaching poachers" and caught the ride to his new life in Nyankunde.

But, not a very new life, since he also went hunting in Nyankunde with a home-made shotgun and was fascinated to see a mother and baby chimp in the trees overhead. Mamma was teaching baby how to grab trees and swing through them by reaching out an arm and withdrawing so the baby would have to jump. He was watching the human-like antics of this pair of "*Soko Mutu*" = "almost a man," or less literally "could even be human." Suddenly, a big male chimp appeared within two meters of André who was sitting under the tree where the chimp's offspring and mate were cavorting above. André reflexly pulled up the shotgun, a home-made contraption, as most are, its previous life having been lived as a piece of outdoor plumbing, and fired.

He hit the big male chimp full in the chest, and he was knocked down but instantly got up to run. They followed him for a day and did not find him. The next day they came upon him sitting in a glade beneath a tree with his head contemplatively on his folded arms, very stone dead—looking "just like a man!" They dismembered him and carried his huge limbs back to Nyankunde where they distributed the meat to all as what Ahuka had called Cape buffalo beef. The Nyankunde recipients were delighted. Later Ahuka asked the people, "Would you eat a *Soko Mutu*?"

They answered, "Oh, no, since they could even be human!"
"Well, you did, now what do you think of that?" replied Ahuka.

After an hour of André's hunting stories—which were not necessarily about "fair chase" on big game species, I told two hours of stories relating to elephants in *Zala,* Cape buffalo near Mambasa, and my encounter with a leopard as I sat through the night, guarding my first bushbuck in the dark jungle.

They still wanted more hunting stories so we kept telling yarns. As we continued reporting what had happened to us before, I subtly asked about recent events. The first little dribble of information about what happened last week in Assa came out. It involves horrors that even these people were not used to seeing. For starters, four men had been made to lie down in the road in front of the Assa crowd and then sprayed with gunfire. But, as any good journalist, I will wait to get several confirming reports before detailing any more about what had preceded our visit. These horrors have made this emotional roller coaster week such a tumultuous one for them. We arrived just in time to help in Assa at the far end of any line of communication, supply, relief, rescue or rehabilitation.

But for now, I am an OR consultant in residence, and am being called to assist in a difficult operation. So, I will leave the ThinkPad to drink in more of what it can hold from the storage battery. I will continue writing this story later, sitting, not quite as Abe Lincoln at the flickering light of a fireside alone in his study, since in my case, the flickering light is the candle sitting on the cover of the ThinkPad. I hope the candle and I can shed some illumination on this situation in the Heart of this Darkness!

OPEN NOW THE LINGUISTIC WORK
IN ADDITION TO THE MEDICAL SUPPLY
AND OPERATING

I was worried that I might never seem to get started on the large volume of work that I had anticipated for Assa. It is now time to get into gear with the linguistic study previously designed for my Ph.D. dissertation. My dissertation committee at GWU torpedoed it, by first changing it all around and then rejecting it. I have decided I would try to salvage what I could of the original project which already has had a great deal of effort put into preliminary data-gathering, both last trip and this one with a good deal of preparation of methods and models in between. I must complete the color linguistics part of my study. On my last trip, in 1996, this was as hard as pulling sound teeth when I tried to round up the informants and have them sit down for long enough to finish just one set of the complete studies. We would either lose the light or their interest, or something else would come up, and they would wander off. That was true of both the informants and the onlookers. They want to be around the action, but feel pressured to come up with information if they are part of that action. So pulling teeth is not a bad analogy for what has to happen now. It is a good thing we have a dentist involved!

André is spearheading this part of the study. He and a number of the others now understand why I am doing this part of the study to get a nonculturally-bound description of their acuity of discrimination, as a measure for the cognitive improvement that has taken place with the treatment program for hypothyroidism. A cretin sits in the shade without blinking as flies crawl into his eyes, is stunted in physical growth and is an imbecile with respect to his mental development. Treating his hypothyroidism is not much of a triumph, if all that happens after treatment is that you make him a hungrier cretin and a better calorie consumer, and change the thyroid hormone levels in his blood without giving him any improvement in quality of life. Even though we observed that several cretins increased their intellectual capacity, such anecdotal testimony isn't scientifically rigorous. We are attempting to gather data to show objective improvement of cognitive function.

DO RESEARCH WHILE THE SUN SHINES, OR ELSE THERE WILL BE NO RESEARCH TO BE DONE

It is and will forever be impossible to test a hypothyroid cretin with some form of culture-bound test, especially based on language. They are deaf-mute generally, and they are subnormal in their mental status when they can be aroused to see some basic simple stimulus, and painfully slow in coming up with any response, especially one that involves judgment. So, the preliminary results of this study were simply dismissed, even though I had supplied the committee of experts with data supporting my thesis. Instead, they called for volumes of library research in other people's theories, saying what I intended could not be done, as though this is not a scholarly work in progress, sitting here on a log in the Congo. The committee called for videotapes of interactive sessions to "contextualize" the color response, while simply dismissing the data already available for review and refusing to read the supporting materials forwarded to them as too voluminous.

With an abstract based on the earlier work submitted to the American Association of Anthropology (AAA)(**Appendix II**), and further data to be gathered at least for that forum, it would seem that I have to go full speed ahead on this tedious, labor-intensive study. I must still do this work to prove a cognitive benefit to the earlier hypothyroidism prevention program. But then, I still must generate a new dissertation thesis and certainly a new committee, since the enormous amount of labor that "invests" this kind of activity is not worth putting into arbitrary and capricious hands. So, after I have worked as hard as I can on this study and its further data-gathering and completion, at least through all the color linguistics part and a few into the discriminatory triads, I will have to return to start all over from zero, on a new thesis

In deciding to forge ahead with the linguistic anthropology project, I am fighting much greater odds than those artificially imposed by a committee in Washington. I am conducting intensive interviews in two very unusual Bantu languages, desperately trying to get these long interviews done by the light of day. Fortunately, the first two informants that I had to interview today were my two hunter-companions, Jean Marco and Kongonyesi. Both are smart and have already done one of the languages, and now we are repeating the color interviews in the other tongue. I am testing them to see if they have acuity differences in Pazande or Bangala.

The next two informants were brought to us as volunteers to be involved in this study and were sitting in wait to be included. They were presented a simple color chip and asked the name of the color, in one of the two languages. Getting a single commitment out of them was harder than pulling teeth, and it was André the dentist at work on it. I had hoped to do several sets of the color interviews, and these two plugged up the entire day. One slow wheel could derail the train. This is almost the equivalent of interviewing the hypothyroid cretins who are stressed to come up with any judgment of any kind. I am typing this in as the struggle is going on at a painfully slow pace under André's tutelage. I will take over for the other language or until the sun goes down, whichever comes first. It is highly likely that it would be the latter, and they would return to plug all of the next day as well.

Progress is being made on my fieldwork for a research project just recently disqualified as any part of my thesis for which I am now "ABD" (all but dissertation). Here in the field, I am dragging answers out of a group of informants who are interested in being part of some happening thing, but are more like an anchor retarding the forward progress of this research in a study designed to entice some support to help them. This is a prime example of the frustration and the paradox in "development assistance" about which we have been talking before and after arrival here at the "end of the beyond."

13 OLD SHOES

A TALE TOLD BY OLD RUNNING SHOES
DESTINED TO BE USED AND REMAIN IN ASSA

July 10, 1998

Now, do not get me wrong. I am not getting sentimental and all choked up about old shoes, or the history of great events that have transpired in them. I brought almost all of what I have with me for a very specific purpose. That, as ever, is to have most all of it make a one-way trip into the heart of African poverty in Assa. Here my old castoffs are the height of fashion when they can be used by those who typically have nothing but scraps of old rags, and even that is a step up from the bark cloth that many were wearing earlier, and some still are. But a thought just struck me as I was looking at what remains in my possession here and will stay here after I leave. I once left Assa barefoot when I had said something to one of the men at the airstrip who had come to see me off with a gift. I looked down to see he was barefoot. *He* was the one giving *me* a farewell gift on this formal occasion. I said to him, "Have you ever worn shoes?"

"Oh, *Bwana*, that is only for Big Men in important places."

I replied, "Well Assa is an important place and you are now a Big Man." I gave him my shoes. I had a chance to feel foolish about this walking back around Wilson Field in stocking feet until I could buy some sandals, but that was a worthwhile exchange.

Now, I have a stock of three pairs of shoes with me. One is leather and was given to me by an old friend named Paul Gibbs, after we had been on a bow hunt at Burnt Pines Plantation. He had given the shoes to me, saying they were too small for him and I should wear them while working in the garden. I have not worked in any garden often with or without them, but I did wear them once to show how little I knew at the time about running. Both of my sons, Michael and Donald, were at my home in Derwood, MD in celebration of Christmas on this happy occasion about 12 years ago. Donald was planning to do the Jacksonville

Marathon, and was in training for it. It was Christmas Eve, and I had arranged to go down to National Airport to pick up some French francs for Laura, a friend of my sons. She was about to go to France for a collegiate study period. Donald needed to do some serious miles on an overcast day. I took Michael, Donald and Laura and dropped them at different points along the Chesapeake & Ohio Canal towpath. Donald ran about ten miles, Laura about two, and I ran from the Marine Memorial to National Airport, about a mile or more roundtrip, wearing these old leather shoes and a heavy sweater. This tells the story of how much I knew as a novice distance runner. I picked up my francs and ran into both Laura and Michael on the way back to pick up Donald, and then drove back to Derwood. I ran my first recorded mile in these second-hand garden shoes.

The next day, Christmas, I was so full of enthusiasm for the idea that I could be a runner that I tried to rouse Donald and say, "OK—let's go!"

"Right!" was his response.

Well, I got out some old tennis shoes, as they were then called. The only use I had for them then was wearing them while white-water rafting. In them, I ran my second time, but this time it was the three-mile circuit around Lake Needwood, adjacent to my home. This remained my standard run for a long time. This was the practice round for my going from first mile on Christmas Eve to first Marathon within the year, in yet another set of shoes, a pair of Nike Air Max I got in Jenison, MI at Standard Sporting Goods behind my sister Milly's house. Thereby hangs the tale of the third set of shoes, which along with the other two sets, are resting here in my room in Assa. I am now typing this up by candlelight and suddenly realize that I will be coming out of Assa once again without shoes. All three pairs will remain here.

NOW, ABOUT THOSE HOARY ANTIQUES—THE RED BALL JETS— AND HOW THEY HAVE GOT FROM THERE TO HERE

When I entered Calvin College in 1960, I was told I would have to take physical education (PE) as a freshman. One of the requirements was a pair of what then were called high-top sneakers. At that time, Red Ball Jets were the top of the line. My mother and I went down Kalamazoo Drive in Grand Rapids, MI and went into a shoe store and asked the salesman for some tennis shoes that I could take with me to Calvin College. He started on a harangue that even had my mother defensive about the college. He said he would not want to encourage anyone to go to such a school and become converted to atheistic communism since I was sure to meet some biology professor who would try to make me believe in evolution.

After the harangue, and not because of it, I bought the Red Ball Jets. I used them not just once, but twice, since I had to repeat PE as the only common course in both the BS and the AB programs I had taken and one course could not fulfill the requirements for both of them. As part of the test for the second taking of this PE course, I was required to run a mile around the Franklin Street Park, and tried to do so in the Red Ball Jets. I probably even accomplished it, but I was lying in the grass panting and convinced that this was the last time I would ever do anything so foolhardy, since I had barely survived this mile-long run at age 21. The Red Ball Jets have since been used for a few white-water rafting trips. I had brought them here to wear them down to the *Zala* Swamps in the rainy season to hunt and stalk with Jean Marco through the mud and then leave them here in Assa.

NIKE AIR MAX AND THE FIRST MARATHON

I was on my way through Michigan on a summer holiday with my son Michael. We ran barefoot along the Lake Michigan beach. This was not a good idea considering what was coming next. We were on our way west to climb the Grand Teton. Glenn Exxum, the first person to summit Grand Teton by the "Wall Street" route, advised us to run to get into condition for the climb since Jackson Hole valley itself was at one mile altitude or higher. So, I wanted to do a bit of serious running and thought I would get the shoes for it. I found two pairs of shoes on sale at the store behind my sister Milly's house in Jenison, MI.

One set was called TurnTech, and I carried them with me to Africa on my last trip in 1996. I ran several marathons in them in South Africa in preparation for the return to Boston for the centennial Boston Marathon. I left the TurnTechs with a young academic surgeon from the Sudan, attending a meeting with me in Zimbabwe's Victoria Falls as I left Africa in September. I also gave him all my running gear I had carried as I attended the conference of the first Pan-African Association of Surgeons.

The other set of shoes I bought were Nike Air Max, state of the art at the time. I knew so little about them, that I placed the arch supports loose in my shoes and did not know they were supposed to be placed under the insole support until my other son Donald told me that later. With the arch support sitting under my sock, I ran the first marathon of my life, only a few months after that run to the airport with the other shoes I brought here to Assa. I did finish my first marathon in these Nikes, and even qualified for Boston, at the Marine Corps Marathon in DC. Incidentally, I recently received the patch for completing my tenth Marine Corps Marathon. I will wear it in this year's running, in three months. This is why I had better get back to running here with Émile Zola and

André. I have just talked them into running tomorrow if we can get our work done by making an earlier start.

The first marathon Nikes rested in state in the back of my Bronco to be available for any "pick-up run," such as the times that Joe Aukward calls. Joe is a blind athlete and I am his guide runner. These Nikes are due to be recycled out as the newest model running shoes come in quite quickly now. I am a test pilot for the new Reebock models. The Nikes are here in Assa to stay as are the others, but they have more history clinging to them than the recent models. These shoes cover the whole history of my running career, from the first mile to the twenty-second marathon, represented here in this brief decade's span. None of these shoes will be in a museum or bronzed. They surely will be worn and used well in Assa for a long time to come even if they would be considered trash beyond salvage back where they came from.

Now this has been typed in the dark except for the light from the screen and the candle guttering at my side. My writer's work has been a source of entertainment to André and Émile. We have made our plans for tomorrow that might even include the promised run. We hope that the lightning and the clouds coming over just now with one of the so-far rare rainy season storms do not wash us out. I am also reluctant to use up too much of our precious daylight when we have so much work still to get done on our projects that require light. After sunset comes the time when no man can work in the land of no electric outlets.

THE MORAL OF THE STORY OF THE SHOES AND ASSA

I would not get too sentimental about some old shoes, except that they got me thinking 38 years back from the first of the Red Ball Jets to the most recent running shoes. I do not have a lot of stuff, but within that span, I have had whatever I need and more besides. And an adult can grow to maturity in Assa without having his first pair of shoes in a place of thorns and snakes and volcanic rock that would seem to require them. I have always had more than I need, and others have never had what little they require. Yet, the generosity is often expressed from their end to me, and it should be the reverse if measured on the abundance of the one over the other. So, it is not much of a gift to leave all my shoes here behind me except for the heavy freight of history that I just recalled. But these represent the castoffs of one and something precious and still useful to another. Each is trying to use what little there might be to comfort and adapt to the harsh circumstances of the world around, with simplicity and gratitude.

The people of Assa always teach me more than I can convey to them. Today's lesson is to use whatever you have, gratefully, in whatever condition it might be presented to you, to the best of your ability rather than whining and complaining that you have been dealt an unfair hand in the game. This applies to old running shoes, to bodies and talents we might have or develop, to the place where one is born or where we find ourselves now, ...and to life.

THE ASSA RUNNING TEAM AND FURTHER LESSONS LEARNED BY ANDRÉ FROM OLD RED BALL JETS

July 10, 1998

Good morning! You would make no mistake about the time of day if you were here as I type this into the still-ticking energy in the ThinkPad's new battery. The surroundings of my last message were a flickering candle in the dark, and a screen I can see since it is illumined, but a keyboard I cannot find except by feel. Now, there is a gray dawn light coming over to allow my seeing where I am placing my fingers, but the "sound track" is much more apparent in announcing the dawn.

Last night we assembled around a dinner table in the dark (always an all male event) and the usual dinner was served—manioc greens in palm fat and peanut oil, over boiled rice. What is this? It seemed like meat? But it was not the little pullet that is the most usual fare. This seemed like real viande. I asked and they said, "*bodi.*"

Now *bodi* is the Nguni word for goat. You can imagine how well goats fare in any attempt at animal husbandry in an area like Assa. Leopards outnumber any other livestock that can be, temporarily, brought in to satisfy the innate desire of the leopard to see just how many times his own weight he can hang up in the trees overhanging the village. *bodi*, as you may have known from reading of my hunting exploits, including those of my most recent visit here, also refers to the antelope, specifically the bushbuck (*Tragelaphus scriptus*). Somehow, these grateful people have risked a great deal in going out hunting. I know well the natural and contrived risks of hunting and am chafing under the interdiction imposed by military edict. Hunting has been forbidden since the incident with the army here within the past two weeks. They have somehow gotten a bushbuck. There are very few "store-bought" firearms here. Even some of the homemade shotguns, made of outdoor plumbing pipes, have been confiscated. Instead of having a clandestine feast with their good fortune, they have offered their guests this highly choice dinner. Once again, I am embarrassed by their generosity and once again, I am "eating first and most of the best."

Last night as we finished our dinner, it had started to flash lightning and toll thunder, which it had done before but without producing much rain. This time, the rain began as a steady soaking downpour, something that had not happened here for a while. Although the OR team was tired and sleepy after we had told stories until quite late, we talked of the consultations tomorrow and beginning the next phase of the linguistic study. Recall that our fieldwork cannot interfere with theirs. They are out foraging by the same precious daylight that we need to have the colors recognized. We cannot have them start here in the early morning, because my research project would displace whatever they might be able to get done from dawn on in their shambas. So, the earliest we might be able to impose on them would be mid-afternoon, by which time we should be finished with the medical work. One of our operations will be the repair of a giant hernia they want to have me take them through. This will be done under local anesthetic, remember, since we have no pontocaine for a spinal anesthetic.

Almost as an afterthought, Dr. Sonny Mwembo said to me, "You speak Spanish." I know that whenever I try to say something in a language other than my own, I slip into "foreign," much of which is Spanish. Then he said, "It is a lot like the 'Romanche' language I had used so I recognize the Portuguesa and the Spanish."

I asked "What?" I thought he was talking about some language here in the Kisangani region, since he already has to use about eight of these African languages apart from the French and the English in which he is surprisingly good, although he is reluctant to initiate a conversation in English. When he said it again, it sounded like "Romanian," which it turned out to be!

It seems he was in Romania for his medical school, since that was the era of the anticommunist Mobutu takeover here and the Ceucescu regime was the only East European nation friendly to the Mobutu dictatorship in Zaïre. So, Mwembo went to school from 1978 to 1984, in, of all places, Yash University! I told him I had been the Visiting Professor there, and asked if he knew my Romanian friend, Dr. Christian Dragomir.

He said, "My advisor!" So once again, from the Heart of the Congo, in a dinner table around an antelope special treat in the dark as the rains come to the rainforest, "It's a small world: part number next!"

THE EARLY MORNING RUN IN ASSA,
EVEN BEFORE THE BIRDSONG HAD BEGUN

I tried to hold the crew to their declared intent to run in the morning, and they all said they would at 5:30 AM unless it is still raining. OK. The rain stopped around midnight. The buzz of insects was then heard followed by a few chirps of frogs, which then went into a chorus and then a frenzy. It kept recurring in "waves" (as in "do the wave" in a football stadium). The silence would be broken by one chirp, then a few, and then a deafening chorus that would decrescendo in the dark to start up again later.

Later this morning I had heard no such sound from the forest, but abruptly the frog chorus started in a loud frenzy from somewhere I could not identify. Awaiting my fellow would-be runners, I had taken a brief walkabout and been met by some very solemn faced youngsters of about six, and eight, a boy and girl who were setting about the serious work they have to do at this age. They were each on a mission. They carried large aluminum pans. They came to the cistern behind the house and moved the cement slab to the side. There in the grass was a cut away plastic jug with a gear as a weight on one side to get it to tilt after it had landed in the water below. The bucket was suspended from a knotted vine that was made supple and rope-like by bending it back and forth. They lowered the plastic bucket with which to fill the aluminum pans that they would then carry off on their heads. These children, barely older than toddlers, were already very accomplished in this rather routine drill.

When they lowered the bucket, the mystery of the off-on chirping of the frogs was solved. Until the slab was moved, it was dark deep down in the cistern. Light entering, along with the descending bucket and the leaking plastic jug being hauled up again, was enough to put the frogs into a frenzy. The echo chamber of the cistern resonated with the chirping of thousands of frogs that I could see as dimples in the surface at the depth of the tank. My drinking water is being "squatted in" by enough frogs to keep a bait shop busy for its entire career. These frogs are not at all happy at having their dark, quiet and wet environment disturbed by a few kids, even if they have serious work to do.

THE RUN FROM ASSA, AS THE ASSA RUNNING TEAM GREETS THE DAWN EVEN BEFORE THE BIRD CHORUS GETS INTO THE ACT

When Émile Zola came knocking, I got into my old running shorts and pulled on the Nikes. André came barefoot asking what shoes he might borrow, so I produced the Red Ball Jets out of a plastic bag that was marked "Hotel Tequendama, Bogota, Colombia"—to give further evidence of both the age and the wide range of my relics. I had used them ten years earlier in Colombia. Émile was going to run in sandals

We set out from the front door on a good even pace. There was no mud, despite the heavy rain, since there is essentially no soil. There is the hard volcanic rock and the pounded surface that can break up into uneven gravelly stone. The humps of the *munga* (this area originally was a cooled lava flow) made tripping in the dark a treacherous hazard, since there are no soft landings. We ran in silence until the light came up with the first orange slivers of the sun.

Now I know why the dawn and the birds that herald it are so important that even the currency in Malawi is named after it. The kwacha (dawn) is the currency unit in Malawi (and Zambia). The kwacha of Malawi is divided into 100 tambalas (cockerels). Thus the phrase, "One hundred cockerels bring the dawn." If anything will be done in the powerless society living in impoverished Africa, it will have to be done after the kwacha.

As we ran a bit further, André said "See that tree? That is as far as we run today, and we will double it tomorrow." We turned around after running for 9:53 minutes, so we covered just under three miles in just under 20 minutes, a good brisk run for starters. My running companions were quite surprised that I was keeping the pace. It hardly seemed fair to complain that I was blistering with something in the ratty old socks I was wearing since Émile was running in sandals. Tomorrow, we will double it!

This is an ideal way to start the day, since otherwise we get up early and not very much happens for quite a while after that. The run enabled us to enjoy the dawn birdsong and to mentally organize a few chores. We might then get an earlier start on the chores of the day. I even had my postrun "shower," using a cup and a bucket. I discovered that I feel well, now that I have accommodated the schedule imposed by the early setting of the sun and the early rising but slow start to the everyday activities. I have shaken my jet lag. The empty, achy, hungry disorientation I attribute to mefloquine has subsided. In fact, I feel downright good!

A LESSON FROM THE WHITE MAN ABOUT THE VALUE OF TAKING CARE OF LITTLE THINGS

Both André and Émile were encouraged also by our little excursion this morning. They were eager to have another go at it tomorrow perhaps for greater mileage. When we came back to the kitchen where the cook was preparing the cistern water for my ablutions, he reported seeing us on the run at dawn. I pointed out the Red Ball Jets on André's feet and said, "I bought them 38 years ago, so that they are as old as you and Émile put together."

André said, "You see—these were white man's shoes; and they know how to take care of things." He went on to say, "If these were black man's shoes, they would have been ruined very quickly." They still would be around of course (as are the fragmented rags of some of the clothes that I recognize from the pattern they had in a former, better life), since they must be if they are the only things available, even after they are broken. Then André continued, "We would never take care of them so well that they would still be useful today for the same use they had at the time they were new."

He is right, at least in the "one tool society" such as Assa. If you only have a knife, it will be used to cut down trees, pry open stuck items, carve out jigger fleas from between your toes, peel oranges, and slice up food. They can never figure out why it seems to be so good at some things and so poor at doing other things. They wonder why is it that you white men have so many things, since all you need is one; after all, all that is needed is to cut, right? So specialized use of things is foreign to them, and therefore one tool serves all purposes until employed in the wrong task for its design, and at that point it breaks. Now this is not a disposable society, so that anything called "throwaway" in the developed world is used here indefinitely, but almost never for its originally intended purpose. Without maintenance or proper initial usage, devices quickly break. Damaged tools continue to be used for all the same purposes anyway, but with less efficiency. They cannot figure out why it seemed to work so much more easily in the hands of the white man than the enormous labor required by them to overcome the deficit in the fact that it is busted. So, I said to André, "Now those are black man's shoes—so keep them and use them in good health and in the furtherance of your own good health for the purpose in which they seem to fit."

He pointed out an aluminum pot in the kitchen as the cook gathered firewood and brought in the cut manioc greens that will be the inevitable ingredients of our later dinner and said, "A pot like that should last for generations."

I said, "Yes it would, if it were not used one minute to pound cassava, the next minute to break up rocks, and to carry dirt away from the rubble. If it were used to carry, boil and keep water or other cooking materials, it probably should be able to be passed down to great-grandchildren, unless stolen, of course." I have had perfectly stable well-used pieces of camera equipment that have met their ends in Africa, and not because they were used to squash bugs or to split open cans of tinned food at campfires. Almost all of these disappeared in airports, and always in official custody. That is a hazard for all such working entities, that may function while they are cared for, but will be trash right after that.

I told André about the comment made to me by a Saudi colleague as he looked over the architectural wonderland of Riyadh's skyline. He said, "What interesting ruins these will make." There is no Arabic word for maintenance.

André said, "But that is true for all black men, which is why you white men can come here with something that has been functioning for so many years, and we can take the newest product and make junk of it or carry it around as useless trash, employing it in other ways never intended for which it is not ideally suited." So, turnaround is fair play, and Assa has learned a small lesson from my Red Ball Jets, probably of longer endurance than the running shoes themselves.

14 COLOR LINGUISTICS AND BUSH PHARMACOPOEIA

ASSA ACTIVITIES AT A PACE THAT IS ALMOST SUSTAINABLE WITH NOTES ON THE GREAT PHARMACOPOEIA THAT SURROUNDS ME HERE IN CENTRAL AFRICA

July 10—11, 1998

This morning we chartered a subdivision of the Montgomery County (Maryland) Road Runners Club known as the Assa Road Runners Club (ARRC). We have set doubled mileage as the goal for tomorrow. By doing this, we have set in motion a plan, that will get us up and mobilized early for whatever action we will then still have to stand and wait for anyway. During today's standing and waiting, I went to the OR and recharged my computer battery. Therefore, I am able to convey these thoughts to you tonight by candlelight. I went to help André pull a few teeth, and he did a rather smooth job of it. His technique was a lot better than the "Bulgarian" (brute force) approach that I had last used in Nigeria at the dawn and sunset of my dentistry career. He has no dental chair, so he puts his leg behind the patient's back and extends their head over his thigh. Then he puts in a dental block and works a probe into the socket until he hears a "good sound," and the tooth appears as if by magic. I was impressed.

So was the first patient, Mawa's wife. Mawa is one of my heroes. He was here last time as the nurse because Inikpio was in Nyankunde still finishing his course in anesthetics. During the civil war, Mawa carried almost everything he could lift out into the bush, including surgical instruments and medicines, most of which are back on the shelves. His heroics made it possible to carry out three operations today, even without the gear I had carried in. Even more impressive is that Mawa went to Kisangani to buy some supplies and carried some things to sell or trade. He did this by bicycle, not *pikipiki*, mind you, but an old "push bike." That is a mere jaunt of some 650 km by way of rainy season paths in overgrown forest!

Mawa's four kids stood looking into the doorway of our little room which doubled as the leprosy treatment room, or at least did before old Doctor Harris was killed while making rounds out here on his tireless and persistent campaign against this biblical disease. Leprosy is alive and continuing here in Assa environs (**Front Cover**). I took a photo of one old man on whom I had once done a tendon transfer when he was younger to see if we might restore some function after leprosy took away most of the use of his hands.

Just to walk across the grounds is difficult without quite a few stops. I am greeted and regreeted by each cretin who remembers me from before, although they do not seem to have remembered greeting me only 30 minutes earlier. On the path, I met a man who had a very obvious epigastric hernia. I greeted him the day before on the same path. I was unaware that he was on his way to the hospital for the repair of that hernia, by Émile Zola with my assistance. Émile was planning to help Dr. Mwembo do this case. Dr. Mwembo washed his hands, but never gowned. It was an easy procedure and Émile was thrilled when I turned the knife handle in his direction, and showed him some small tricks that make such an effort much easier. He has done the first subcuticular closure of his life, and went back repeatedly to admire it. The closure under the skin appears to be magic, without any visible sutures to be removed later.

PUSHING HARD ON GETTING THE LINGUISTIC ANTHROPOLOGY BEGUN

Yes, the study is linguistic, despite my dissertation committee's interest in keeping it from being called such so as not to have any obligation imposed on their attention. This work may be harder than any other research I could have attempted. We are making up the methodology as we proceed, in a place so remote that no one can imagine what these circumstances are like. Rob MacLaurey had advised, "Just work on summarizing the data collection of each day when you are collating it at night as you are having a beer and chart the results so you will have all that ready when you are back here to be analyzed." Right! My biggest problem is daylight and I have to keep fighting the inevitable, a big black curtain that falls just before 6:00 PM. Finding my way to the refrigerator for a "brewski" is not my biggest problem.

Today, I came over from the theatre, while Mwembo and Émile did the other few cases, and found no one here. The two people who should have been here at noon showed up at 3:00 PM bumping back both Jean Marco and Kongonyesi, my hunter-colleagues, who might have been able to finish the entire series if they had not been forced to wait. As it is, JM and Kongonyesi may be the first ones finished after all, since they are going out to their shambas about the time the Assa Running Club takes-off at 5:30 AM. They will return at 8:30 AM after I have had a chance to use the water that will be heated up over the fire during our 40 minute, six-mile excursion.

Lunch had been prepared and was waiting, but by now I had a full house of informants to be worked with and I did not want them to sit and wait while I went to eat. So, I organized teams, and when André came back from pulling a few more molars, he went to lunch and I waited until he could take over. I ate a fashionably late lunch about the time it would be called supper, and made it possible for the cook to skip the second preparation of the same things. I pushed so hard, that I got nearly all the tasks that should have been completed at least three fourths done, and made a firm plan to get the remaining parts (at least with this group) completed tomorrow. If I keep pushing this peanut up the mountain with my nose, I may get to the point where this impossible study is at least stocked with enough data to make reasonable conclusions on what more should be done or abandoned. I can feel my backside getting numb from sitting on the log dampened by the light rain that fell in the middle of the afternoon. The rain delayed the color interviews for a while of the four hours each typically takes. I hope everybody there would have patience enough to still have the team around at the end of such a lengthy engagement. Forget about my tedium as I had already "been there, done that" many times on this drill.

Furthermore, I am not at all eager to be pushing hard on these suffering people. They are still literally shell-shocked. Many are just now gathering back in Assa after having been scattered out in the bush where they have fled spattered with the brains of four of the Assa residents who were riddled in front of their eyes as they made them watch. People coming back with the wonder of gratitude for my return to help so recently after such an experience, all within the space of ten days, are probably not well-suited for concentrating on the cognitive color discrimination difference between home and market languages. This project seems as frivolous to them as it does to me, in view of the other larger needs for understanding here. I know their circumstances better than the pedantic advisors a world away from any reality even remotely resembling this one.

I actually got done much of what we had hoped to do today under frustrating conditions of prodding and pulling in both the medical and anthropologic work. Now if only we can keep it going at this rate and not stop now with the first view of a part way finish line ahead. Maybe I can gather data from the many folk who have yet to complete the whole process as opposed to the two informants who are just now closing in on a complete study after two years of data gathering.

A ROMANTIC CANDLELIGHT DINNER FOR ONE!

At dinner-time, I was still full from my late lunch. I communicated in two languages that I used and two that I had borrowed through others and declined dinner tonight. But, no, here it comes so I have the opportunity to dine in royal solitary splendor, "carbo-loading" for tomorrow's early run over the hard volcanic rock of the *mungas* just as dawn arrives. It occurs to me that this is the almost ideal situation for them to make dinner for me. The dinner may be designed not so much for my benefit even if in my honor, since I will not be eating much of it, and what do you think happens to the redundant food that I will not consume? It is *they* who are hungry, and it would not do for me to decline, since they would have no crumbs to fall from my table. So, I thanked them with good grace, and tried to make a show of eating before passing on the whole loaf (metaphorically speaking), since it is the same *pondu* that is almost every meal ever served except the light snack of breakfast. My favorite part of breakfast is the fresh pineapple chunks and not necessarily the sliced fried cassava.

THE PHARMACOPOEIA AROUND ASSA

I look around this green curtain that surrounds me and see a lot of seemingly nondescript botany. But not so, for those who live here. Today, I learned about two new products and one I had heard of before. I gave Inikpio a notebook and pen and asked him to record the ethnobotanic information I am trying to learn. Here are three items I learned from Inikpio.

1) When I prepped and draped Pastor Bule for his hernia repair, I noted a lesion on the shin of his right leg, which looked like it had been an open wound, but now was a green plaster. "That is bush medicine." Inikpio said at the time. "It comes from a root they make into a paste to put on open wounds." Bule seemed embarrassed about the attention to his own relief of a wound that was incidental to the reason he had come, but I was more interested in the ingenious response to this circumstance of his own resourcefulness than his garden-variety hernia. Subsequently, I have learned the name of the plant is "*Nzawa*" whose root is pounded into a resinous paste and then rubbed as a gel into the wound. It hardens into an impervious plaster. Healing in the skin wound occurs beneath it. Dirt and bacteria can't get through it. Water does not wet it. It is a coagulum that contracts, reducing the wound and allowing cleaner scarring. I will mark this one down for later wound care notes! Any agent that aids clean healing amid tropical pathogens eager to invade is a major medical benefit.

2) Residents of Assa use one plant specifically for the treatment of fractures. The leaves are cut into strips and put on the broken limb. There is

perhaps some anti-inflammatory effect of the leaves being applied to the skin. This reduces the pain associated with the fracture and is said to promote healing. The local pastor knows the name of this plant and is going out to fetch some for me. It is not an aloe or any other kind of topical broken skin care but appears to be therapeutic for the deeper fracture within the unbroken skin.

3) One plant called "*Babadi*," found in the forest, is said to stop diarrhea. An American missionary in Assa developed horrendous diarrhea on a trip through the bush to Ndamana. It was Kongonyesi who went out and got the plant and gave it to him with a reported cure.

ANOTHER CURE OF ALL EARTHLY ILLS IN A CEREMONY I AM INVITED TO ATTEND TONIGHT

Kati told me that there would be a death in the Assa village today. An older woman was preparing to die. This was not a medical event and did not happen in the hospital but in her hut, where she refused food and was lying on a mat as her family gathered. One of the family members was a son who was a schoolmate of André, so André went to visit the family tonight just at dusk, when they buried the old woman only a few hours after her death. A reception was held by the old woman's extended family and friends around a big fire in the middle of the space within the Assa compound. They gathered to sing songs and to offer prayers. It seems it was time for her to die, and the old woman knew it. This natural event was incorporated in her family and village life.

I was honored by a special request from the family. They wanted me to share in their joy of her life now that it is over. I headed into the night with my little Mag-Lite, somewhat less powerful now on its fading battery than the candle it replaced. After receiving permission from the celebrants, I taped some of the proceedings and took some photographs with my trusty Nikon flash camera.

So, the day began with a run, continued with operating and linguistics, and ended with me as a "contextualized anthropologist fieldworker" after all. Graduate student advisors would be so proud of their star pupil in the Heart of Darkness, holding a candle at a ceremonial death ritual—the participant/observer making a hut call! It has been a long, full day and I am ready for sleep.

LIFE AND HEALTH:
DEATH AND DANGER
RITUALS AND ROUTINES IN ASSA

July 11, 1998

I have two amazing observations to report from my experiences last night. These experiences are related in a way that expresses the rhythms and rituals of life and death in Assa, theirs in Azande culture, and mine in my somewhat hybridized American-African world.

THE OLD WOMAN, VULANGI, "TIRED OF LIVING," "*KUKUFA*," AND BRINGS TOGETHER THE AZANDE FAMILY AND THE ASSA VILLAGE IN A RITUAL OF REJOICING IN LIFE RATHER THAN MOURNING HER DEATH

A woman in the village, whose name is Vulangi, picked this time to die (*kukufa*). After the recent terror of the soldiers and then the tumultuous reception of our arrival even if constrained by the bittersweet recent events impinging so close upon it, she made a decision. She reported to her son and others, that she was now "tired of living." This could be a case study for a natural death. There was nothing medicalized about it. She had attained a very long life. She took to her bed in her hut and visitors came to wish her farewell in "going back." She neither ate nor drank anything and just died, simply, quickly and serenely. It is important to recognize that this was not in the hospital, and she had no known illness, but expressed her wish to die as a rather natural and inevitable part of life. She would now be taking her leave of life, thank you, and she had no fear of this event, which, after all, is about as natural and commonplace as any individual in this life can identify any experience.

Yesterday, Kati announced that there would be a death in the village, and André went to see the woman and learned that her son was a fellow student when they were in Dungu. So, he returned again in the afternoon, when a file of visitors passed by to view the body. Within hours she was buried in the same small plot where Pastor Tanda had been buried on March 31, 1998.

I was typing on the fading strength of the IBM battery here at candleside, having paused briefly for what was a perfunctory and redundant dinner, largely for the sake of being sure there were abundant leftovers for those who had prepared it, when André came back carrying his fading torch. He was dressed in full Azande robes and conveyed the message that there would be a special death ritual tonight around a big fire, and they would count it a special honor if I could attend the death ceremony and pay my respects.

This ceremony, as would have been pointed out by anthropologist Émile Durkheim, would be paying homage to ourselves, to humanity, the common link between us, and our shared faith. So, although I was about ready to turn in for an early start in the morning, I hesitated only briefly before eagerly assenting. This would be the dream of any working anthropologist, to be participant/observer at an important component of the community's life and social structure. It would give a rare and direct glimpse into the culture that had patterned this ritual for their use in the mythic explanation of the events that shape and give meaning to their lives. I packed up my tape recorder and pocket flash camera with notepad, and set off to what we would call a wake. *Contextualization*, here we come!

KUFA (DEATH), A NECESSARY, INEVITABLE, AND INSTRUCTIVE PART OF LIFE FOR ALL THOSE OF US, WHO, FOR THE MOMENT, GO ON LIVING

There were no tears, but quite a bit of singing and clapping and dancing and a serial feast in many courses. My arrival interrupted one of these courses. I made formal rounds of all those present, and thanked them for inviting me. I passed them greetings in the few Pazande banalities I could muster with a few French phrases thrown in. The ceremony was almost all conducted in Pazande, with one pause, with apologies, by the song leader, who said that he did not have a songbook with this song in Pazande, so that they would sing in Bangala.

There is a full moon over Assa now, but we have not seen it very much. There is a heavy cloud cover from which the infrequent rains have been falling this rainy season, mainly at night instead of the usual pattern of a midday soaking. The large full moon came out from a break in the clouds that later came together again to put us back into the blackness. The night was lit only by the large roaring fire and the pitch torch that was carried to a small table and periodically trimmed by Kazima, as he sat in solemn splendor with a headcloth wound dramatically around his head and neck. These garments were not an everyday feature around here. They were more like some ceremonial vestments. The celebrants were wearing all the clothing they had, which is not too much, on the equator. They were reflecting that this was a special occasion, and they would have put on another layer, such as a cloth coat, if they had one. Only the little kids and some of the older women were in rags or less. I was making rounds in tee shirt (issued, as colorfully noted in red and white, by the Long Island Marathon), Bermuda shorts and knee socks with a red band that matched the shirt. I am a virtual slave to fashion, in this group only. I was comfortable, while they all seemed to be somewhat chilled.

Mine was hardly a surreptitious appearance. I was ushered around the circle, and shook hands with each attendant in the front rank, and also shook hands with a selected group of the women who would be the *chanteuses* of the choir. The orchestra consisted of a good drum with a bushbuck skin mounted over a hollowed log segment and a series of dikdik horns used as percussion instruments. My arrival caused a pause in the forward progress of events. They found a chair suitable for my rank and station, which they parked in the front and center of the elder males.

Having just arrived, it was time for me to rest, so that the women of the choir "took ten" and adjourned to an adjacent hut which was the Assa meeting-house. Here food was served by a group called the "good sisters of the church," a beguinage of women who respond to celebratory occasions by making the preparations of food and other things to bring to the needy when required. Vulangi had been a member of this group. I was interested in the ceremony and participation in it, but did not want to consume their food, which would require someone else going without. I made a ritual pass through the food hut, and sat and waited, something Africans do a lot more, and better, than I. As I sat, others would come and go, always for some purpose, and always in some rank order in the community.

Kazima came to sit on the stool behind the small table and placed the pitch torch on the table over a plastic wrapped Pazande Bible. Then he put his head in his hands as though he were deep in thought, or was going to take a nap, while events were unfolding later. Another of the pastors stood under the overhanging thatch until called upon. Then he moved slowly forward, and delivered what was translated to me in *sotto voce* by André, a very moving and quite biblical sermon on the questions placed, "What say we, then, brethren, about those who have gone beyond?"

My favorite, of course, was the singing. The choir was led by a dancing young woman who would start out as shrill foresinger, and give a lilting counterpoint to the rhythm section of drums and dikdik horns in percussion. The choir would swing in a dance rhythm and used energetic gleeful tones singing lyrics that André would translate to me as quite somber text. For example, one spirited rendition was said to mean: "Man is evil and all his intentions are bad. Only God is good and he chooses only a few to be redeemed, and only by faith is that redemption sure." Quite biblical, and nearly perfect Calvinism, I would presume, but hardly a "joyful noise" to make before the Lord, dancing with timbrel and sackbut, while being overcome with a cheerful spirit, somewhat like André's African name itself.

The song leader then led the group singing in what were recognizable hymns, a few of which I had been able to sing along with from memory. It is always wonderful to hear a familiar piece sung in an exotic tongue, a throwback to the era of Babel and an adumbration of heaven. I cannot help thinking that many more of these people will get to heaven from here than those who are weighted down with the effort it takes to stoop and get down through the eye of the needle.

Their simple faith is one that gives one of two responses. The first, from someone who would be getting to know them for the first time or from a very great distance in time, place and culture is that these are very primitive and superstitious peoples. They are not far removed from the *Witchcraft, Oracles and Magic Among the Azande* about which the early anthropologist, Edward Evans-Pritchard had written. They have simply substituted some of the missionaries' magic and myths into their own, and used them for the same purposes, as "opiates of these poor people" who are suffering in such desperate deprivation. It makes life just a little more tolerable to adopt something bigger than themselves and cling to it in hope in their otherwise hopeless entropic condition.

A second perspective is that these are people whose simple faith has been tried and proved in a crucible most people could not even imagine. There are no missionaries even close to this place. This is an indigenous *Communauté Évangélique Centrale d'Afrique* (CECA) church. What I heard was no mere social salve applied to a grieving community for a loss that today seems much less grievous than the four killed by soldiers previously. It was a genuine declaration of a faith much more sophisticated than that of a crutch in hard times. These people have a few customs that may be unfamiliar to me, but this is no sham ceremony. It is a dedication of life to a purpose with carefully scripture-based thought as to its eternal significance.

ANDRÉ SAT AT MY SIDE, INTERPRETING THE SIGNIFICANCE OF SEVERAL PARTS OF THE RITUAL AS THE "AZANDE INSIDER," GIVING HIS OWN VIEW OF HIS SIMPLE AND PROFOUND CULTURE

André had an idea. As he pointed out to me the component parts of this funeral service, he told me that he had wanted to have such a ceremony as a memorial to his father. André has a sister with a grown daughter in Assa, and that may make enough of a quorum to have the service here. We will be in Assa sufficient time to prepare the gathering for his people. His father died in Banda.

Last time I was in Banda, I could see then what was going to be coming shortly and I believe his father understood and appreciated that even more than did André who was unaware of most of the times I had photographed them posed in filial embraces (**Figures 23 & 28**). Those precious photos actually made it through the post to arrive in Nyankunde at the most horrible part of the civil war as the Nyankunde CME was overrun. The photos are in a small album that was in the first bundle taken to the bush hideaway with the color linguistic kit and forms. André evacuated them from the CME compound on the first day that Mobutu's soldiers came through on their shooting and looting rampage.

Much of André's family, including his brothers and his father's surviving second wife, live in Banda. We would not have time enough for the ceremony to take place there since we will only be overnight and will be busy. We have to restock the OR, do consultations, and operate on anyone waiting before running for the plane waiting to return to Nyankunde. For that reason André would like to have the celebration ritual of his father's life and a commemoration of his passing done here in Assa where he has enough family and a lot of Azande community to make it meaningful. He will have enough time to have it set up right. We will not be rushed here in Assa, as we would be in Banda where his father died. Banda is also much too far to travel to by any means these people have available to them (except those lucky three hitching a ride with me.)

The reason that André still has a stepmother in Banda is of interest, since it seems that Dr. Sonny Mwembo has a similar situation. Both of their fathers married early and had wives who kept on bearing children, in André's case, so many that he knows only the seven who survived. André recalls that there were at least eleven others who died. In fact, his mother was pregnant near term when she went out into the forest to gather wood. She was chopping down a tree with her *makute*. André said simply, "The tree it fell," killing her and her unborn child instantly.

101

During the previous visit to Assa, André told me another horror story about his "last hunt" in the Banda area. He told me laconically, "I borrowed a *'fabricacion'* (home-made muzzle-loader) to hunt, and was unaware that my father-in-law and I were stalking the same animal. I shoot; there was an accident; and my father-in-law, he died." That should be enough of that story to make me less than eager to go hunting again with André, I am sure. Nevertheless, we may still arrange an excursion over the mountain near Nyankunde to his hideaway in the bush where many of the things I had sent him had weathered the storm. While there we may look about for antelope, carefully!

Now, let me tell more about André's stepmother. His father married quite soon after his first wife, André's mother, was killed by the falling tree. He did not want a good thing to stop, so he married a woman quite a lot younger. Just how much younger we had to stop and calculate, since he knew his father was born in 1929, and subtracting from that his step-mother's birth date, we came up with a 33 year age difference. André went on to say, "She then kept having babies, too, so I believe there were ten more, and most of my sisters are older than his second wife."

When we discussed this at the dinner table in the dark the previous night, Sonny had added, "Oh, that is the case with me as well, since my father's second wife is 34 years younger than he, and the children of his first wife are older than his second wife and all their children." That means Sonny's father's grandchildren outnumber and are mostly older than his later children. I said to them, "This gives me new hope!" I believe that this small joke failed cultural translation.

THE FATE OF ANDRÉ'S FATHER
AND THE FATE OF THE CHIEF BENEFICIARY OF HIS LARGESSE,
BOTH STORIES ARE FOLLOW-UP EXAMPLES
OF AFRICAN CULTURES

During my last trip, I wrote about and photographed the reunion between André and his father upon André's return to Banda. This was André's first return since he left for school and had studied as a *dentiste* in Senegal's school for dental assistants. This school is a major dental resource for the Central African bush. André was the first of the breed at Nyankunde. André's younger brother was dispatched to fetch his father on the back of a bicycle, and I was aware of the significance of this homecoming event. First, I was wearing a jungle safari outfit and André was sporting his only coat and tie. Second, I had carried some cyclophosphamide, a drug that may be used to treat cancer. I had given the drug to André to be carried in his dental kit. I had learned that his father had had an "African melanoma," a black skin cancer that occurs in Africans in the areas of skin that are *not* heavily pigmented, e.g., underneath the toenails.

André's father had been operated in Nyankunde at CME for an African melanoma. Amputation of toes and the adjacent tissues to which the cancer had spread did not control the advance of this disease. The melanoma had progressed to "cutaneous in-transit metastases," apparent all along his lower leg and involving the lymph nodes at the back of his knee and in his groin. With that degree of local spread, I could tell without a chest x-ray that it was systemic and had spread to his lungs and other viscera. This was the end-stage of this disease although he was up and about in good spirits. The only chemotherapy available at CME was the cyclophosphamide, and that is not very good against this cancer. It was all that we had so we brought it and gave it to André's father.

THE HEART-WARMING GENEROSITY OF ANDRÉ AND HIS FATHER

When I was in Banda in 1996, I operated on a number of individuals, in our short stay there. As we started to leave the OR, a woman carried in her daughter who had an obvious and advanced case of Burkitt's lymphoma (**Figure 8**), a jaw tumor named for my late friend Denis Burkitt. This tumor was studied and described by Burkitt while he was a missionary surgeon traveling from his base in Kampala, Uganda. He traveled throughout East and Central Africa in an old Ford station wagon, on his "research safari." He was always proud to point out he had never spent one day in a laboratory, but has two major lasting research contributions named after him. All this was accomplished on a research budget of 125 pounds, with which he bought the old Ford. When I was studying in England, I visited him often at his Cotswold cottage in Bisley. We co-authored several articles and I made videotape of him on commemorating his achievements on one of his visits with me at GWU.

One unusual feature of Burkitt's lymphoma is that it has all cells synchronized in the same phase of the cell division cycle, making it exquisitely sensitive to chemotherapy, even the simplest sort that can be administered in the bush far away from laboratories to monitor blood counts and chemistries. So, I had told André and his father that as little as a single dose of the cyclophosphamide has been known to make the Burkitt's lymphoma tumor fade away, dramatically in most cases, and sometimes nearly overnight.

Father and son went away a little distance for a consultation held in Pazande with their arms around each other. They made a touching picture, the proud father in the bush with his son made good, now a professional, speaking

103

not only French but a little English as well, and traveling back to Banda with an American Professor. "Did the American Professor say that this drug I have might save that little girl's life?" asked André's father.

When he returned to me André passed back to me what his father had given him to pass along, saying "It is all for the best!" (**Figure 28**). André's father was giving up his use of the drug that might help him but that would surely help the little child. Who else would be this heroic under the same circumstances?

AND NOW, THE HEART-COOLING STORY

I told the child's mother that this drug could save her daughter's life and that we could administer it immediately. We found some water for the little girl to swallow the pills and she took sips of the water. Mother said she would take the pills along with her. We tried to impress upon her the benefit of immediate treatment. She was probably convinced that she had on one arm a doomed little girl with pencil-thin extremities and an enormous tumor. In the other hand she held the one set of pills that represent one of the few cures for cancer on earth. Both of these miraculous concurrences were here in this most remote spot on God's green earth through the extraordinary circumstances of our visit much less than through the generosity of André and his father. They were passing this chance for life along, from one who had the pills in his possession, but had had a long and good life and did not have much hope extending from them, to another who had only got eight years into life but would not go eight days more without some kind of miraculous treatment.

Now, this is an African story, so after the heart-warming generosity of André's father, you will have to hear the African conclusion. The mother is a woman. In this African culture, women do not make such important decisions, even when they concern whether their own child lives or dies. Such decisions must be brought up before the elder males who will decide whether she takes the treatment or not. In the Congo, there would not be the equivalent of litigation on behalf of the minor offspring of Jehovah's Witnesses (such as we have in the US) requiring treatment. For a more immediate context, you should be told that the last other person operating in Banda theatre last year turned to see not a cockroach, not a mouse, crawling through the window over the sterile field, but a Black Mamba (**Figure 11**), one of the world's deadliest and most aggressive venomous snakes. Medical risks also vary with circumstances.

The young girl's case was presented to a council of the Azande males who would determine the outcome. They recognized that notwithstanding the wonderful coincidence of visitors from another planet dropping in, she was an

Azande girl, and this would have to be resolved the Azande way. Fair enough. Go with what you know, but be quick about it. There is not a lot of time for deliberation, since her life would be short. These were my last parting words and "consultation advice" as it is called on our initial survey of the problems we find on arrival in any area where they trot out the people who have been waiting with some "*malad*" or have been literally "drummed up" for the doctors' arrival.

I was curious about her outcome, of course, since there are so few cures for which there is such a spectacularly successful outcome following relatively simple therapy. Let's admit it. The real gratification for the healer's encounter with an exotic ailment is the rare but genuine magic that can be worked. I said, "So, André, report to me the result!"

"She died," André reported stoically.

"How come? Was the treatment given too late?" I asked.

André informed me that "The treatment was not given. The Azande way is that the elders have to have a ceremony to determine why this young girl has this serious problem, and identify who it is that gave her this disease. They were going to do the divination to see first who was the cause of her disease, then to see whether it is right to have her get this treatment or another that might be more appropriate. While they scheduled the ceremony to find out the answers, she had died." So, another score for the etiology of illness and its understanding: Africa = one, modern medicine = zero.

We took our leave from Vulangi's Azande death ceremony during a break for the others to get food to eat in the main hut, somewhat complicated by the lack of water to drink or wash. We walked along the path toward the house, with long cold shadows of the tropical vegetation cast by the full moon, reminding me of the funereal march I had made up the slopes of Kilimanjaro at midnight two years ago last week. As we were walking in the silent shadows thinking our own thoughts, an explosive rustling sound was heard above us, as dozens of huge fruit bats burst out of the palms overhead and circled around the aura of the full moon. Assa can be a place of very moving experiences.

A SECOND INTERESTING EXPERIENCE OCCURRING AT DAWN THIS MORNING

This experience relates to a culture of health that is mine, if not Western, and how good and healthful practices, however conscientiously applied, may turn out to be hazardous for one's health. This is a brief story about *nature* more than *nurture*.

I turned in late to get up early. Not as early as others had to and not as I once did as a resident or physician on call, when I had to rouse myself for any call for every kind of reason. The emergency call last night that roused Inikpio and one of the others related to the young pregnant woman I had seen over in the room that serves as the labor room. Her mother was feeding her the same *pondu* that was my dinner, as she was propped up naked with her big belly giving evidence of what she was doing here. She was in late labor, and delivered as I was in and out of hernia repairs. The stir last night was caused by the new mother's failure to pass a placenta. The attendants thought of doing something like a dilatation and curettage to help that process along. At about 3:00 AM, her mother gave the new mother some kind of herb that worked quickly. Score another for the pharmacopoeia of the bush!

I rolled out at 5:30 AM, wearing only my running shorts and the Nikes, nursing a blister on my left big toe. I had heard it rain gently from about midnight to 3:00 AM. When the others were stirring under torchlight it had stopped. The clouds had gathered again over the full moon, which peeked out occasionally, as we set out on our doubled mileage run, just André and I since Émile was late. Note three facts to start the pattern of this story from the morning's adventure. It had rained, settling the dust on the hard volcanic *munga*. There was intermittent moonlight but it was mostly misty dark and warm. Émile was not with us, but ran alone to catch up with us, as André and I, two middle-sized men by African standards, were running down the path just outside the compound of Assa. I carried the small disposable flash camera "Fun-Saver," in the event that we encountered anything of interest. Right! Or as is the Bangala equivalent "*Solo!*"

AND NOW, A "PAWS" FOR REFLECTION

Very few of my fellow Assa residents would consider running, wasting energy to no purpose, not even trying to get out of the way of something frightful. These are not Kenyans, who also, I suspect, do not run for the sheer joy of it or the health of it, but as a way they have found to make a living in a sport that can support whole villages. The winner of the 1997 Boston Marathon returned in triumph to his home village carrying the substantial prize money. He was seized by the police, beaten unconscious, robbed, and left paralyzed. The 1996 Olympic Marathon winner returned to South Africa in triumph. He had been previously shot in the face in a hijacking of his pick-up truck. Life is not always easy for the winners in Africa.

The early morning run was progressing smoothly, when André looked back, having heard a noise and said, "Oh, good! Émile!" I too looked back and saw Émile running in his sandals, alone behind us, trying (we thought) to catch up. There was a discrepancy in the direction from which Émile was running, and the direction from which we had heard the sound, which did not sound like the slap of sandaled feet. Ah, well, no matter, we three were on target now to get to the three-mile turnaround tree, for a total today of six miles, doubling yesterday's distance. At this rate we would be passing Assa Village on Sunday, Digba on Monday, and would be in marathon range by Tuesday.

"Oh, Oh!" said André softly. He did not need to say a good deal more. Under our running feet, in the dust freshened by the rain, there were fresh tracks. They were pugs, the size of my outstretched palm, but without visible toenails. André did not need more than a glance, and Émile recognized them also. Lion tracks!

We reached our destination tree, and I jumped up and swatted the leaves of the tree as an announcement of our arrival at destination. We turned and ran back toward Assa and home, this time listening carefully, and we heard one very nonhuman noise, as if something with a very big set of lungs was taking in a deep breath.

I remembered several things about dangling a bait in front of big predators, such as the slow-moving, easy prey of a human runner. A lion roars when coming for you, sending an alert that it is about to hit, lowering your chances of being eaten. If he does "close," you are dead meat because of the power of this massive carnivore. In Nyankunde, a lion lifted a cow over a cattle fence, as an example of brute strength. The leopard is far more likely to make contact with you since he will make no noise on the rush of the final charge. He is not invariably successful in killing when he has made contact, however, for those of you seeking cold comfort in some small facts. I once saw a very large greater kudu (*Tragelaphus strepsiceros*) bull hanging five meters off the ground in a leopard's *(Panthera pardus)* larder tree in Botswana. A kudu bull can weigh over 300 kg. A large male leopard can weigh up to 90 kg. To get an idea of a leopard's strength, try climbing a tree with more than three times your own body weight clenched in your teeth. Under usual circumstances, leopards prefer prey that weigh less than they do but I would not consider the leopard a "wuss" in the brute strength department either. I had every intention of staying out of trees this fine morning. For one small indication that I was human and not much of a prey species, I kept the button depressed on the flash charger of my "Fun-Saver." If I heard the roar, I intended to start triggering off flashes of light that so terrified the small boy in the "recovery room" when I had made rounds yesterday.

We crossed over the fresh lion tracks again on our return run—the same number of pugs, heading in the same direction, with no new joiners. We said little but just kept plugging along, having rather quickly forgotten previous large order distractions such as my left great toe blister. I was wet when we all arrived back at the house, and gave high fives for our return from yet another memorable run in the heart of the Congo.

As I soaped up and tried to dry off with the towel that had been left out overnight to "dry" on the bush in the rainy season rainforest, I realized that I had so thick a film of unrinsed soap from my bucket bath that I was leaving a spoor of my own, just walking across the floor, and on the smooth surface this constituted a slip-and-fall hazard. Right. Bucket bathing is dangerous, and should be OSHA regulated!

My morning run reminded me that this is not Rock Creek Park, a wooded park in the middle of Washington, even though the possibility of sudden death might be about the same in either venue. At least it would be a bit more colorful to meet my maker in Assa than in DC, and one would have fewer reasons for outrage over such unnatural savagery. Who is ready to go out for a few more miles tomorrow morning?

16 RAIN, RUN, RICE

THE SOUNDS OF SILENCE IN THE DARK

JULY 12, 1998

The last two sounds that closed my evening were the bleep-bleep of the computer saying it was going to close down since the battery was flat and the sputtering singe of the proverbial "moth to the flame" as my candle was extinguished by a kamikaze moth. Later these sounds were replaced by the soothing sound of a soft gentle rain that went through the night and has continued until this moment in the morning when the sound of the Azande drum is beating out its rhythmic "first alert" that there will be a church service coming up later. I brought my tape out to the cistern to record the chorus of ecstasy as the frogs are enjoying the dark damp infusion of fresh rain water until disturbed by this presumably bird-like intruder.

THE RUN IN THE RAIN

This time there was no such single line of tracks of a prowling lion in the fresh spoor along our running track. There were a whole pack of them. This time I stopped to examine them and saw the marks of toenails. They were only a bit smaller than the lion pugs, particularly for one of the larger specimens. These were so fresh that the water had just begun to trickle into them, so we no doubt spooked them ahead of our run in the gentle rain, beginning in the dawn dark of 6:00 AM. I recognized these could not have been made by cats. The cheetah is the only cat with nonretractable claws, accounting, in part, for its traction on acceleration for short spurts. All other big cats leave only pugs without nails. Nail points on pawprints are a feature of the Canidae. There are only a few dogs in Assa and they are the tiny basenjis the size of overgrown rats. These dogs are kept by the pygmies and the Azande for hunting, driving *kangas* (guinea-fowl) and *bodi* (small antelope, such as bushbuck and duikers) into ground nets. Yesterday, I watched Bule weave such nets in the shade of the courtyard tree as he is recovering from his hernia operation of two days ago. André and Émile came up upon me in the lead of our running string. We all immediately whispered, *"Fisi!"* (Kiswahili for hyenas). The hyena is a more efficient hunter than the lion. The pack is much more organized and cooperative than the pride. Once the group of hyenas starts their tag-team pursuit, their chances of success are much higher than the lions' daytime ratio of 10 charges for every kill. Don't take comfort that we are not running like lame antelope through a pride of prowling lions. We are, this time, in much more efficient gang territory.

As I ran further than we had before, we got into some hill country. The area of the Assa station is built on one of the volcanic rises—a *munga*—of very hard lava flow. The hardened, red, igneous rock is pounded to cinders over time. Without much in the way of soil or spongy capacity to absorb water, the rain runs off the red rock rapidly if it does not puddle along the path. These cinders were cooked in the furnace of the long-dormant Ruwenzori Volcanoes, the "Mountains of the Moon" that Richard Burton longingly looked over as their European "discoverer." I have been eager to climb these mountains at some point, when there is not the inconvenience of a shooting war on either the up or down slope. Such a felicitous situation has been absent for the decades since I have been coming to the Congo.

Going uphill on the hard rock surface should be harder work than cruising downhill toward the Assa River that was our goal. I noted, however that the downhill run was tougher going. Then I realized that my feet were getting heavier with each stride. The cinders that get ground to dust are washed downhill by the perpetual cycle of rainy and dry seasons, and this red gumbo accumulated in sticky clods on the soles of my treaded running shoes. The clay stuck to André's and Émile's feet was also thickening their soles with a "cuirass," and providing unwanted protection to their already callused feet. I could only shake these clods off the bottom of my feet when I had hit the up slope and could grind them against the abrasive cinders.

I also noticed that I was slipping a little. That would be understandable in this sticky stuff, but it was not the mud that seemed to cause it. I looked down and saw white streaks in the red clay, in rivulets running down through the clods underfoot. I had tried my "bucket bath" yesterday after the run, and a soapy rinse left me with a film of soap that was at last getting rinsed down by the rain, and I was causing my own traction failure. This should teach me to avoid dripping soap into the small amount of water before rinsing. This precaution will keep me from being an even whiter man on the run in the rain.

I remembered frightening folk several years ago near here on emerging on a run from the river below the Malitubu Camp having lathered up in the stream, and not having rinsed off when the nondirectional roar of a lion echoed in my ears. I ran for the rifle on the river-bank. I believe, under the circumstances, that I was entitled to look a bit whiter than usual.

We reached the log bridge that had been dropped over the Assa River, a small river, but very full now compared to when I had seen it in the dry season. The river is full of fish, André had explained. I knew about the "*barba*" (catfish) we had eaten from there, but he said there are also tilapia. I am still looking for the opportunity to catch the tigerfish, a sporty long-toothed running and jumping game fish, which I hear is in the Uele River not far from here. Tigerfish are also abundant in the Kariba area of the Zambezi River where I will be in two more weeks in transit from Zimbabwe to Zambia. I made a mental note to add that trophy sport fish to my experience one day. We turned at the Assa River to begin our return run home.

RICE, AND THE LABOR-INTENSIVE PROCESSES THAT PRECEDE EATING

On the subject of experiences unique to me but everyday occurrences to residents of Assa, I have been invited to pound rice with Inikpio's daughters. I stopped dripping wet from the run in the rain, and visited Inikpio's kids in the hut behind their house. We ran the eight-mile run in about 70 minutes, and came "bearing gifts." One of the Assa families had spotted us on the early morning outbound run and collected two pineapples that they prepared and presented to us on the return run. There was a moment of embarrassed shuffling as they tried to decide which was the bigger and better one, so that they would present that one to me and the other to André; yet, I must not be made to appear to be carrying it, which would be the function of one of the bearers. There is always a subtle attention paid to precedence and protocol here, and my egalitarian dismissal is not "on" for their own face-saving.

Precedence and protocol relates to my rice-pounding experience with Inikpio's family. I went to pound rice with Inikpio's daughters to get more of a feel for everyday life in Assa. I did so in my friend's family because this sort of activity is normally not done by grown men. This is a task normally restricted to women and girls; even boys, after becoming teenagers, would not be doing this work. It is by no means easy. Two of us—for starters, Inikpio's eldest daughter and I—would each have in hand a heavy hard wood pestle with a smooth rounded end, and worn smooth of slivers in its midshaft by a lot of hands doing a lot of work for a long time (**Figure 14**). They are made in several sizes to be

111

appropriate for the person wielding it. The rhythm is easy to get into, but one should not be distracted or it will trip up the process. We stand on either side of the mortar into which a half dozen handfuls of rice are thrown. The rice has been harvested by knocking the heads off the stems into a cloth the person (most often a woman) was wearing at the time. This unhusked rice is then pounded in the mortar by what looks and sounds like a reciprocal piston engine, with each of us alternatively going "thump, thump" into the carved bowl of the mortar, with enough force, yet not tipping over the vertical mortar and spilling any of its contents. After thumping for a while, the rice is "shucked" and it is winnowed of the chaff.

This exercise explains the muscular shoulders of most of the women around Assa. One older woman here looks a little like a middle linebacker, at least in the shoulders. Soon after my arrival, when I visited her home, she had smiled and swept up two of the heavy log mortars and put one on each shoulder to move them out of my way. I went back to try lifting one with both arms, and it was heavy. This exercise made up for the bench pressing I like to do daily at home and have not done since I arrived in Africa. I was worried that I had gone a week without running, but that, at least now, seems to be a solved problem, since the inaugural meeting of the ARRC. Now the rice pounding exercise used up half the calories the rice intake was worth. I got to appreciate the effort that the big bowl of rice served to us at each meal represents.

In Assa, they are far away from any industrialization, but that does not mean that fresh air is still not at a premium. Indoor cooking fires in windowless huts bite the eyes and lungs, and blacken the areas around the indoor spaces. I returned to the house to pass through the kitchen, where Tasamu was bending over from the waist. This is a classic posture of African women, who never seem to squat or to lift things with their knees bent, but put their "backs into it" in high-risk lifting. She was fanning the fire in the cooking stove, which was billowing out smoke, but no fire. When it burst into flame at last (probably a consequence of all our combustibles being rain-wet this morning) the choking smoke diminished. I could hardly see or breathe. The cooks were going about their business as if they had not noticed anything unusual. They were probably wondering what was wrong with me.

This cooking fire heated the water from the cistern in spite of the chorus of enraged frogs protesting the removal of my bucket bath water, and I have dressed for the formalities of Assa church services, in which I will be greeted all over again. For the occasion, I have taken out a brand new tee shirt. My clothes that I have been wearing through the week thus far had been washed, but hanging them out to dry on the bush over the last 24 hours did not seem so successful as a clothes dryer. All of my wardrobe will be on display here for a long time, not only now until the sun comes out to dry it, but also for a very long time after I am gone. I wonder how many of my former gifts I will see today as "Sunday Best" finery?

I continue to feel not just "not unwell," but great, and elected today to forego my weekly mefloquine as malaria prophylaxis. The rains have begun in earnest in the last days. I should be on an antimalarial of some sort, so I will substitute 250 mg of weekly chloroquine, even though the plasmodia lurking within the mosquitoes over *Zala* marsh zeroing in on me for later attack are probably resistant.

I have been storing up some information about the first long visit and talk with Jean Marco yesterday, and will tell you what I learned from him after I have recharged my computer battery in the OR.

JEAN MARCO COMES TO VISIT
AMONG A LIST OF OTHERS WHO ARE AT THE DOOR

The list of people who have come for a "*Hodi Hodi*" (generic "Hello," to attract attention) at the door has included Jean Marco, a scheduled visit in his instance. A very persistent young lady with a lilting African English accent has come to see me several times, each time when I am least able to speak with her, e.g., once while I was carrying out the first color interviews on Jean Marco and Kongonyesi. Her name is "Siaduwe," and she is 27 years old, unmarried and has "not yet" had any children as she says.

"Please, I want to speak with you. I have three problems, and you will help me with each." First was that she wanted to write a letter to Diane Downing and needed paper and pen. That was easily done because I had brought out a stock of about four dozen pens. When that had been resolved on the first day, two problems still remained.

She went on to explain her second problem by saying, "Please I want to go to school. I have no money. There is no money for the pens and notebooks, and for the books and school fees, and the food I would eat while I am in school. You will help me do this." André determined that her complaints were that the school here, even if she got in, and even if she had money to stay in, was most often not functioning. The teachers are poorly paid, and rarely show up. They, too, must go searching in the fields. What she would really like to do would be to go to school somewhere, wherever school is in session. She wanted transport to such a far place and money to keep her while there. Diane had once given her some help when she was here, but without Diane, she knows no one, and I am the manna from heaven that will solve her problems. If only it were that simple.

André explained that schooling is a big problem for him since he pays a total of $10.00 per month of his $76.00 salary for school for his several children, ranging from about $1.50 per month for the elementary and $5.00 for the eldest daughter in secondary. It should be noted that of his $76.00 salary, André saves out about $6.00 to help the people of this region, and I use that as an example for those of us who have somewhat more. I obviously cannot support her in a place like Dorima, the place where the hospital is where André was born, 425 km from here, so maybe the support of Lazunga's son on the occasion of my last visit was a precedent that unbalanced things here.

The third problem is that her head is "*découverte*." Say what? After we had been through this several times, I called in André's assistance. The *découverte* issue turns out to be a high fashion item. She wants me to supply her with the one thing she wants most, a decorative scarf for a head tie. Now, I believe I can spring for that, but I would not be the most likely person to ask for such an item of apparel. Only after she left did I remember that when my camouflage shorts were confiscated in Bunia, they went through the pockets and returned to me the folded Kleenex, the foldable toothbrush, and the bright red bandanna that I had in the rear pocket. Now if she would not mind looking like a Wild West cowboy or a Midwestern, kerchief-clad farm hand, I may be able to help her make a high fashion statement in Assa! When I presented her later with the bandana, she had her *echarpe pour sa tête* (**Figure 26**).

THE MENDICANT PARADE HAS JUST BEGUN

I had a string of requests for everything from batteries to cameras to money for specified purposes. The list runs to a bit more than what I have available. Jean Marco came to report to me, and apologized that we were not able to go hunting because of the current situation. He had been out scouting, and had found the bongo (*Tragelaphus eurycerus*) that I want to hunt. This is a large, beautiful antelope with a reddish-brown coat with prominent vertical white stripes. JM told me not only where they are hanging out, but also he found a big one that was going to be mine, if we had to put a guard on it and follow it day and night.

Alas, the vagaries of politics and military action require some shifting around such primary priorities as hunting. We did a quick inventory of what was still here. The Winchester Ranger shotgun that I had once got for my son Michael no longer is. Neither is my most reliable gun, the Sako .375 Weatherby that was airlifted out of Assa to Bunia by Dave Downing's request somehow mystically the week before my 1996 visit, to be transferred to Bunia. This rifle caused great consternation at Bunia Airport where it was quite a surprise when pilot Tim off-loaded it from the Cessna. It was planned that it would be made available to a MAF missionary there. No luck there. I could go on in a much longer inventory about all the things that have been stolen by the soldiers. Basically, next to nothing has been overlooked.

JM had hand-carried a letter he had written to me last year, and then made a special trip by bicycle across the border to the Central African Republic (CAR) to deliver it, along with the disposable camera I had given him last time to Don, an AIM Air pilot based in CAR. JM's letter appraised me of what was needed here and what I might do before coming this time. Unfortunately, the recent plundering by the soldiers had changed all of the details and made the hunts for which we were going to be prepared impossible. I gave JM a disposable flash camera, and told him to take all the photos he wanted to take in the next two weeks, and get it back to me before I left, so I could take the exposed film back with me and give him the prints on my next visit.

JM's "store-bought" .22 rifle is here, but the scope is "pranged" as they might say in Britain. I was going to try to get a scope for it and for the old .458 Golden Eagle that has had a home-made stock carved to fit under the action. These were the only guns that had been available, along with one box of the .458 *cartouches*. I have about 200 rounds of these huge .458 cartridges at home in Derwood, but there would be no way at all of mailing, smuggling or getting them here without major hazard of getting people in trouble, or even killed. I had hoped to get a cheap scope and barrel sight the .458 also, but a piece of innocent clothing like my camo hat was enough to put the customs officers into orbit. A telescopic rifle sight would not likely be greeted with affectionate terms of endearment.

So, somehow, I have to get a reliable and reasonable piece of firepower into Assa before launching a big game hunt, wandering in less than innocence among Cape buffalo and elephants and with evil intent on a bongo. It seems like the chances of this are slim to none.

André's actions provide a good example of just how badly terrified these people were of the soldiers. When the fighting was at its worst in Nyankunde and the blood was rolling in the dirt streets of Bunia, he took his only firearm, his "very good" pump .22 rifle and threw it in the river. Then he went home to see that on his dental laboratory stand was a set of the *zigba* tusks that I saw last time and which I took a picture of as Jean Marco was holding them next to his wounded leg. These tusks had ripped open J M's leg before he killed this giant forest hog with his *fabricacion*. We ate the *zigba* at the *fête du chasseurs* held last time in 1996. André knew that if he had *zigba* tusks, they would think that he had a gun. That held also for the one set of elephant tusks he still had. Then he remembered that he had a beautiful leopard skin pelt. He took all of them and threw them into the latrine septic pit at the approach of the soldiers. "I was very afraid," he said, and you can believe that statement, following the previous ones, and the high regard we have for the hunting implements and trophies we have seen and appreciated.

JEAN MARCO'S DAUGHTER
AND, AS I ASK LATER, HIS WIFE

During my last visit to Assa, J M asked me for some help. He planned to build a new house. He tried to get the plaster and other building materials he could not produce locally from Nyankunde where I had established an account for him. He had started on the house, and worked it up to a frame house awaiting the bricks, when someone came and stole everything he had done that far, and he abandoned hope to start over. Besides, things were very dicey around Assa. His wife had a mental break and ran away into the bush. She was a stalwart workhorse of the house, field and church, producing yet another child with each year that had passed, and had next been heard of at Dingila, where she was from and her family still lived. He visited her one year after the breakdown, about the time I was here last, and then again last year. She said she wanted to come back, and would, but nothing happened and he does not know why. He went to see her six months ago, and they had a good talk, and apparently she said she would be coming back even before my visit this time, but she has not shown up. She had seemed "better" but is still under the influence of some evil spirits. This condition is a prevalent diagnosis among the Azande.

I said, without a lot of expectation of how much understanding it might receive, "I wish I knew a lot less about all this than I do!" I helped raise two sons as a single parent while working as a busy academic surgeon, so I do understand something of the obligations of single parenthood under adverse circumstances.

Meanwhile, JM is trying to raise the large family alone, and do the garden work his wife had done before. He has his sister and his family including his father Bule to help, but it is hard. He has several entrepreneurial ideas about things that could be produced here, and had been trying to collect and export palm fat when I knew about his business interests three visits ago. His latest venture is making soap.

I had made an exploration of the local soap-making process that I watched at Nebobongo. JM has a way of making soap that actually looks like soap, is in cakes instead of blobs, and is even impressed with the label "*Savon ☀ Assa*" (**Figure 19**). It has three features that should be improved. First, it should have color added to make it attractive for personal use. Right now it looks like the tan-brown Fels Naphtha soap cakes that are supposed to be for washing out your mouth if you use bad words or for scrubbing your skin if you contact poison ivy. I can still remember the important things I learned as a kid! Second, it should be perfumed instead of smelling like lye soap. And third, it is quite caustic. If a set of clothes is washed several times in it, the colorfast colors fast disappear. So, these little R & D problems are being worked on. On the other hand, he has a captive market. There is not a single store from here to the CAR in one direction and for 80 km down the road in the other. JM is a self-starting entrepreneur. He aims to develop a positive attitude in the people here to help get them out of the grinding poverty that has trapped them. He usually does not need or ask for any handout, but he is almost beaten by one more thing, going wrong with his good ideas.

In Africa, especially here, when anyone works hard and comes up with something for his efforts, someone else will simply come along and either steal or wreck it. Someone came to the only health care resource in the whole area and stole the only source of energy that was perpetually renewable to light the incision that they may need to have in their belly sometime soon. Furthermore, the solar panel probably is not even being used to power some other clandestine energy user, but is probably being used as a grille to smoke poached meat, like the IBM computer keyboard that I was told during my last visit had been used by a Congolese for this purpose. For another example, JM started to build a new house. This is an accomplishment that would make him that much better off than those around him who had not invested such time and labor in a similar effort. Jealous neighbors destroyed his effort before it was half-finished. Africa is not kind to "tall poppies" of African origin.

NOW A SHIFT OF EMPHASIS: THE NEXT GENERATION IS THE ONE ON TO WHICH TO PASS THE HOPE

JM has not left the area recently, nor for very long, since he is staying close to home to guard Assa and his own family. It is a wonder that he was not one of those killed by the soldiers last week, showing that they were from quite another area, unfamiliar with leadership in this community, and had pulled out their victims of violence randomly. JM's oldest daughter is 18 years old, and he wants her to study medicine, like the *Bwana*, and go to school. The school here is currently nonfunctional. Who can blame them? Doing sums is not the first priority when Assa residents are being shot in the dirt path outside the school building. She should go away to Nyankunde to learn about medicine. This is as far as I have come. It was neither easy nor cheap to come here.

Here is JM's proposal and next is André's. It reflects far more generosity on André's part than mine. JM will take his 18-year-old daughter on

117

the back of his bicycle to Isiro. He will wait there with her until she can get on the mission flight by MAF to CME. This is the first expensive part, and that is where I might be coming into this story. She will go to live with André and his family. She will not cost too much to feed since they have a garden, but she will need some school supplies. She will go to shop for clothes, probably just once, since right now she is a child of the bush and would need something to present herself in a real village like Nyankunde. Here she will see light bulbs for the first time, even if, as at my arrival, they are not always brightly shining.

So with these items requiring foreign aid in some exchangeable currency, the irony of the situation is that the "stopper" here, as well as in the US, is one looming and forbidding expense: *health care costs*. If she should get malaria or some other illness and require treatment, that would be the straw that would break this bongo's back. Heaven forfend that she should become pregnant, since then even I would be off that trolley in supporting her further with a family in tow like the others. André's kids are covered by *assurance*, a CME policy he has, to take the edge off any unexpected emergency. She would not be, so I would have to add some further funds to the balance they still hold from my last contribution to cover this contingency as well as the fixed expenses just outlined. So, as you see, JM has shifted his priorities, and is not going to try to restart the building project that has been frustrated before, but to invest in his daughter, if I could help get her up and into a self-supporting position. As you can also see, I am the front-end contributor, but the continuing expenses and support are through the generosity of André.

JEAN MARCO'S REQUEST FOR PRAYERS FOR PEACE AND FOR THE WORKING OF A WILL THAT IS NOT HIS OR OTHERS, BUT THAT GOD'S WILL IS DONE, IN HIS COUNTRY AND IN YOURS

JM said to me that perhaps the damage and death that the renegade soldiers perpetrated here on his neighbors and friends reminds us that we are not in control of the circumstances of our lives. This calamity is viewed as a lesson from God, not necessarily just another kick in the face while we are struggling again to get up from under the weight of this oppressive poverty and despair. It is not through our own efforts that any peace and prosperity can be achieved or any contentment in life obtained if we are acting out our own agendas. He asked in a very pure request that whatever God's will for this messed-up Congo, or for wherever it is that you find yourself, that His will is done, using your own best efforts or overcoming them if they are based in contrary self-interest. This is quite revealing on JM's part, and is quite representative of the community as well. They are poor, desperately so; but they have the dignity of being better people than we are often, and can teach us a lot from their better-exercised faith.

Neither you, nor I, are *compelled* to give anything to Assa in the Congo. We could each probably continue to ignore this, one of the prime examples of the bottom of the world's human pyramid. But we might want to take away at least one lesson they have learned in a course of much greater intensity than most learning curves we have been through.

17 GIFTS FROM THE POOR AND "EPHEMERADAE"

GIFTS FROM THE POOR

July 12, 1998

It seems rather easy to be generous when you do not need the excess that you have, or if you are entering a bargaining position in expecting reciprocity (as in Marcel Mauss's *The Gift*, given in anticipation of some exchange of equal or greater value). But what if you happen to be the sole representative of the "Haves" dropped into the middle of the world's "Have Nots?" The result is an unexpected and overwhelming generosity of response, and not from the end of the deal that would seem likely.

When we ran on Sunday morning, I spotted a family squatting in the mud floor of their hut without walls around a smoky fire looking through the rain at us; a trio of bizarre individuals was *running* toward the Assa River with nothing clearly in pursuit. Any sensible person would know that running through the jungle is a good way to attract carnivores, particularly hyenas. Hyenas hunt in packs, as those tracks beneath their feet show. Hyenas are always looking for something to eat. And that one man, why he is so very white that he virtually *foams*? Surely those two black men should be able to pound some bush sense into him or warn him if we do not.

I recalled on one occasion when I had gone for a dawn run alone on one of my prior visits, a concerned group of Assa *citoyens* got together and delegated one of the elders to approach me with some advice based in their concerns for my health. Was it about the threat of my running into danger amid big game? I waited through the preliminary pleasantries. Then, with a bashful reticence and clearing of throats, I heard the advice transmitted to me, based in their perspective of caring concern. The designated elder spokesman said, "You know, *Bwana*, if you keep running like this, you will just never get fat and have a really good body!"

Instead of questioning our sanity and dismissing our foibles as a cultural aberration, they recognized that the *Bwana* and his team were here for some sort of benefit to the people of Assa. Despite such puzzling practices as their running, they really are all right fellows with their hearts in the right place. When we got near the Assa River, André pointed in the downstream direction and said "See, that place; that is where we were stalking the *zigba* when they spooked and leaped over us, followed by two lions in pursuit." This is the story André had told the other night as we were swapping hunting stories. I told them about the close encounter in which the urban African, Ahuka (whom they all know well), had the occasion to see his very first lion at a range he was not interested in ever testing again. This is prime habitat for prowling lions, and those that were the subject of the story André told were probably the progenitors of the one who made the tracks along our way just yesterday morning.

Nonetheless, the family responded to our fleeting presence by going out into the rain to prepare something for us. They knew where two ripe pineapples had been waiting, and they just needed a special occasion to put them to use. When we returned on the back half of our one-hour run, they were waiting for us, and presented the fresh fruit to us as a gift.

When we got home, there was a file of people at the door, bearing firewood, bananas, and rice that had been pounded. Having tried my hand at the mortar and pestle arts, I can assure you that this skill is neither automatic nor easy. All of this effort was to feed the larger appetites of the visitors. The people here have more easily supplied needs. They neither eat as much nor as often as I do, nor require such luxuries as boiled or hot water. What high-energy consumers these fellows are!

Next came an old hunter to the door to greet *Bwana*. It was Hoko. He wanted to say "*Merci mingi*" (many thanks) for the *Bwana's* return visit. He carried something he wanted to give me—a small clutch of eggs, quite a bit more protein than Hoko had consumed this week. He also reported that he had been scouting in the area of his shamba because he knew that *Bwana* wanted to get a bongo some time. He reported that there are many bongos near his shamba and one very big one. It would be an honor to show the way so that the *Bwana* could shoot the bongo, thus making life easier for him since the they have eaten up very much of his labor.

Next I went to church, a simple and sincere service. An offering was called for, so that people came forward with their gifts. A few had rolled up dirty 20,000 NZ notes, the currency that is being replaced by the Congolese franc. I owned a large bunch of old notes, but André loaned me some new currency to give in exchange for some Kenyan shillings. Others proffered carved log basins of peanuts, a straw basket of rice, and then a heart-rending portrayal of the biblical Widow's Mite. An old woman, half dressed in old rags, with long flattened breasts slapping as she bent over, came down the aisle with a home-made crutch supporting her tortured walk. She carried a wooden bowl, and in it she had several full ripe ears of corn, and placed them on the collection table. She slid out the side door of the church along the cinder track barefoot without looking back, and disappeared back into the forest.

I went to visit Pastor Bule, who is finishing his ground net for hunting *kangas* as he sits under the kapok tree outside his "private room" in the hospital. There, Inikpio told that the young hunter who was talking with him had brought me a special treat. He risked a lot when he took his *fabricacion* out this afternoon. He came upon a *zigba* with long tusks, which JM knows from the business end, and killed it. He brought back the first chunks of this very good meat for —well, who is it that is always expected to "Eat first and most of the best?"

The generosity of these people is overwhelming. It is also embarrassing, since they are concerned about our welfare when they have not had a very good break on their own. I sometimes wonder what they expect in return. But, you may remember what JM said yesterday, and consider that they have had much of their "dross consumed" and the refiners fire has left them with a very genuine gold which they are more than eager to share—even with those who have so much more of what they need that it would bring tears to try to decline their gifts when they give it all.

"EPHEMERADAE":
REFLECTIONS ON RUNNING THROUGH
THE BRIEF TRANSIENCE OF LIFE

July 13, 1998

Since it did not rain, at least not much, last night, the path over the *mungas* had not had the diurnal slate wiped clean to show us what had passed recently, just before the dawn when we went running this morning. Émile Zola and I ran alone this morning. An old injury had incapacitated André despite my passing him the whole Tylenol bottle. How he injured his left knee is the subject of a whole other story. I have not even so much as thought of the femoral fracture and left knee cartilage injury that I had nine months ago in the snowy Colorado Rockies, kicked while loading elk quarters on a packhorse.

This is a story they would readily understand and appreciate here if it could make it through the language translation and cultural gap, such as trying to explain "snow," "horse," and big-racked "elk." There are enough other distractions while running here that I have not worried about my own "old injury," and just now thought of it while packing away the Cosamin (a dietary supplement alleged to prevent traumatic damage to your joints). I will run out of Cosamin during this trip. No, there are other distractions to occupy one's thoughts. Here are a couple of them from the creepy crawly, invertebrate department.

ENTOMOLOGY:
I AM AN "EYEWITNESS," RUNNING THROUGH A HATCH
THAT WOULD BE A FLY FISHERMAN'S DREAM,
OR, A RUNNER'S NIGHTMARE!

There were far too many tracks for me to tell old from new. I saw hyena tracks again, probably the same as yesterday's since there are the scuffings of bare human feet over them. Skilled trackers can determine the chronology of superimposed tracks but I am unable to read the signs at that level of expertise. There are aerial events of interest here at dawn.

The first show was the termite hatch. These big ungainly insects are otherwise terrestrial except for this brief aerial mating frenzy. This species has these large detachable wings but they never get enough practice time to learn to use them well. After a frenetic cruise off *terra firma* for breeding, the wings fall off, usually in mid-air. The wings flutter down like petals. They scatter along the volcanic *munga*, glittering like isinglass as the sun comes up. The airborne termite whose wings were clipped in the mid-flight glories does not similarly flutter, but crashes unglamorously to earth. It plays a frivolous part in this play to keep the termite world moving forward to build the grand palaces that arise everywhere along the *mungas* like the "fairy castles" of Cappadochia.

I can see them in flight in the subdued light of dawn, since they are big and ungainly. I dodge to miss them, but when they are too thick to avoid, I can feel and even hear the "swick, swick" of my collisions with them on the run, as though I were a windshield, clearing a swath through the air.

The ground is littered with many shed wings. There are even piles of scattered wings. I can see a sign being hoisted for the very large market represented by the millions of termites I am running past every few minutes: *Good Condition, One Owner, Low Mileage, Mint as Flower Petals, Used Only Once on Courtship Flight!* The previous owner has returned to a more mundane terrestrial existence. For one brief shining moment, he was soaring, and for most of the next part of his laborious life, he will not be playing at hang-gliding, but will be burrowing underground, forced to hard labor for the good of the collective mass of termitehood. *Sic transit gloria mundi, et, breve, coeli!*

The second show comprised large land snails, sliming their way across the path and looking like stones in the darkness that rolled out under foot if kicked inadvertently. I don't think that there is an African equivalent of the Neotropical Snail Kite (*Rostrhamus sociabilis*) here, but there ought to be because a bonanza is awaiting him in this cafeteria line. I did see a pair of Hamerkop (*Scopus umbretta*), an odd, brown, stork-like bird that builds an enormous arboreal nesting hut out of sticks and mud. The Hamerkop has a head shaped like a hammer, thus the name. I also spotted a trio of *kangas* "droving" ahead of us, one owl, a few passing ibis, and a myriad of LBJs (little brown jobs), obscure song birds past my counting as the light streaked the sky.

Columns of army ants are on the march at ground level, to be seen and avoided when there is light enough to notice. Stomping in the middle of them would be a mistake that would be realized some time later as the hangers on would be in lockstep marching order, pinching their way along, trying to regain their column, wherever that crossroads should happen to be upon one's person. This is most often on a considerably more tender parade ground than the volcanic rock of the *munga*.

Swarms of gnats delivered the heaviest hits yet. We were running toward the tree that I had marked on our second day's run as the three-mile turnaround, to be reached at around 20 minutes, when I hit the first wave. I had seen nothing ahead of me, and never did, even as it got lighter on the return run for the total of the 40 minute/six-mile run. But, like a wave splashing over the boat in making way into a heading sea, a slap of particulate stuff like rain hit me in the face. But rain does not stick to all mucosal surfaces such as lips and tongue, nose, and worst—the eyes. I put my head down and breathed forcefully out, wiping the layer of these gnats off my sweaty skin. There was no way to avoid them, and we must have pushed through about 20 swarms so thick that they stopped us. Stopping in the middle of a cloud of these biting dots of airborne protein does not seem smart, so sneezing and coughing we lunged forward with heads down.

Now, it is not for reasons of vanity that I wish there were at least one small piece of mirrored glass or reflective surface left in Assa. I am not trying to check on Carl Dees's last haircut, or trying to see if I am having a bad hair day. I have to wipe these pesty little brutes out of my eyes, particularly my right eye where one was still trying to wiggle free. I rubbed my eyes and ears, and actually was crying, from my right eye at least, but it did not wash out the intruder whom I carried back to Assa. After my run, I poured my "bath water" over my head. I left my eyes open, hoping to irrigate the detritus of the gnats out, along with the smoky burning sensation from having passed through the kitchen to get the bath water in the acrid atmosphere of wet wood smoldering more than burning.

I had brought with me a head net/hat, which I thought I might need if I were down in the marshes hunting, to both obscure my white face, and to reduce my mosquito exposure a bit. But I might now have thought of carrying it on the run, and putting it on as an emergency piece of running gear tomorrow. The rains have returned to Assa and brought about what are clearly much more "normal" events for this time of year. The rainy season is said to produce this profligate life of a myriad species, most of them creepy crawly and some quite nettlesome when inspired on the run.

A QUICK TAKE FROM THIS PERSPECTIVE
ON "LIFE ON THE RUN"

But both these little creatures and we, only somewhat larger ones, have this very brief shining moment to make ourselves known and take our places in the sun for the instant of a passing day. They are doing what they can to be good little gnats, and the termites are doing their very most cooperative social best to perform for all termitehood, and may there be lots more of it. That is presumably what the medical, surgical, and public health care work I am doing here is all about as well. My work here can be seen as a brief flurry in the dawn before whatever larger events sweep along on the run. It might be an AIDS pandemic, genocidal soldiers, or the grinding poverty, oppression and neglect in which this whole area (and, for that matter, much of the Dark Continent) is caught up. These trials will work their way with whatever life can survive as a residual.

The army that came through last week and the army ants that marched along this morning are both mindless groups moving in the sweep of something much larger that may ultimately be mindless as well. Even the empires that come and go are "ephemeredae." In the Central African Republic (CAR), the "Eternal Empire of Central Africa," declared by Jean-Bédel Bokassa, (who later crowned himself Emperor Bokassa I), lasted only a few years. Neither running programs, medical regimens, surgical operations nor public health grand plans will provide permanence to this society. Despite the vaunted claims of each, all are transient. Life is disposable out here, as quickly extinguished as a gnat in the eye.

My runs along the *mungas* near Assa have been a good time and place for reflecting on the ephemeral – insects, humans, and empires. For reflections on any permanence that life may hold, I would refer back to the conversation with Jean Marco and his hope that *all* human plans are forever frustrated, his own included, and that we seek to know and do what is God's will to the best that we can understand it. That understanding may be easier to accept in Assa than in some bugless air-conditioned luxury condo elsewhere in the modern Western (but equally transient) world.

OUT OF ASSA: HEART OF THE CONGO

BLESS THEIR GOOD HEARTS!
THEY ARE ALL TRYING HARD!

July 13-14, 1998

When the civil war came calling upon Nyankunde, and the CME was evacuated, the carefully collated sets of color linguistic interview forms were salvaged and spirited away into the bush. I copied these in Washington. I carried half in my luggage, and posted the rest to Nyankunde. My plan was to have all the forms ready for filling out when I arrived. I had to write some numbers along the margins of some of these forms since the copier missed them. This is laborious, mindless, yet attention-requiring detail. I presume this is what a good graduate student is supposed to do, spend day and night maintaining his instruments and working with his data-gathering forms. There would be more than enough forms at Nyankunde for the immediate study.

Then came the civil war. The staff grabbed all the papers that looked official and hurriedly stuffed them into a wicker basket. That included all the forms copied late into the night at GWU. They had my name on them and a GWU "foreign appearance," looking important enough to get them stolen, destroyed or at least (and best) sequestered in the bush. André's tusks, leopard skin and .22 did not fare so well. These papers were carried on the heads of good-hearted and not necessarily deep-dish thinkers whose job it was to hide all of *Bwana's* papers in such a way that they would neither be captured nor destroyed and still might be available for him if anyone and anything survived the war engulfing them. The papers ended up in fair condition. Many are soaked with precious bodily fluids, and all are scrambled—shuffled beyond any conceivable order. The paper clips and rubber bands did not survive burial. A random stack of air-mailed kindling paper was returned to Nyankunde in the last few months. I paid the freight for a bit of this otherwise trash to be carried out here to Assa.

As André worked with the shapes and colors with the third person to finish, I set about trying to unshuffle all of these reams of paper, about two thirds of the nonmedical loads we carried here for this study. Otherwise, these forms would be nothing but some of the world's more expensive, air-mailed, well-traveled jet trash. It now is destined to became quite a bit more expensive yet, since *it will* make a global circumnavigation, now that there is value added in being recollated (despite quite a few missing pieces and parts that are scrambled past recognition) and new data added thereto. It took me only two and one-half hours of our daylight, and the others could see that *Bwana* was working diligently on the unglamorous parts of his work as well.

We have the tabulation of the data to go through. This task will also take daylight but that might be possible anywhere; whereas, the test subjects who speak Pazande and Bangala are here. A lot of willing labor is also here for this mind-numbing task that requires total concentration. I would like to do part of it while training some of the standers-by. Several seem interested in taking part in the analysis now that they have been color interviewed and might want to see how all of this is patterned out. It would at least hold them here available for the next step in their testing so that they might be able to be started on the last parts of their own particular study before the light fades. Much of this data tabulation, of course, would be done under the lights—if such there were. Kerosene is inadequate, besides being in short supply. Without light, bedtime for me last night was an absurd 7:30 PM after both ThinkPad batteries were flat and a moth extinguished the candle I am trying to conserve anyway.

Most graduate students involved in library research projects (of the kind such committees seem to understand better from having pursued them themselves), probably do not have to contend with or even imagine such constraints. But just consider what life is like for an Assa student, who has to study as well as forage for his food, both of which require some hard and rapid work, for the night is coming.

STUDY TARGETS IN SIGHT
IF WE CAN JUST "STAY THE COURSE"

I am beginning to believe that we can finish the interviews to obtain the desired data. If we keep on it consistently and do not fade out in the effort, we may be able to carry back data from twenty informants, including all three component parts in both languages, and have some of that tabulated for analysis. Who knows, it may even result in a good show at the American Association of Anthropology meeting, and at least give me the "I-told-you-so" option for the committee that will have to be replaced anyway to start all over with a new thesis proposal.

The *Chef du Médecine du Zone* has requested Inikpio and the visiting Doctor to come to Ango to discuss what has been happening here. I suggested that Dr. Mwembo should carry out this formality. I am trying to emphasize the indigenization of the medical work, and am only helping indirectly. I do not want them to think that a white hand is guiding or even doing most of the medical and surgical work in Assa. This story may be most forcefully communicated by having a Congolese doctor meet the *Chef du Médecine du Zone* as I am sitting in

♦ OUT OF ASSA: HEART OF THE CONGO

Assa working over old buried linguistic anthropology forms recently unearthed and only now getting "value-added" data applied to them.

18 PROGRESS AMID MENDICANTS

A MAJOR ERASURE

July 13, 1998

This may be the first time you read this chapter, but it is the second one that I have typed. While trying to recharge the ThinkPad, I had brought it over to plug it into the OR battery and returned to do color interviews. I cleverly (I thought) removed the disc for safekeeping, just in case the ThinkPad disappeared. Later in the afternoon when I realized that we would have no lunch, and as there was a bit of a pile-up among the linguistic informants, I returned to theatre. While watching in support of a hernia repair, I typed up a story about the forward progress on several fronts, while trying to ignore the many cries of "*Hodi Hodi* " from mendicants seeking a private audience with *Bwana*. I saved my work to the C-drive alone. On later return to put together a new chapter, the computer asked if I should want to replace the story already there, and forgetting the number that I was on, since I had not stored it on this A-drive disc, I punched in *YES*, thereby deleting the whole prior chapter. This is a significant loss to me, since I will not repeat all I had written, but also because it soaked up daylight and computer battery in vain with nothing at all on the far side for the effort. I tried to spare the A-drive disc from possible loss, and instead caused the loss of a full chapter and about three hours of typing and about six hours of battery. Basically, I bombed the village to save it, as they used to say in Vietnam. Alas—another African story in miniature.

PROGRESS ON THREE FRONTS

My presence in Assa is vital in encouraging the population to do something for themselves with the reminder that someone else knows about them and cares about the troubles they have been through. I am traveling with Dr. Sonny Mwembo, a Congolese from Kinshasa originally and then from Kisangani later, who knows no Pazande. He has ability as a surgeon, but no skill or particular interest in the anthropologic work. I am also accompanied by Émile Zola, a local boy who made good, and he would prefer to be seen on return after eight years at Nyankunde as a visiting surgeon. I have not discouraged either of these two in taking the visible lead in the surgical work, since Inikpio himself is here with Tasamu and they do a good job on the medical/surgical front, not only for Assa, but for the whole zone. I am eager that everyone knows who it is that is doing the operating, and am pushing the recognition that patients are receiving Congolese competent care.

I am critically needed in the linguistic anthropology work, and am continually pushing the progress on that front. André is the other key person, since he understands and appreciates what it is that the project is trying to do, and is the one person directly involved who is bilingual in Pazande and Bangala. Besides, his heart is in the right place. He is interested in serving his people. He would be a superb co-author for the study. He is needed for the explanations of the color/shapes similarity/dissimilarity tests since the instructions must be given consistently and in both languages. So, I have taken on more of the mind-numbing and time-consuming color interviews, although there are some informants who are standing around after having completed the study already who might be good to train in this repetitive part.

The one thing that no one can or would do is to tell my story, of the observations I have made and the unique perspectives that come from this view on the world—a good number of which were just recently erased! I have to keep trying to get enough daylight, or enough battery to be able to do what I can to put in time at the keyboard. Later I will write by candlelight until the dying battery beeps or the candle sputters, and I turn in, surrendering to the darkness. Then I will rise again for the predawn rendezvous of the ARRC, the one unique idea of this trip that has really made it a hit. The early morning run is a way to get me out into the bush when I cannot hunt on this visit, although it is not clear to me why there is this prohibition. After all, we are feasting on *zigba* at breakfast. Running gives me a chance to make wildlife observations and to think about the meaning of life in this quarter of the world where issues are in clearer focus than in my home territory.

On a less lofty note, running also gets me back here at the house to have my "bath" at the right end of the day and clears me out of the competition for the water to be heated by volunteer wood gatherers and water drawers. The others prefer their "showers" in the evening. Unlike the case during past trips, there is no rush on the bathroom since there is no functional plumbing here just now. Since everyone is up and about when we finish the run, we can make plans for the day balancing out the first two objectives—the study and the medical work. André is a prince about this and is most helpful.

Regular formal meals consumed lots of time, even though we almost always ate the same required feast menu. It was served three times a day, even if lunch was delayed until 5:00 PM. Yesterday I suggested as I had before, that the evening dinner could be skipped since we had just dined at 5:00 PM, and would not be needing them to stay to fix a later dinner. The last time I had tried to head off a meal, they fixed it anyway. This time I succeeded. There was no supper on Sunday night.

Breakfast was late this morning even though we were all back from the buggy run early so I spent the waiting writing. When we finally gathered around the breakfast, I realized why it was late in coming. It was last evening's dinner, in all its *zigba* glory! Unlike the fresh pineapple slices, fried cassava, bananas in peanut oil, and a little coffee, this was a large dinner for our *petit dejeuner*. I was working hard and fast later today and the informants were getting exhausted in the study. I invited them to eat our lunch, since we did not need it and they did. I became a hero much more than if I had tipped them all for their efforts on behalf of the study.

While running at dawn, we came upon some heavily laden porters walking in the opposite direction. Obviously, they had started early. They were not carrying the usual daily head loads, but had made pack frames, as my hunters and porters had when I had gone out with them and we carried back large, heavy portions of quartered game animals for meat. These men and a few women were bent over double sweating at dawn as they shuffled barefoot along the cinders. They were headed to CAR, explained Émile Zola, and were en route to deliver something salable to Zemio. These raw products of forest gathering were going to make this trip on the backs of Azande porters who have half my hemoglobin, trekking all the way to the CAR. This is *only* 100 km in the direction they were headed and then they would need to cross the Uele River in a dugout canoe if one could be found. There is no ferry there.

Something interesting happens when you are in a society not as complex as the one I am usually in on the other side of the world. Here we are, each of us at dawn upon the cinder path, and it is obvious what we are about. *No explanation is needed for shared experience.* After all, are we not on this same pathway together? Can they not see we are running, even if they do not know why? Is it not obvious that they are working hard carrying heavy loads? What more need be said, than "Hail, fellow traveler on life's road! Well met, and right on as you were!"

MENDICANTS SEEKING A PRIVATE AUDIENCE FOR FAVORS

Several pages of the vanished chapter had to do with a note handed to me by Lazunga written in stilted English from his son, whom, I believe is eager to make an appointment for a private session to go back to the well another time. He struck it rich on the first hit. "Please, Sir, I urgently need conversation with you alone, with no one else to hear." It would be very inconvenient for anyone else to translate and learn his separate plans for escape from the grinding despair and poverty of Assa, through his fortunate discovery of the one stop shopping for the single foreign aid resource this community can apply to; *C'est moi*!

I may have set a bad precedent the last time I was here. I acceded to the tearfully moving request that Lazunga made that I support his son in his attempt to get schooling. Not just here, but there is a special program, at Bunia. That is as far as I have come and for the same rate. It is not just for the tuition, schoolbooks and supplies. Play me a few lines of that tune. I believe I recognize the chorus on this one. He will also need money for a place to live and food. "Oh, and it will not be just for him, but also for his wife who must go with him. Oh, and the children, and the family members who must also go with them to take care of them." So, I seem to have been the chief sponsor for a special education project that was allegedly to return Lazunga's young son in service to Assa in some special skill that was never quite made clear. I said I would help, but could not give everything he asked for in shooting the moon in his request. He indicated that the special accounting sort of work he was trying to qualify for would take several years. I am not interested in such a disproportionate recipient of aid when all the others of much greater need and higher priority would not get anything at all like this rather presumptuous request. And of what "account" is Assa?

Compare this request with the selfless and community-spirited requests made by JM and by André who have meant so much more to Assa and to me and who have done so much to help. I do not even know Lazunga's son, and have heard nothing about what he has done for Assa except to try to get out of it. Well, he is coming back again to hit me up one more time. I think I should prepare myself for a request for a Land Rover. I am not inclined to pursue this much further, since it seems in the example of Lazunga's son, I am not being asked to save someone from abject poverty and life-saving intervention in a one-time problem, but required to support him as an adult dependent. I will see what transpires when he comes. I did not make the appointment he wishes to book so urgently.

For one thing, when I had met Lazunga at the airstrip on arrival I asked about his son. Lazunga replied, "Oh, he is living at Ango." So, he did make good his escape from the community I am interested in. Perhaps the next request is to seek to emigrate to the US. I will not be eager to extend too much aid in a single direction, and this last recipient soaked up more than half of all the others' gifts last time.

So, I have put down less than half of what I had eliminated from the day's typing in trying to rescue some of my own erasure. This time the total loss was my fault. I hope it is the only example. This manuscript is just one third of the effort I am putting together here at Assa: the last third that you may think has already overstuffed your incoming e-mail box, before coming to a bookstore near you. The medical/surgical part is well under way and nearly running on autopilot with the medical resupply and the personnel we have specialized in that department among our visitors, supporting even better people who are here and will remain. The anthropologic project is progressing steadily, and may even result in some complete interviews.

The report of progress and events here in Assa will be communicated to you by the "Author in Africa" function, if only there is energy enough in the theatre battery that can still be hot-wired to charge the computer. There may be light enough to write if the computer-supernerd *Bwana* in his computer naïveté does not delete it all once again. Then there is the additional requirement of sufficient renewable energy in the author.

The wonders of this machine have been a great attraction to passers-by who come to read each line as it is spelled out, and spell-checked. They stand behind me in candlelight's fringe with full bellies rumbling in each of my ears, a phenomenon I have witnessed before elsewhere. This is a distraction somewhat greater than someone reading the newspaper over one's shoulder, without the additional hazard that the newspaper can disappear into ether forever.

19 EX AFRICA SEMPER ALIQUID NOVI

STORIES OF LIFE'S RAW MATERIALS, *SEMPER* OUT OF AFRICA

July 14, 1998

Africa is a wonderful, never-ending source of raw materials for the stories of life. I am sure that you believe I just make many of them up. Right! With a never-diminished supply of exotic events rolling over me on the double-quick, I should strain my imagination to fabricate any when I am in the cornucopia everyone from Pliny the Elder on down recognizes as a mother lode of rare and fascinating secrets? Try a few of these as "throwaways."

GETTING THE MONKEY OFF THEIR BACK

Sonny Mwembo's family kept a pet monkey. It was given to them when it was very small. It lived in a small box with a blanket over it since it was often cold at night. They grew attached to him. They fed this pet well and so it grew.

Once, they travelled back from Kisangani to Kinshasa where the family is originally from, so there was no language barrier or cultural gap involved in the misunderstanding with a local official who stopped them in Kinshasa, and wanted to take the monkey from them. He made up lots of regulations on the spot, as seems to be the habit here. It needed to be quarantined. There was a fee associated with the movement of primates. It required numerous vaccinations. Get this for sensitivities to the Convention on International Trade in Endangered Species (CITES) and other straws that can be clutched by the urban elite: It was an *endangered species*. Now normally, the Congolese have not been known to be especially bleeding hearts about such problems. Mobutu, the former head of state, was the one who could flagrantly wear the leopard skin cap and claim to be the only one entitled to do so.

In other words, and to shorten any number of similar stories, with which the reader of my pages already has familiarity, as you have followed me in and out of the kleptocracy: Sonny's father was showered with the hassles that mean "Caution—Big Payoff Ahead." He resisted this familiar drill, partly because although the monkey was their pet, it was only a common vervet, the kind that is a plague in many backyards, especially in the urban African compounds. He refused to come up with the payoff, at least in time.

So, the "officials" cooked and ate the vervet!

SOME FURTHER ANECDOTES FROM ANDRÉ

Many of André's stories are so precious as he tells them, that you should hear them directly, especially in his understated African English. They have a suspense-filled build-up, and then a conclusion that you can only imagine, following recurrent themes: "Then I fell down."; "But, she died."; "'Twas not very good."; or "We try to make an escape." There is the bone-chilling story of the last time he had gone hunting out of Banda where his father and father-in-law lived. This expedition ended in the death of his father-in-law, just one of those unfortunate happenings that have a habit of recurring in these parts.

One of the stories I taped in its entirety, since he was telling the story of being near Assa in July 1983 "apprenticed" to a hunter, learning how to track and kill elephants. The story took 45 minutes to tell, but considerably longer to carry out. André was part of a group of five hunters. They tracked elephants, following the spoor wherever it led them in the vast wild bush around Assa. When they finally caught up with the elephants, they ambushed them while taking great care to maintain escape routes to avoid stampeding elephants. After a barrage, there were five elephants dead. These stories of animal survival, and, indeed, efforts at human survival out here, are not for the conservation-minded. Well-meaning conservationists may often watch people starve, and that is not the way these folk out here typically vote.

It took the five of them a full day to butcher the carcasses and to carve out the ivory. Now, which way back? They all realized that they were hopelessly lost, without a clue on the route home. Aside from the raw elephant meat and the ivory, they had nothing with them except a rifle and a few cartridges, some of which were marked in red, indicating that they were military tracer rounds with incendiary elements. They staggered around with their heavy burdens in great circles for over a full day, and were making no progress in any known direction after a second day as well. They had water from the river, but no food, and were getting hungrier with each step. They tried lighting a fire by shooting the tracers into a pile of tinder, but no luck there, of course. So, they ate a little bit of raw elephant meat, trying to carve it with the *makute*, their large, all-purpose hunting knife. The carving provided them with pieces of meat but it also served another purpose. They used the meat carving as a divination as to which way they should go depending on which way the meat should fall from the carcass.

After the third day of aimless wandering, André came up with an idea, saying he knew they were between two river systems, and if they followed any water down stream they would get to a larger river and then could recognize it by the color of the water within it. This was dismissed as schoolboy prattle by the more senior hunters, and they separated, but after a few miles of further aimless bush-bashing, the hunters tracked back to André and followed his plan since they conceded they had no better idea of their own. They were exhausted and fell asleep, each leaning back against opposite corners of a termite mound, hungry and worn out. André got up and prayed for a vision of a way out. He cut a slab of elephant meat and threw it into the air asking that it land as an oracle pointing in the direction for them to get out. This method, Evans-Pritchard would have noted, is a typical solution by the Azande to help solve their dilemma. He did so and told them all in the morning the direction down the river they should lead the next day. They followed his lead, but not without a lot of disagreement.

They plodded along for another day recognizing nothing, but finally they reached the first artifact they had seen in five days. It was an old bridge. One of the men said he knew the bridge. He had been there with "Pastor Piesey" referring to Pastor Pierson, the original trek missionary here. One of the hunters said, "I know this place, and if we go that way we will find the road to Assa!" So, they did, and it was right, but there was a further problem as they went on. There would be a soldier guarding the area of the kind that were called "game rangers" and here they were packing elephant meat (quite obvious after five days trek under the hot sun) and ivory. So they hid their stuff in the bush and made it to the posted soldier. He recognized them and said in good Congolese fashion "I will feed you, give you matches, and let you pass, but only if you pay me 50 *cartouches*." They gladly paid the tariff and that night they feasted on the first *cooked* meat they had eaten in over week. Have you ever been hungry enough to eat raw, "aged" elephant meat?

That was not the end of the troubles. Since they were coming closer to Assa, André was the "bag man." He was carrying two pairs of tusks to dispose of, one pair weighing 10 kg and the other 14 kg. The animals had probably been cows. This is the pitiable story of the ivory trade, as old bulls are poached off they have to take younger bulls and cows. He then had to go on to Digba to see a man who was buying ivory. He saw the man who gave him half the money and took all the tusks saying that he would go to get more money and return. Right. André was warned in the night that the man had not gone to get money but to get the soldiers to come and seize him, not so much to get him for the elephant poaching as to plunder the ivory. So he had to leave in the middle of the night, and to content himself with just half the money after this heroic effort which nearly cost all their lives several times over. He arrived back at Banda, in time only to tell his family that he had the school fees but would have to be leaving right now, since there would be some soldiers coming along shortly behind him. When the soldiers arrived, André had already made his getaway. And thus it is that André had financed his ascent to the position he has today as a senior citizen and leading light of the community, and one of its chief indigenous benefactors.

ZIGBA AND LIONS

I had long since run out of audiotape, and was swapping stories about Cape buffalo hunts that I had made. I also told them the story about how I had taken Ahuka out into Nairobi National Park to introduce him, an urban African from the big city, to the wildlife I knew better, as one of the adopted bush *cognoscente* from uncounted safaris in the African bush that I love. Ahuka said, "I never see a beeffalo, and now I see them here. What if I should see a lion?" Ahuka had a chance to remember that line and that lion very well, since we had reminded him of it after I came upon him at Malitubu Camp with his eyes larger than any saucers to be found around here. A male lion had brazenly walked through the camp just ahead of me to pick up a quarter of my first Cape buffalo next to the meat drying fire, not two meters from Ahuka sitting in the screened gazebo for protection from bugs. He looked out from under insect netting to see a considerably larger pest, about which, now, at last, he could truthfully say, "I have seen, and very close!"

This story reminded André to tell about the *zigba* hunt with the same Assa hunter who taught him the ways of the bush. I believe the hunter was Hoko, the older man who came to greet me and presented me with eggs, with apologies that the bongo he had found for me could not be hunted this trip. They had scouted down near the Assa River and walked for a day beyond it in search of game. They eventually spotted two *zigba* across a *munga*. They were crouched in cover while watching the *zigba* rooting around far away, trying to figure the wind and terrain for an approach within shooting range.

The *zigba* began moving closer to where they were hidden downwind, so they let them come. Suddenly the *zigba* burst into high gear and ran directly at them. This would mean a very easy shot, so the hunter positioned himself for a dead on shot as they came to within a few meters. Then the reason was apparent why they were on the run. A pair of lions had worked behind the *zigba*, and both were crouched with the cat-like springing stance for the charge. The first lion sprang directly into the air and ran at the first *zigba*. The terrified *zigba* suddenly barreled right at the hunter. The hunter was shaken and did not know what to do. He raised the gun and fired between the *zigba* and the lion as the former overran him and the latter jumped clear over the heads of the crouching men. At the sound of the shot, the second lion jumped, also clearing the heads of the hunters lying in ambush. So, André has also had lions pass very close to him, as close as they did to me or to Ahuka. But his distance was measured vertically, whereas ours was at least horizontally! In each case, we were in the middle of the lion's business of getting fresh meat. In the lion's case, it was the *zigba* meat that the human hunters also were trying to get, unsuccessfully. In my case, it was Cape buffalo, that both human and lion were ultimately successful in getting, each in his own way, and one still the king of this particular jungle with no argument from me.

WHAT I SEE, AND WHAT I DON'T
ON THIS VISIT TO ASSA

You may get the idea that everything I see here is exotic, and that may be more nearly true than not; but there are some common things here that would be recognized in the developed world, and for me what is startling is what I do *not* see, though expected. For starters, the goiters are, if not gone, much diminished. I took a couple of pictures of two of my former patients, one of whom I had operated on during my first trip and the goiter has about half regrown. Yes, there are people here with large thyroids, and some with firmer smaller nodules, but the *huge* goiters are absent on this trip.

So are the new cretins, although my old friends, the adult cretins are still very much around. I see the former Chief's half brother, Sasa, and his colleague Bodo, the fellow who would wander around hitting people with a stick to let them know something was of interest. One day, Bodo stopped hitting people with a stick and it was soon discovered that he was desperately ill with an incarcerated hernia. This was fixed and soon he was back to much his old self again, running around awkwardly and hitting with a stick to express himself in substitution for his deaf-mute aphasia.

Sasa keeps following me and greets me on every entry into the courtyard. He has taken to circling his eyes and ears with his fingers, designating eyeglasses. I remember on one of my earlier trips, he was sporting home-made eyeglasses, made of twisted vines and cut out parts of old surgical gloves for lenses. I believe he did this because they added distinction to his appearance. I photographed him then and now. He seems to be mentally sharper since his iodine injection and he may have seen me after I had treated Lazunga. Lazunga came up with bad trachoma (inflammation around the eye and eyelids). I have observed that there is a lot of that around here at this time of year. I had my own Bacitracin eye ointment, which I got from the GWU Ophthalmology Clinic. I put a squirt in each of Lazunga's eyes and gave him my sunglasses to walk outside with since he would be photophobic, making jokes about his being a celebrity incognito. I believe that Sasa saw these glasses and is eager to have a pair like them.

Soon after I treated Lazunga, other patients with eye disease appeared. I had a full eye clinic of waiting patients. I treated Yuni's daughter for the same disease. Now there is a young girl with a history of trauma to the left orbit with a very large swelling there and granulation of the conjunctiva, which seems as though she may have an old foreign body that needs to come out. We will probe and drain that in the OR soon. So, we now have a regular eye clinic going, something I thought would be part of the dry season, not the rainy season.

Assa's church is carefully segregated by gender, almost as though it were a mosque, with all the men sitting on the right side and the women on the left. The children are in the rows between, with girls on the left and boys on the right. At one point during the church service, one of the small boys in the front row was thought to be misbehaving, in the opinion of Bodo, an adult cretin. He got up from his seat on the far side of church, and staggered over in his cretinous station and gait and swatted the small boy (whose IQ is probably twice that of his disciplinarian). But a chuckle went through the crowd since the social order and respect of elders was served, even though this adult is a little bit of a special case, and even the small boy looked over in my direction with a grin.

It appears that no new cretins have been born since our widespread Lipiodal therapy blanketing the area, even though the effectiveness of that treatment of two years ago should be wearing down over time and new untreated people would be giving birth by now. The new Congo is participating with the rest of African nations in outlawing un-iodized salt. Great! A fat lot of good that is going to do this far away from any supply line whatsoever. I had taken a photo of a bag of salt that Kati had brought back from a recent trip on his bicycle. He was once the driver for the missionary nurse Ruth Powell, and had been the last driver of the last vehicle in this station, now several years ago. The bag of salt says on it that it is the *PRODUCT OF NAMIBIA: 100 MG IODO/KG IMPORTED, DOUALE.* That is the seaport of the Cameroons.

This bag made it up from the Skeleton Coast of Southwest Africa, around the Bight of Benin by sea, and then by truck inland in West Africa. It was probably transported on the heads of a dozen porters before reaching the only town deserving such a name around here (and a delightful name it is) Bangassou, in the CAR. This is the river port west of Zemio, the CAR border town closest to Assa. Zemio is about one quarter the size of Bangassou. It was toward this town that the porters were struggling at dawn under 20 liters (= a *bidon*) of palm oil that will fetch perhaps 5,000 CF (the new Congolese francs, about $10.00 US). The barefoot porters that we saw earlier while running still had about 100 km of this back-breaking trek to go. I say "about" because the map distance is 100 km but the trail is winding and goes up and down hills. In addition, how does one calculate distance exactly on a rutted and often slippery trail? On their return trip, they will carry back all this largesse in soap, salt, matches, batteries, kerosene, and a bail of old used clothing. This is what Bangassou is good for. It is the last point at which such imported salt could get here. Far closer are the poor quality local salt-mines that are easier to carry from even if the freshly dug up salt is a bit dirty. No resolution, passed 12 countries away will ever cover these multiple sources of local salt.

Also, I am happily surprised that I do not see lots of *malaria*. I expected a lot more malaria in this rainy season. I am encouraged by not encountering much in the clinic, nor have I encountered swarms of mosquitoes as I had in Mozambique at the start of the rains. Now, do not misunderstand, I do not miss them, nor is there an absence of biting insects. The bites on my ankles stand as mute witnesses to the truth of this assertion. But the singing of mosquitoes thick in your ears and eyes as you trek through the tall wet grass is absent, and I might encounter more of them in Alaska's North Slope next month than I have here in Central Africa in the rainy season.

I would figure *diarrhea* to be a common rainy season plague. Nevertheless, I was not even asked to produce my cholera vaccination report on entry into Bunia. Of course, the intense officials there had other distractions to attack in my equipage. I have not been in the swampy marsh-like areas of *Zala* myself this time catching up with who-knows-what incubating out there in the culture plate of the Dark Continent. Assa has not seemed an altogether unhealthy place, despite marginal nutrition and severe repression and isolation with occasional political violence thrown in. There is less pestilence than violence from renegade bands of bad guys with guns who, because they are far enough away from any authority structure, can grab whatever they want. These are the conditions that made a cesspool of the Eastern Provinces of then-Zaïre, and Goma and other places have still not returned to a semblance of the neglect that has isolated this place from such epidemic contagions.

I have not yet heard of anyone this trip who, in the interval since the last visit, has experienced "death in the tall grass." There were regular squashings by elephants and enraged Cape buffalo on prior trips, sometimes quite close around me, and possibly from buffalo of my brief acquaintance that I may have put into bad humor. But, either because people are still lying low to keep from provoking any such similar savagery as that which was seen earlier, or they are still gone to bush and not returned with such stories, or they are very intent on still not telling me what has happened, I do not yet know. But the ragged army band is still fresh in everyone's minds. These soldiers with government-issued automatic weapons were brought up on the killing fields of Rwanda and Burundi. So what if they momentarily forgot that these were their own people (don't all those desperately poor folk look alike anyway?) So what if they happened to want something they could reach for over a few dead bodies and the automatic means for grabbing it were at hand.

SHUTDOWN/BLACKOUT TIME FALLING UPON ME IN THE "HEART OF DARKNESS"

I have quite a lot more to tell. Night has fallen and the keyboard is black under my fingers. I am exhausted from a full day of pushing my study at the halfway point in my stay to nearly half the data collected (not, of course, analyzed) through a heavy effort involving every hour of the light today, wearing out whole teams in my full court press. The falling curtain of darkness only just preceded the beeping sound of a dwindling battery that warns of imminent shutdown. This is probably a fitting noise to represent the high technology intruder from civilization, wearing itself out against the entropy of Kurtz's "Heart of Darkness" while Marlowe is at the scene making observations to report back in literary form to civilization.

NEWS OF BUSHCRAFT ON THE RUN AND
LATE BREAKING NEWS OF THE ASSA "FRONT"

There is a lot of news today. There might be on a regular basis if only Assa were not so isolated. The "phonie" has been down, and is unlikely to recover with the solar panel "gone missing" and the storage battery being put to so many uses that is draining its life without being recharged. When it goes down, Assa's last electric energy source will be lost, along with the ability to write to you about these late-breaking events. Assa will be isolated even further, which seems most likely now from the news that returned with Inikpio and Sonny Mwembo on the *pikipiki* from Ango, the administrative capital of this entire zone—and, as seems always to be the case these days, that news is *not at all good*!

Let me start with much more direct, personal and cheerful news, from the resumption of the ARRC this morning. We were slugs yesterday, sitting out the dawn rain. We were back in action today, intending a semi-long run to make up for the lay-off of one day and a try for *presque la Rive*, nearly the Assa River, which would make it eight miles. We did. We ran seven good miles, over 10 km in 57 minutes. We waited while trying to spot a large owl. Could it have been the Giant Eagle Owl *(Bubo lacteus)* I have seen in Africa before? This huge owl was making hooting noises at me from 5:00 AM onward from the tree that is outside my window, and we could almost see as we left as the dawn began. I am used to owls outside my Derwood windows, so I was going to try to tape the sound to give it a bit of balance between my Old and New World friends. Like the pitch of Bule's drum, it seems the owl's call, which is very haunting and clear in direct contact, is not picked up very well on audiotape.

WATCHING TRACKS
WHILE MAKING TRACKS
ON THE ASSA ARRC TRACK

I spotted them first. This may not seem too much of an accomplishment for an old African bush master such as I, and I was not out with my crack hunters but urbanized paramedical folk who have lived in Nyankunde for quite some time. Both André and Émile were born in the bush, either near or in Assa, so they were good at confirming my findings when I literally "ran across them."

For the first I needed very little help. No, today was not the day to run over fresh lion tracks or even hyena. These big boys I know: *myati* (Cape buffalo), several of them. The Cape buffalo were probably moving slowly, even before they heard or smelled us.

Next I came across a delicate track in the mud along the side of the volcanic *munga* and saw that it had been made in the night, and correctly identified it (according to the confirmation with André) as African civet (*Civettictis civetta*). The next one was so easy I did not even bother to ask or point it out. I saw *bodi* tracks, the bushbuck (*Tragelaphus scriptus*).

We ran cheerfully along, seeing no one, nor encountering the "buggy" clouds that plagued our last run. I looked ahead at the downhill slope where the tall grass closes in on the slope toward the Assa River. Just before we got there, as I was in a long lead over the other two, I hit the brakes. There in a long line were smoking fresh tracks headed away from us. The maker of the tracks was probably alerted by the sound of running feet and, at the same time, attracted to them. The animal was perhaps slinking its way toward the heavy cover of the closing tall grass with riverine trees for perches. We saw the unmistakable tracks of a big cat, *chui*, the leopard!

Both André and Émile confirmed the impression: this was a leopard and a big one. We heard something coming up from the river on the road and looked to see a man on a shiny new fat tire bicycle, heading, as it later turned out, toward Assa Hospital to bring some money for the woman who had had the hysterectomy two days ago. He also saw the *chui* track that gave him pause. I had carried the Nikon and shot a photo of the ARRC considering this hazardous running track condition.

We then heard a swish in the grass, made by the leopard we feared, and our run had abruptly reached its "turnaround point." We loped along back the way we came accompanied now by the fellow on the bike, keeping pace just behind me, as my rear guard, more like the sacrificial bait, if old *chui* makes his stealthy attack.

143

I put a fair amount of space between the two other runners and myself, something you might understand if you were in the slipstream of a pair who do not have the same access as I do to the bucket bath with a bar of store-bought soap. This was not so much a matter of avoiding their admittedly impressive aroma as it was of slipping out of the scent plume that trailed over their departure, toward old *chui*, who probably had been watching us from some "bait tree" at riverside, fixing us with his cat-stare.

We returned to Assa in time for the water to be pulled off the smoky stove for this crazy *Bwana* who has been out working up a sweat. As I was getting ready, Émile came back in a rush, "Come quick!" What wonder of Africa "*aliquid novi*" awaits me this time? I grabbed the camera and recorder to go through the smoky kitchen to see what was up.

THE MONKEY AT THE DOOR

There was a flurry of leaves as the monkey swung from one tree to the other over the *choo* and climbed for cover. Apparently the lure of the banana peels thrown out back, and (another of my favorite French names) the *anana* (pineapple) leavings, was the attraction for the monkey. What was attracting the crowd including the cooks was that there goes *nyama* (meat), almost falling into the pot! I stayed long enough to see it, shoot an inadequate photo, and then turn to "greet" all those who were stirred up to come by at this hour as I stood in my soaked shorts and sweaty skin.

THE BAD MILITARY NEWS, BROUGHT BACK FROM ANGO BY INIKPIO AND SONNY

André and I had just sat down to eat a *kanga* (guinea-fowl), with our heaped bowl of rice in the dark only smudged a little by the kerosene lamp on the floor. The recommendation for this hearty "*Bon appétit!*" given by André had gone as follows: "My uncle caught the *kanga* in a net. It was still alive. We were going to save it, trussed up, for later. But the *kanga* died. So, we eat it now!"

"*Bon appétit*" indeed! This automatic preprandial salutation in French-speaking parts is frankly unnecessary. Having a good appetite is never a problem in Assa for those who live here, hungrily most of the time.

"It was very difficult," said Inikpio in answer to my question. They had returned after dark, when we had not expected them. They would rather not have returned, and risk the rainy season paths by night, but for a bad "security problem" in Ango. They had to return and could not stay the night even if they had planned to. "We fall down four times," Sonny had said simply. Once going out, by daylight, and three times coming back in the dark, the Honda had gone out from under them in the cinders and mud of the track. A double red line on the map marks this "road" to Ango. Ango is the administrative headquarters of the zone in which Assa is located. There are only seven districts in the entire Congo, each of which has a few zones. Ango is a major administrative post. The friend and schoolmate of Sonny, whom they were going to visit, is *Chef du Médecine du Zone*. This social call and point of interest would make good protocol sense, and they carried it out as planned.

A surprise greeted Inikpio and Sonny. Ango is not under civilian rule, and the situation is not normal. The same renegade military band that had swept through Assa two weeks ago apparently is now controlling Ango. The people of Assa still will not tell me very much about their recent encounter with this group until it is time for me to leave. Several have explained that recounting these horrors "...would make us very sad and put us in a bad mind to tell you of the things that had happened to us, and we want to rejoice with you and be happy in your visit." It had been reported that this maverick group of the old army of Mobutu had been disarmed and disbanded (and its leaders probably executed) by the regular army under Kabila before my arrival. Not so, apparently, since these brigands, who make up their own rules and follow loosely whatever command and appetites they have on their own, retreated from Assa and went on to Ango and "took over."

There is martial law in Ango, the only kind that is recognized universally here (or elsewhere from time to time), the man behind the gun makes the rules and does what he jolly well wants. There are many such men in this world, who can do only two things according to André: "march and shoot." These are the same people who "trained" in eastern Zaïre, when the Hutus and Tutsis were in the middle of one of the most immense recent genocidal holocausts. They were busy bashing in the heads of women and children and clubbing whole villages, regardless of whatever national citizenship they or the army clubbing them were alleged to represent. The killing fields of Rwanda have spilled over into the Congo. The ultimate death toll from this genocidal horror will probably never be known, but there were millions of deaths along the way, such as those here at Assa just last week. Philip Gourevitch's excellent documentation of the Rwanda genocide: *We wish to inform you that tomorrow we will be killed with our families* (Farrar Straus and Giroux, 1998) should be consulted for further details.

When they tried to get to the Ango hospital they were held up by a military barricade between the doctor's house and the hospital. They had to go through the hassles and the permissions (always a costly process) to make rounds to see the sick patients who are either not intimidated enough or are so sick that it does not matter that there are the universally feared shouts of danger ahead, "Soldiers!" The soldiers most to be feared are our own.

If they were an invading army, they would be far more disciplined than these rowdy street gangs of orphaned punks and small boys who become terrifying when clutching a Kalashnikov. The hospital was nearly empty of patients except for those dying. They cannot make the getaway or survive the hardships of the bush into which the rest of the citizenry of the town of Ango had fled, leaving a ghost town of plunder bait for the irregulars who were picking it off at leisure.

ADMINISTRATOR BUTA IN THE BUSH

The deposed *Chef du Zone*, named Buta, has fled from Ango. He was the *Chef du District* as well. This official covers the four zones in the district of Bas-Uele. This high-ranking government officer is very much like the population he serves now. He is a fugitive in the bush along with much of his population. The reason he is on the run, it is widely surmised, is that he reported the incident at Assa that caused the Kabila regulars to come to discipline the perpetrators. They will conduct an investigation coming over to Assa to see if the grave for the chief is dug here as it was reported and then fill it with a few new corpses. Kabila himself (or the new District Governor, if security risks make it too dicey for the military dictator head-of-state) is supposed to come to Ango tomorrow to see what is happening up here. This news further increases the anxiety and prompted Inikpio and Sonny to get back onto their precious *pikipiki* and leave Ango as fast as they could make their escape.

"Why is this happening now?" the people out in the bush who have evacuated from Ango in terror are asking. They say that they understood the army of Mobutu, since Mobutu did not pay his soldiers and they had to get whatever they could by stealing, shakedown, bribes, and looting. The population was always terrified of "soldiers." They did not mean invaders, but their own, since the parasitic pestilence that crawled along on the land here had no supply line except for the *cartouches* that they expended freely in the reign of terror in "living off the land" and its thoroughly cowed citizenry. André had said to me, that in other countries if you were lost or needed help, you would go to the nearest policeman or soldier and ask directions or seek help. They were typically not busy and would actually be happy to do something constructive besides stand endless guard detail. Often a major use of military sentry time here in the Congo is guarding clotheslines, so that laundry did not disappear. Going to ask help of a soldier in old Zaïre, or apparently, now, new Congo, would be like dragging a broken limb in front of a hungry carnivore. Such weakness would quickly be winnowed out of the population. The Big Men had private armies, sometimes better armed and better off, and possibly better disciplined, than the "irregular regular army."

But why now? These soldiers of Kabila's army are even *paid*, and not just a little. A solider in Kabila's army gets paid the equivalent of $100.00 US per month. To give you an idea what that means, the whole of the Assa health effort here takes $ 130.00 per month, and that includes the budget for salaries, supplies, equipment, operations, "bad (essentially all) debts," and transportation. The entire operation would have to be shut down for a year to pay for a replacement solar panel. Inikpio and his team would have to go into the bush for a year just so that it might be stolen once again.

Despite this largesse in a heavy payment to the army, Kabila's soldiers are taking even more than Mobutu's army used to. They are getting comparatively rich with the loot they are able to garner with the guns they have been issued. If the guns are not used, at least the threat of their free usage gets them what they want. To give one passing bit of evidence that sits upon the table before me——I can see the boot prints of the army right at my elbow. Here is my water bottle. What is it? A bottle labeled "Johnnie Walker Red." There never has been any "urban trash" I have encountered on my frequent forays through the bush, since a tin can is such a precious commodity it would be used forever as a tool even if it had holes in it and it were rusted nearly into oblivion. A soldier has obviously passed through, and either drunk to oblivion with the booty snatched from some wealthy urban spot previously looted, or so well-fixed that he did not recognize the bush value of this commodity, he dropped or discarded it on the march through Assa. Now it comes to be used here to hold my drinking water, bearing mute witness to the passage of plunderers.

NO GOVERNMENT BUT THE GUN
AND HE WHO HOLDS IT IS, FOR THE MOMENT,
THE ABSOLUTE RULER OF ALL HE CAN GRAB

There is no government left in Ango, the capital of one of four zones in the entire district of Bas-Uele. From here over to Banda (our next stop) there is no government. No government but the gun, and the heady thrill that rushes into an orphan's head when he realizes he can grab anything he wants with this weapon. This thrill will last at least until someone else comes along with a superior weapon and takes his booty along with his life.

André expressed all of our anxiety when he said, "When the MAF pilot hears this, he will be afraid to come to get us since he could lose the airplane and a lot more if he comes into the territory that the renegade soldiers are claiming as their own plunder." We might be marooned, according to André's concerns. We have work to do, right here and now, and are in a communication vacuum, so let us be about it and quickly!

21 MARKET DAY

MEMORIAL OF A CHILD WHO DIED
BRINGS ME TO AN ENCOUNTER WITH THE
"ASSA WEDNESDAY MORNING MARKET"

July 15, 1998

As I walked over to theatre with the ThinkPad to make the precarious connection of one crossed copper wire with another lashed by an OR cotton sponge, Kati called out for my help. He and Kazima have been very helpful in rounding up informants and keeping them in line to help with the linguistic study. Kati asked me for a favor, and showed me a photo of an 8-month-old child being held by a family member. Kati wanted me to see the child's mother, I thought to take another photo. I had just wrapped up a roll of film to replace the one in the small Nikon I was carrying, and as we walked over to the mother's hut, I looked up along the way we had run this morning and saw a crowd. Abruptly I realized that this is Wednesday morning, and this is the time of the weekly Assa market. What a colorful scene! I should have had the other camera with me, but I did not want to run back for it. I had another roll of film in my pocket so we went on to the hut to see if the mother of the child in the photo was at the hut.

She was not, but Ngasyi was. He was returning from the shamba where he had started early in order to go back for further help on the linguistic project, bless him. So, I took photos at the hut, and thought I had done what was requested, but, no, the young mother was at the market. Perfect! Let's go see the market and find her there.

MERCREDI MARKET IN ASSA

So, I went to the market. I would have caused quite a stir, except that people there already know me well. They know the eccentricities of this *Bwana* whom they saw half-naked and sweaty running back to a perfectly good house he left before dawn this morning. You see? These people are far more intelligent than they are given credit for being. I furtively began snapping photos, some from the hip, as I surveyed the *people* (far more interesting than the *products*). There were pitifully few "goods" on sale, and almost all were simple commodities. I saw pounded cassava root on large green ("*kpe*" as I now know well from Pazande color terms) leaves. I saw a few spongy green compressed messes of unclear purpose. Kati told me that this was someone's homemade soap for sale. This looked even worse than the gook I had seen being made at Nebobongo. Still, this soap got the cleaning job done. JM's regular bars of "*savon*" would compete favorably with these in a moment, even without color or scent added. There were a few pineapples, plantains, and small mounds of a few handfuls of peanuts. These people subsist on pitifully small quantities of *anything*.

One dude had come from a distance with a fanny pack and a bail of old clothes. There were women clustered around trying things on as though these were the aisles of Filenes's basement! Some of the garments they thought were quite impressive had seen earlier service as items of not necessarily *haute couture*. I especially like nonclothing worn as clothes. I remember chasing a woman all around a market in Nigeria to take a picture of the wonderful terry cloth head cover she was wearing, with a neat bow tied under one ear. The head cover had, in an earlier life far away, been a *toilet seat cover*!

One especially clever fellow had obviously just come in as a hunter from the deep bush. He was the picture of the *Forest People* come in to a village. He was wearing bark cloth and a special hat. The hat was the better part of a discarded plastic bag, no doubt rain proof, with even a little visor made of the bag's carrying handle. I think he would have been proud of me if he could have seen me in the last Marine Corps Marathon, starting out in what he would immediately recognize as the rainy season, wearing a plastic trash bag as a raincoat. I am into *haute couture* as much as anyone in Assa, so I thought it was appropriate for him and me to shake hands, as I was dressed in a Long Island Marathon tee shirt, which might be a garment at least as labor intensive as his bark cloth suit.

The woman we sought was young with her hair neatly done up in four braids projecting from her head, what I called the "four-poster surprise" style. When the photo that Kati carried was shown to her, she explained to him what she had wanted and he made it known to me in return. This was a picture of her child. It had been taken by Mr. Wayne Watkins, a volunteer retired mechanic. He and his wife had come to visit in Assa for several months when he had been a friend of David and Diane Downing. He had come to help repair the Bronco back around 1990. I believe I remember that time, since I drove Diane Downing to

Baltimore-Washington International Airport to get a KLM connecting flight for the Congo out of Amsterdam. She was carrying "truck parts" which were heavy as lead and cost a fortune in excess baggage fees. Mr. Watkins had taken this photo of her child, and sent it back to her, and this is all she had to remember that event and that child who had died subsequently.

She would use the photograph to prove her fertility to increase her status in this community. The only witness to her having been able to produce a child is the small part of this picture showing her with her child. She would like to have this blown up and returned to her. Since Kati has helped me a lot, and this is a favor to a relative of his (not his wife), I will carry it back and try for cropping and enlargement.

I had taken photos of Kati at several critical moments in our lives. One photo was taken in 1990, when I shot the two male waterbucks and he had posed by one of them with the *makute* spear. He asked me on subsequent visits if I had remembered that event. I found the photo and got him copies. Another was taken when he posed with his father. I took their portraits at what turned out to be at a critically good time. His father died soon after the picture was taken. As is the case for many of the photos I have returned to Assa, they have become precious since they are the sole remaining memorial to those within them. Save those old family pictures to preserve the memory of your ancestors or offspring.

MY GRAVEN IMAGES DISTRIBUTED
AROUND ASSA

The population here is getting quite trained by my photography. They used to hoot when I would show them a picture of themselves, and deny that they looked anything like that. Right now, I would probably feel the same way, since fortunately for me, there are no fragments of any mirror anywhere left in Assa. Several times people would turn the photo around and ask, "How was it that the little animal or person could crawl in there?" Now, I have supplied JM with a flash camera no less. And each time out I have given him a disposable camera that would go back with me, except for this last time, when he had given it to MAF Pilot Don from CAR along with a letter to me, which I have not as yet received. This time I gave him the flash camera and told him to shoot it up, and give it to me as I leave, and that way I will be able to carry it along and hand-carry pictures back with me. The disposable camera/film technology has come along just in time for my use here in Assa.

Both Kati and Kazima have asked me slyly how much a camera costs. They had been thinking about getting something like the Nikon 8008. This costs approximately ten times the net worth of Assa and surrounding District. The

Nikon NTT I had used surreptitiously in the market is still the value of all expenses for the Assa health center for over a month. I have told them that the disposable camera could get down to about $10.00. I am leaving one of them, the waterproof underwater variety for the rainy season.

FLASHBACK THROUGH THE EYES
OF A FRIGHTENED CHILD

There is at least one little citizen here who is not yet used to me and my technology. I had gone over to the dark and very gloomy "ward" to shoot a photo of our postoperative patients. When I entered there was a toddler sitting at the door looking up at me in wide-eyed wonder. I made rounds, and returned. The child even toddled up to get another look at me as I paused in the doorway and turned around and shot a flash photo. I was not even pointing in the direction of the child, but the sudden flash of light so terrified the child that he screamed in panic and could not stop crying and scrambling to get away. This reaction was far out of proportion to the kind of surprise one might expect of a first exposure to photography or anything else. This was an anamnestic response. Perhaps this child had seen and heard the recent events, and was expressing the terror that the rest of the population also felt and still will not express.

There must be more than a conspiracy of silence, since there is a persistent troubled look about the people, which does not quite go away when I come upon them and they burst out with smiles and greetings. They will not tell me the names of the fallen, since one of them had said, mysteriously, "You know him." Still they say, when the sadness of my departure will be upon us, then they can speak of many things including the horrors that preceded my visit immediately before all their tears and anger turned to such joy.

I believe that this little boy saw in the flash what the rest of the adult witnesses had also seen earlier. They are still thinking about the differences between one week and another, of the native soldiers who came to kill and steal and the outsider who came to live and help. They are still overwhelmed and are quite muted about the comparison. They are working hard with me on the linguistic anthropology study, harder than would be expected as just a feature of humoring *Bwana*. One of them, Ngasyi, yesterday asked me "When will we know the results of this test and whether we have passed?"

Meanwhile, they are giving the "contextualized response" that would be an anthropologic fieldworker's dream.

"This color is a friend to that one."

"This one is father to that one."

"This is the color of the *Paipai* leaf."

"This is earth after the rains have not come."

"This color blue is the same name as sky," and they will look up to the (rainy season cloudy) sky for comparison. These should be good data, and certainly on the basis of the all out effort I am making, I have communicated that this is important to me, and they are trying to give back as good as they get.

A RETURN TO DOCTORING
AS "BUSH SURGEON"

Now, I have to go to the OR, and not just to charge the battery, since it seems I am the eye clinic doctor with the others reluctant to do much involving the eye. I have used up all my own Bacitracin ophthalmic ointment on the apparent trachoma outbreak around here. I do not remember seeing this much before. I have an orbital abscess to explore and drain, and possibly probe for a foreign body, a four-year-old wooden sliver. So, the "Author in Africa" must suspend for the moment his *œuvre*, and the tropical doctor must once again take up his tools of another trade. While that happens, I am going to try to delegate a continuation of at least data tabulation, so that we are using up the time of daylight for forward progress. André, and this morning independently Sonny, had said to me, "What these people need to get is the 'mentality' that something can be done about their problems!" This phrase I have heard repeatedly about the effect of a visit such as ours. I am such a prisoner of the Western hegemonic mind-set that forward progress is an essential ingredient in it.

22 *"IT IS VERY DIFFICULT"*

A SUMMARY STATEMENT AT THE HALFWAY POINT IN ASSA
MORE FOR THEM THAN FOR ME

July 15, 1998

Today it is Ngasyi. He and most of the other test subjects have been coming very diligently to get their chance to work on the linguistic anthropology project. They received no promises in advance for any substantial reward. They know full well that I am the sole source of any kind of "foreign aid" in Assa, and that they have to try to get close to *Bwana* because he is the one external "sky hook" that could lift them out. After all, Lazunga and Jean Marco had got close to *Bwana*, and both of them had benefited substantially, at least to their view that Lazunga's son managed to disappear from the Assa community and get himself and spouse and kids to Bunia just after my last visit. I was the only upward mobilizing happening thing that has transpired here. Now *Bwana* is in theatre, and we know that the only people qualified to follow him in there have been to school, such as the young Émile Zola as he seems to be known somewhere else (although we knew him as an Assa boy back then). Émile has good used clothes and a transistor radio and even a flash camera now, so the CME school in Nyankunde *must* be the road to ready riches, and the only access ramp we have to that which we see for the likes of Inikpio is the *Bwana*. We cannot follow him into the theatre until after we have been to school far away, so therefore, now, we should humor him and help with this crazy color test and the languages and see if this will result in a magic carpet lifting us out of this misery.

TODAY: THE CASE OF NGASYI
ONE AMONG MANY MENDICANTS OF ONLY THIS DAY
AMONG MANY OTHERS STANDING BY

"It is very difficult," said Ngasyi, as preamble to his request for help. This same phrase was used earlier by each person who has considered one of the many problems they face at every turn here.

In fact, I wanted to shout at least once, "It is *not* difficult. It is *bloody impossible!* "

Today's request from Ngasyi, lined up in a queue of four more for the day, is to see me privately after he has worked on the tabulation of the color linguistic data. I am grateful, so I will hear him out. He had gone to his shamba early, and had come over about 10:00 AM after I had seen the market and before I had started my major cases, and he was patient until the light began to fade, and then we went outside for his story. His story is helped by his fairly good command of English. He does not stammer around or try to gloss certain ascertainable facts that render conditions just *difficult*.

"Please, sir, I need you to help me," he said. Really he does not need me; he needs something more like the UN Development Agency. He continued with, "You see, I have been working here in Assa as a teacher for 12 years. I need to go to school in Nyankunde at CME to learn medicine, but it is very difficult. I need you to think about it and help me get there."

So, let's run the numbers. It will be $450.00 per year for an as yet unknown number of years. It sounds like a bargain, but wait. He must also get to Nyankunde, and the only way he can do that is by air. I talked with him about a bicycle and going up to Bunia, since he mentioned making some money by carrying *bidons* of palm oil. He could get over $100.00 if he could carry five *bidons*, which would be 100 liters of the oil, as I had once seen enterprising men do on bicycles at the Ituri River bridge as we were on our way back from working with the pygmies in Lolwa. But Assa is very remote, and it is (I know, let me guess) "very difficult" to get these to Bunia any way but by air. So, could I help get him and the palm oil to Bunia by air, where he would wait until the next windfall came along that could get him into school at CME in Nyankunde, since he might have money at that point to start.

Well, let's see. The freight charges for the mission personnel, not I, who must pay a higher rate, and certainly higher for the *commerçants*—is $1.50 per kg for a one-way transit from here to Bunia. That means I would pay $150.00 US to get his palm oil (without him attached to it yet) to Bunia where he is in hopes of collecting $100.00 US if the market is still holding, right? Yes, "It is very difficult." So, can you see that making money by air transport of palm oil to Bunia is what the British would call "a nonstarter?"

"Now, how about getting you there?" Well that too, is very difficult since, you see, he is not alone. I would be undertaking the carriage of him — and, let me guess again, a wife—"...yes, of course..."—and, hold it just a minute, some children—"…only five…!" Well that as I see it, is a total of seven "…only if my sisters cannot come…."

I thought, "You may count that in as a given!" I am going to have to get you all to CME at Nyankunde, which does not yet get you into CME, understand, without a wisp of a plan about getting you back, in what sounds like two chartered plane loads. This would be twice as much air traffic as Assa has had in the past two years since I was last here. Are you with me so far?

The mendicant would reply, "Yes, it is very difficult, but I want to go."

"Roger, that. Now, I calculate several thousand dollars before you get into school, without any support once you are there for the fees or living expenses for a family that is unfortunately, a great blessing while you are here, but totally unaffordable, for me, for example."

HOW TO DIVIDE VERY FEW LOAVES
AND EVEN FEWER FISHES

It is very difficult. I had planned to make a contribution to the unfortunate people of Assa that might help them get started into something that would generate some yield that they themselves might be able to use to leverage themselves out of the grinding poverty that afflicts them right here. But I am not for sponsoring refugees, who are interested in my sustaining them either here or elsewhere for any indefinite period of time. With four mendicants lined up for the day, I could not face another after doing the math with Ngasyi. I had done this for a number of mendicants on my last visit. They were eager to tap into me again, with a few others who must have heard that it was worth a shot. It is probably even true that I am the sole source of any aid they can hope for, even unreasonably.

What I had planned was to leave some funds in Nyankunde for distribution through one or more of the good, wise, and compassionate heads to support Assa projects. I cannot be the bridge to the good life arching over the vast Ituri that carries these people to a better life that I will be inventing for them. Somehow, a few folk have gone from being overwhelmed by my generosity in giving them my old shoes to expecting currency that apparently oozes out of me for the asking.

The original pair of hiking boots I left behind last time look better than ever on Kongonyesi's feet yesterday. They even look better than they did when they were new and my then three-year-old son Michael and I went overnight tenting in the Shenandoah Mountains with our matching hiking boots and backpacks. After all, if I am wealthy enough to give away perfectly good shoes, with only a little more luck, I could make them wealthy enough to buy such luxury items and others as well.

Quantification is not one of their strong suits, and it seems that one thing is a lot like the other, except better and more to their liking. For me, for example, living without plumbing or power is *difficult; not very difficult*, just inconvenient. For them, going without these "essential utilities and services" is not a big problem, since they have never known otherwise. This is like finding an unsurprising absence of complaints about the lack of such services in sixteenth century writings. But now I am here, and they have seen cameras and would like to have one as a gift. And others have been to school, and it surely would be good if those that have been could make it possible to have us go too.

Let's run the numbers again. Ngasyi has a salary from being a teacher at the primary school here. You might say that it is not much, but you could also say it is a service that is not worth much. The students will come to school, leaving all the tangible chores for which kids are needed, e.g., fetching water and wood, pounding rice, or tending siblings. The daily excuses for lack of attendance on the part of the teachers will vary. Most recently it was "There is no chalk for the lessons. Come back again in two weeks when there may be chalk—if it has not been stolen then." Recently it is the case that the teachers have uniformly not shown up since they need to work their shambas. That one has a job as a teacher does not mean that one can live off that source of support. In fact, Ngasyi reports that his salary from school over the twelve years he has worked there at Assa has never come up to the two items he required money to buy, salt and soap. So, if he did not work his garden, he and the six or more other mouths dependent upon him would not eat. So, he has not exactly bankrolled a lot, and is trying just to live day to day and dream of big plans for the future based in faith. Some of that faith is in God, and some of it is in hopes that *Bwana* is mathematically challenged—like those who play the lottery. If I just overlook a couple of very inconvenient sums, it not only becomes possible, but with a little faith, all such difficulties can be overcome.

If I say unto that mountain, be moved, and it is, then just possibly this immortal Ituri Forest will be paved over as a highway for me and palm oil and a raft of dependents to get to the rumor of the Promised Land in Nyankunde, nearly as far from here as Disneyland for all practical purposes.

While we are running numbers, I have another idea. Why don't we recover the billions of dollars that Belgium's King Leopold II (see Adam Hochschild's bone-chilling history of the "rubber terror" under King Leopold's boot [*King Leopold's Ghost: A Story of Greed, Terror, and Heroism in Colonial Africa*. Houghton Mifflin, Boston, 1998]) or Mobutu stole from these people and build some schools, roads, and health clinics? While we are at it, we should throw in some family planning information, a decent diet, money for school construction, salaries for teachers, development of rural agriculture, clean drinking water, and some hope for progress out of this grinding poverty. Surely Mr. Kabila (or his replacement) should want to help his own citizens.

The really poignant part that these people are probably thinking without getting bold enough to say it out loud is, *"With just a little bit of the luck you have had, I could get to be like you."*

And you know, they probably could!

23 CONGOLESE LINGUISTICS

THE BABBLE OF BABEL,
AND MANY MORE TONGUES TO GO

July 16, 1998

BATS IN MY BELFRY
AS DAWN RAIN WASHES OUT THE RUN
FOR THE SECOND TIME THIS WEEK

I am sitting in the area of the window in the cacophony of dawn, having had a light sleep through the night as I listened to the various sounds around my room. The gibbous moon lit my bed, and I heard a lot of sound from the trees just outside. There are large bats that make a raucous amount of stirring in the fronds of the tall royal palms in the courtyard, and I thought I heard one closing in. Something large was moving in the attic crawl space overhead. It made a sound like that of the bats in the palm trees. When I went out to pee in the moonlight, I was buzzed on three passes, like the pursuit of the star fighters from the Millennium Falcon, by three bats, smaller than those I heard in the palms. There are lots of prowling mammals in nocturnal aerial and ground surveillance.

I got up early to get ready for the run. So, I am now sitting here all dressed for the run, and have no place to go. I was up at 4:40 AM and almost immediately the soft, gentle but soaking rain began. It has put the resonating chorus of frogs in the cistern into high voice. I thought I should go to bed and wait for it to stop or my ARRC colleagues to come by. The first happened, but the second did not. So, this is our second washout in a week. Today I was planning on taking the GPS out on the run. I wanted to measure how far we had run and also get a fix on the Assa River, our planned turnaround point. The GPS could give me an estimate of our distance as the Malachite Kingfisher (*Alcedo cristata*, there are no crows here) flies. I suspect that we run as far in that opposite direction as our airstrip is from the other side of the Assa station.

159

♣ OUT OF ASSA: HEART OF THE CONGO

THE BABEL OF THE CONGO
A FURTHER SOURCE OF ISOLATION IN THIS REMOTE REGION

Assa is near the center of the region of Pazande-speaking tribes, in one of the few areas of the Congo where there is not much linguistic overlap. These Azande people may number over a million and a half in the northern part of the Congo, the CAR, and the southern part of the Sudan. The Azande originally came from the Sudan and then spread out in conquest of the more peaceful peoples of various Bantu stock that they assimilated.

The only "universal languages" in Congo, as in many other parts of the once colonized world, are European imports. Here it is French because of the Belgian colonization. French is still taught in school here. This means, of course, that you have *to go* to school, if school there were, to learn a European language, or else be very active in the markets where it is spoken. English is widely spoken in Africa and throughout the rest of the world since everyone wishes to *go* to school and to *do business and communicate* with the largest marketers of modernity.

This European overlay of languages has reached even this far into this remote corner of the Congo, and if for no other reason other than that I am here now, there is an interest in greeting me with a "Good morning!" rather than "*Bon jour!*" or even "*Mbote!*" In those three steps we have just paid tribute to the colonizers in, respectively, English, French and Lingala.

FOUR FAMILIES OF CONGOLESE LANGUAGES

There are four big language groups in the Congo, and to say that someone speaks Kiswahili does not mean that each Swahili person can understand all other Kiswahili speakers. The tongues are quite different, even within language groups. These four groups are: 1) Lingala (or Bangala, a more recent European missionary variant construct of Lingala), the dominant language grouping of the north; 2) Kiswahili, and only a derivative of that language, not all variants of which are mutually intelligible, dominant as a market language in the east; 3) Chiluba, the spoken tongue of the Luba peoples, dominant in the central and southern regions; and 4) Kikombo, the language of the west and the capital area of Kinshasa.

With these major groups established as indigenous African regional language divisions for starters, things will get complicated since there are areas of overlap and also some outside forces that put pressure on the languages to convert to dominance some tongue that was not the major one before. For example, Kiswahili is the market language of both Kisangani and Nyankunde. This is not the same as the Kiswahili that is one of the official languages of Kenya and Tanzania. These are mutually unintelligible languages with the same roots perhaps, and the same name, but different usages. They are not the same in the sense of someone understanding what is said or written.

Further, the Kombo people of the capital area of Kinshasa had used Kikombo before 1960 and the rule of Mobutu (from a small tribe in the north and therefore lingalaphone). He made Lingala the official language of the capital. After all, it was his government, and it would jolly well speak the language in which he felt most comfortable. Far more important, *Lingala was the language of Mobutu's army.*

"COMMON MARCHING ORDERS" IN THE ARMY AND IN THE MINES UTILITARIAN INSTRUCTIONS IN A NEW LINGUA FRANCA

When I was in Pakistan, and looking over the Mogul rulers' relics, I came to an important realization. The Moguls had swept through the northern areas of what would become India with an army of conscripts from all the areas they had conquered. The strains of Persian, Hindi and many other distinct languages were spoken by soldiers who were commanded to all march and fight in the Mogul ruler's common cause. So, *a language of the army*, Urdu, which literally means "army," was created. Urdu remains the official language of Pakistan today. Lingala was Mobutu's "Urdu."

The same kind of forced communication utility occurred in South Africa. Here a "language of the mines," "Funagalu," evolved from Bantu strains, numerous Nguni tongues, a few pieces from Portuguese (from the Mozambicans and Angolans), a little Afrikaans here, and a little English there. Funagalu was a language that might be common to all, and would consist largely of orders for action and safety precautions that could be understood by every miner in South Africa, regardless of geographic, ethnic or linguistic origin.

Even before Mobutu, there were reasons that Lingala, the market language of the north, might spread to both the capital Kinshasa (colonial Leopoldville), and to the second city of the Congo Kisangani (colonial Stanleyville), over 2,000 km away up the navigable Congo River. Remember Joseph Conrad's description of the steamer plying the long passage of the only river on earth that crosses the equator, and this mighty one does it *twice*, the River Congo. The steamer that Marlowe took to get into and through the *Heart of Darkness* passed through the tribes that spoke Lingala. To trade with or make war on these people would require accurate intelligence and knowledge of their language.

There are two ends of the navigable Congo as it passes through the rainforest, the Ituri of Central Africa. The mighty river collects the rain that falls off the scarps of the plateau that is the main body of the African continent, its "shorelines" over 200-km inland, having been defined in ice ages long past. The Congo flows west past Kinshasa, the capital city, and then passes over Juey Falls, a series of tumultuous cascades that carry the great river to the Atlantic about 100 km downstream from Boma, at Pointe-Noire in the People's Republic of the Congo, which is more than 300 km from "Kin" as the inland capital, is known. Kinshasa is sited above those falls at the beginning of the navigable river, the only road into that impenetrable rainforest. The other main city of the Congo, Kisangani, is located at the "upriver" (= "Haut-Zaïre") end of the Congo River. Just east of Kisangani, the river also "falls down" (to use a favorite African expression for most accidents), this time off the scarp and into the Great Rift Valley, the tectonic division of the continent slowly separating the east from the continental body of Africa itself. These are the Boyoma Falls. When Kisangani was called Stanleyville, these were known as Stanley Falls, named after the infamous explorer/journalist Henry Morton Stanley. Stanley found David Livingstone in his travels into the interior, coming upon him in what is now Zambia where I will be exploring myself in two weeks. There, Stanley said, "Dr. Livingstone, I presume?"

The MAF pilot Lary Strietzel chuckled when I had landed at the remote Assa air strip with him, he for the first time having touched down anywhere nearly this remote. He asked with a laugh, "How will I know you if and when I come back after you?"

I said, without even considering the truth or implications of having been now repeatedly in this interior outpost of the Congo, "I may be the only white face in all of Assa!"

He laughed, and said in response to André's comment, even if inaccurate, "Try 500 km in any direction!—I should be able to find you." Therefore, if someone is out here searching for me, I hope a competent explorer and friendly type like New York Herald journalist Stanley (as opposed to, less happily, the soldiers currently occupying the administrative capital of this zone at Ango) reaches me sitting under the *Rauwolfia* bush as I type. The person who finds me might ask with the same degree of probability that Stanley had in asking his question under the remote and grueling circumstances, "Doctor Geelhoed, I presume?"

Stanley Falls still fall, but their name has been changed to Boyoma Falls and Stanleyville had been renamed Kisangani. Stanleyville had been a town that spoke Kiswahili learned from the porters that had penetrated this far in from the earlier Arab traders and later the British explorers of East Africa. Each of these *commerçants* and adventurers was outfitted in the Indian Ocean islands of Lamu and Zanzibar off the east coast of Africa. Twice a year, the Islamic (Middle Eastern Arabic and Omani) traders would make passage on the trade winds up to the Gulf, as I had in retracing the route of the dhows on Air Tanzania's one 737 named *Kilimanjaro* in 1996. These Kiswahili-speaking islanders, picked up as porters first by Arabic then later by British traders, were heavily involved in the ivory and slave trade that made the East Coast ports an exit for the largest commerce the continent had seen, the traffic in human chattel. With the porters came their language, as far as Kisangani, until now the limit of the Kiswahili incursion. All along the way from Kisangani on the east, west to Kinshasa, as far west as the Congo River is navigable, Lingala could be used as the market language throughout this northern Congo. Lingala got mixed with the other market languages at either port on opposite ends. At the time of Mobutu's despotic rule, only ended recently, this commercial dominance in the north was both *de jure* and *de facto* because Mobutu came from a northern tribe. His army kept that dominion for more than three decades and its "Urdu" was Lingala.

BANGALA:
CODIFIED CREATION OF A "SALVATION ARMY"

The army of "Christian soldiers" marched into the remote bush just ahead of or not long after the explorer/exploiters. The missionary soldiers required an "Urdu" of their army also. With *Two Thousand Tongues to Go*, the book by Colonel Townsend's Wycliffe Bible Translators and the work of his disciples in the Summer Institute of Linguistics, the Bible has been translated into nearly every spoken language on earth. There is no spot so remote or so few people speaking a fading language that they cannot reach it. The missionaries in West Africa took on Hausa and Fulani, large language groups there. Smaller divisions of these and other home languages were being worked on in West Africa when I was there 30 years ago this year. I remember working with college mates Rob and Esther Corry. They were working on creating a Bible in the Nigerian languages Jukan or Kuteb while I was doing medical work in Nigeria's Benue River State east of Biafra near Takum. Similar developments of the written word were completed all across Africa. The first written text derived from Lingala was the missionaries' written version of this spoken language, which is called Bangala.

Bangala, therefore, did not exist until after the European missionaries codified it to communicate with these peoples of the northern Congo. The

Congolese physicians from Nyankunde, with whom I have been working, come from elsewhere in the Congo. They know that they will be speaking to the peoples of the north in *Lingala*, although the people respond in the tongue that the missionaries wrote their gospel and hymnals in, *Bangala*, a variant of an African lingua franca as filtered and codified by Europeans. There are insubstantial differences, so that the people, who came from some place such as Nyankunde (and, each, before that, both Kisangani and Kinshasa) like Doctors Ahuka and Mwembo, are recognized as coming from some place else, but can be "heard." Their Lingala is well-understood, even if as a market tongue. It is a somewhat sparser language than the people of Assa's own home language, Pazande.

THE AZANDE: FROM THE FIELDWORK OF
EDMUND EDWARDS-PRITCHARD TO THE PRESENT
TOILER IN THE ANTHROPOLOGIC FIELD
IN CONDITIONS THAT HAVE CHANGED
LITTLE IN NEARLY A CENTURY

One of the first of the new field of anthropology's professionals was the British anthropologist, Edmund Edwards-Pritchard. He advocated getting out into the remote isolated community and being a participant/observer in fieldwork. He studied and wrote about the Azande and the Nuer in the Sudan. His original work, *Magic, Oracles and Witchcraft Among the Azande,* was one of the first books I read on this group of Sudanese conquering warriors. The conditions of his fieldwork over 75 years ago cannot have been too dissimilar to the conditions I experience today in this spot. I am making notes as a participant/observer during a circumcision of a small boy. I am writing with a ballpoint pen for the moment. I am recharging my battery in the OR.

The Azande, who speak Pazande, are the group I have been working with here and may be working with in the next station at Banda. The people and their language are spread across the Bas-Uele region over into CAR and Sudan from which direction the original warriors with their Azande blades came conquering before Europeans ever heard about them. But, because of the large size of the group, and the early work done by such legendary trek missionaries as "Papa Dix," their language was written into Bibles and songbooks. There was even a "Jesus" film produced in Pazande. This film was carried through the region by a team of itinerant bush evangelists. They toured with a projector and a portable Honda generator balanced on their *pikipiki.*

So, Pazande is the "home language" of this group of northern peoples who are the amalgam made from the Bantus assimilated under Azande conquest.

Papa Dix, in fact, knew only Pazande, besides his Nebraska farm-boy English, but neither French nor Bangala. Once when he went to Kinshasa to apply for a permit to shoot the elephants that were marauding the shambas of his Azande communicants, he explained to the bewildered officials there about the peoples' predicament, unaware that these cravat-wearing officers had a problem of their own. They did not understand a word he said, since he naïvely addressed them in Pazande rather than Bangala. An interpreter was found for him, and he got his permits. Eventually, he killed over 500 elephants: André had witnessed one of the killings. André reported that this animal's tusks were five meters long and a half-meter across at the base (this sounds exaggerated) but they were clearly so large that two men could not carry one.

So, Pazande is the base language of my study to compare against the northern lingua franca of Bangala, a codified variant of the official Lingala of the long dictatorship of Sese Mobutu.

LINGUA FRANCA OF THE OTHER REGIONS OF THE VERY RICH NATION OF THE CONGO, DESPITE ITS DESPERATELY POOR PEOPLE, WHOSE LINGUA FRANCA DEPENDS ON WHO IS IN POWER

The Luba peoples are in the southern and central areas of the Congo. Their territory includes the Kasai province, the only place where Chiluba is spoken. The Kasai is important because it is the center of the diamond mining enterprise that was once the business of a couple of well-placed Congolese. The diamond mining operations were nationalized with the Simba Revolt, and are a collaborative part now of the DeBeers Consolidated cartel, which may explain why many diamonds are cut and polished in Antwerp, since the Democratic Republic of the Congo (DRC) as this country is now called was once the Belgian Congo. At one time the Congolese cartel was the largest producer of diamonds in the world. It has now fallen to fourth because war and political instability do not cause such an industry to thrive in the uncertainty of whether you will be able to take your high-value portable wealth out of the country while cutting more deals than diamonds. For 100 years, DeBeers has run the most successful cartel in history. It keeps prices high by restraining supply and raising demand by prestige advertising. This was the model for the OPEC oil cartel that fell apart from too many unconstrained sources of the product. The Congo could have been a wildcat producer of diamonds to the point of selling them by the kilogram, if the cost of doing business in this area (trust me, on this one!) were not so forbidding. International economics of monopolies aside, Chiluba is the language for the Kasai region.

There are also the abundant mineral riches of the Congolese "copper belt" in Katanga Province. Part of the Katanga Province, in the eastern region of the Congo, is the home of most of the unrest (a very mild term for the mass genocide that has stained this border, and the world, in perpetuity). The long-standing Hutu/Tutsi conflict made basket cases of Rwanda and Burundi near the Katanga border and contaminated neighboring Tanzania and Uganda. The overflow of Hutus from the Rwandan conflict was the major factor in toppling the government of Zaïre in bloody civil war. The first anniversary of Kabila's rise to power was "celebrated" at the time of my arrival. The war crimes tribunal meeting in Arusha, Tanzania is looking into the role of Mr. Kabila in perpetrating the very atrocities he said he had sought to end.

A NEW LANGUAGE FOR A NEW ARMY UNDER A NEW DICTATOR, EVEN BLOODIER THAN THE LAST

The military marauding going on will be a key element in not only the linguistics, but also what happens to Assa, and to my projects. Kabila's "*Urdu*" is *Kiswahili*. And that is not just any Kiswahili, but Ugandan/Tanzanian Kiswahili. There is no major mystery as to why this should be. His rebel army was sheltered, trained, and supplied from rebel bases in Uganda and Tanzania. His army gave support to whichever side in the horrific Hutu/Tutsi pogroms happened to have the upper hand in beating up the forces of the army of his own *bête noire*, Generalissimo Sese Mobutu, *All-Conquering Hero, He Who Goes From Triumph to Triumph*. No, I am not kidding. That is only part of his official name, which had to be saluted after the national anthem each day, along with a final salute, which had to be given in his small northern home language: "He is cock among chickens!"

To curry favor with the shorter agrarian Bantu Hutus, against the taller, nomadic, Nilotic, herdsmen Tutsis, a cattle culture of the Rift Valley side of the Ruwenzori Mountains, Kabila was not above generally allowing, or encouraging if not actively participating in massacres of whole populations of Tutsis. Kabila exploited these ancient ethnic rivalries for his own political agenda. His own plans consisted of a series of campaigns to sweep from the east through all of the richer parts of Zaïre to oust Mobutu and to create his own "People's Democratic Republic of the Congo." He was persuaded (as was Mozambique) to drop the "People's" appellation since it was only labeled on communist countries and that might sour potential international donors on reconstruction aid. So Kabila followed the money. He recognized that client states of the former Soviet Union (such as Cuba) or the People's Republic of China have not fared as well as those who leaned toward the West and thus attracted capitalist investors. Thus, this pitiable excuse for a nation (in the perspective of the region where I now sit) is called officially the "Democratic Republic of the Congo."

No matter that there is another completely separate nation and government across the Congo River that had prior claim on the name the "People's Republic of Congo." This other country is now often called "Congo-Brazzaville" to avoid confusion, using the name of its capital city across the river from the other Congolese Capital of Kinshasa. In 1993, my Air Afrique plane landed in Brazzaville's chaos en route from Jo'burg to Senegal/Gambia by way of Abidjan, in Ivory Coast. My through-checked bags and their contents are still in circulation, presumably somewhere in or around Brazzaville. Kabila believes first and foremost in the proposition that brought him to power: He who has the guns makes the rules, and the rules are changed to the benefit of the man with the guns. Long live the new "President-for-Life Kabila!" Kiswahili will be the language in which he is saluted.

During the long kleptocracy of Mobutu, Kiswahili was the unofficial language of Goma in the eastern region. While Mobutu set the rules and his army was present to enforce them, Lingala was used all through the nation, in spite of the fact that it was the lingua franca of only his northern region. Other than along the River "Zaïre" (at that time, now "Congo," again) and its two principle cities Kisangani and Kinshasa, no Congolese spoke Lingala. The majority population and the people of the centers of extractive wealth neither spoke nor understood Lingala. But Mobutu had his army and it had his language.

Now, the new kleptocracy of a different military dictator has emerged and he has a different army with different rules and a different language. Kabila's "Urdu," is the Kiswahili language of his benefactor camps in Uganda and Tanzania and in his earlier successes in the eastern region in the smoke screen of the Hutu/Tutsi chaos. Kabila's army includes the core of his own mercenary gang, rag-tag misfits who are very accomplished killers from the Ugandan camps, and the recruits from the small boys with Kalashnikovs who have joined in. The remnants of Mobutu's army and Kabila's army with which it is supposed to be assimilated after recently doing all their dead-level best to annihilate each other (and are occasionally doing so still on a case-by-case basis of old scores to be settled), *often cannot even speak the same language.*

This is the new and "integrated army," two parts of which passed through Assa two weeks and one week before my arrival and are threatening to return, either together or in pursuit of each other, through Assa from occupied Ango. The only thing worse than an army of soldiers heading for these poor people, is two armies of marauding soldiers. Each army is pillaging their way through the destitute countryside in pursuing their own bloody quarrel. While devastating the locals, they do not understand one another, because of differences in language, culture, and command and (lack of) control functions.

Kabila is in the capital Kinshasa, speaking a language that is gibberish to the command structure that he has vanquished, and the confusion is understandable at that end of the country. He is *paying* a Kiswahili-speaking army, who have learned only one thing from the Mobutu Lingala-speaking army, and that has not been the language: the whole population is ripe for plucking, and whoever shoots first has a far better chance of running away with the loot.

The new army's Kiswahili is quite different from the Kiswahili that Sonny Mwembo or Ahuka learned in Kisangani, which in turn is different from the Kiswahili they are using in Nyankunde. Areas of overlap are not very broad unless there are commercial interests—like the River Congo that had linked Kinshasa and Kisangani, the two biggest cities in Congo, and nearly the only ports of consequence other than Pointe-Noire in the People's Republic of the Congo on the Atlantic. But there are two things that travel well together, without cultural, geographic or commercial constraint. One is the arbitrary edict of the Head of State (by definition, the one with the most guns). The other is the army that he can command in marching orders that they understand. Armies have intruded into the lives of these remote and poor people who would otherwise not have anything of interest to an armed band of marauders intent on spoils. But, this area is also so remote and among a people no one much cares about, that anyone with a gun can do jolly well whatever he wants, marching only to the drummer of his own "Urdu." The thunder around Assa is in a polyglot Babel that has caught these poor Azande in the crossfire.

DOES THAT EXPLAIN THE DYNAMIC JOY OF MY BEING HERE IN THIS CHAOS AMONG THESE VERY SPECIAL PEOPLE?

This geopolitical/linguistic dissertation may be a prerequisite for the rather mundane detail work of explaining to you in a later discourse the meanings of color terms in two languages. Look for the color lexicography of terms in Pazande/Bangala (**Appendix III**) as we get closer to analyzing and displaying the data of this arduous field research process, and the reasons for undertaking it in the first place. One overall reason may have been best expressed by Mohammed Akhter, whom I had met in Pakistan and who is now Director of the American Public Health Association in Washington, DC when he said to me, "It is a special privilege in life to joyously participate in the miseries of mankind."

PAZANDE VS. BANGALA
WHAT AM I TRYING TO DO HERE ANYWAY?

July 16, 1998

A scientific study, you say, amid all this entropic collapse? You must be kidding! Go to a library or a laboratory! It certainly would be a whole world easier, and under circumstances that are more user-friendly. I believe that my fieldwork is the only way to find out quickly whether the medical interventions have enhanced the mental capacity and quality of life of the people of Assa. If so, the indigenous medical staff would have further support to continue the therapy to reduce hypothyroidism and its effects. This simple and inexpensive treatment would be immediately beneficial to a very needy people. I am trying to raise their profile from the very malignant neglect they have suffered generally, and at warp speed recently.

So, let me explain the basic details, and then get to the reasons for trying so bloody hard to pull off this anthropologic research beyond the ends of the earth. I have given the broad strokes of the general picture of the linguistic divisions of the regions of the Congo, and the peculiar (not to say, diabolical) circumstances of the civil unrest continuing during my current visit.

THE WORKING OF THE STUDY PLAN IN PRACTICAL DATA COLLECTION

The linguistic study attempts to compare the discriminatory ability of Assa residents in their home (Pazande) and market (Bangala) language with respect to colors and shapes, measuring how analytic they are in cognition and expression. Colors are universal stimuli for recognition of some kind of experience to which a name is given and distinctions are made. I am presenting 330 different colors (Munsell chips) covering the entire color spectrum visible to humans, to the informants, asking them to name the color they see in each language. I also elicit the focus (the one best color with that name) and range (of all possible colors with that name) from the set of colors.

I have also made it a point to find, observe, and often photograph, the substance (e.g., a cassava leaf) that may share a name with the color they have designated in either tongue. I have put that into the context of their use, often on the simplest day-to-day basis, of their simple, harsh lives.

Then, on separate days, I have shown them a triad of color chips and asked them to arrange these in a triangle according to the *similarity* of these colors when instructed in Pazande. They have then been asked to arrange them in triangles of *dissimilarity* using the same language.

This same process is repeated next for a series of triads of simple objects, whatever their color, that they may arrange them first in order of their *similarities* and, with another series of objects, arrange in triads of *dissimilarities* when the language of instruction is Pazande,

The whole process is repeated in all its parts, on another day, with the informants instructed in Bangala, and making the distinctions they see in this market language

LABOR-INTENSIVE PROJECT FOR INFORMANTS AND INVESTIGATOR

This study is difficult. It must be carried out in the 12 hours of daylight in the equatorial tropics where we have no artificial lighting. The informants are not always available for interview because their opportunity cost is high. They could be out gathering food, so we are sacrificing the time that they need to keep themselves and their families alive. The data-gathering that must be done here is formidable, as are the obstacles to our success. We will do our best under these trying conditions. All the tabulated data will then be carried back to Washington, D.C. for further analysis by the investigator completing this very labor-intensive study.

The informants are unpaid for participation in this study. Their reward is a contextualized one. They became familiar with my efforts over more than a decade of providing volunteer medical and surgical services to this community. They have seen the community benefit that the prior projects including the goiter/cretinism work, which essentially eliminated highly prevalent hypothyroidism, which severely constrained their development potential. They have benefited when I provided medical and surgical equipment and medication resupply. There is also the direct benefit of clothing and other goods dispersed to some. Also, I set up a fund for special needs such as educational projects. This fund does not provide the sole support of any given individual. Rather, the fund was spread out over the entire community to benefit study participant and nonparticipant alike.

Appendix III is a simple list of Pazande and Bangala names for the colors of the rainbow. This is not the way they name colors. Instead, they use colors that share the names of familiar objects. i.e., the color of the object and the object itself often have similar names. During the interview, they may even look around to see the passing clouds or the sky, or look for a leaf, sometimes a specific leaf or a part of it, like *kpe gadia* (= the cassava leaf) or *kpe ndunda* (= the violet stem of the leaf). Their modifiers provide excellent specificity. I have tried to watch them in naming the colors since the more discriminating utilize more real world comparisons and referents than the less discriminating.

USAGES IN COMPARISONS IN TRIADS

Our informants express innovative insights about colors or objects and their relationships:

"This color is a friend to that one."

"This is the father to that one."

"These two objects are fish and that is a leaf, but this fish has no scales so it is very dissimilar to the other even if they are both fish."

"These are two animals and that is an object, but this animal is an elephant which is like no other animal, so they are dissimilar."

If I listed the narrative in each interview (and I have taped a few of them), they would seem all quite individualized, since their reasons for including or excluding something in a similar or dissimilar way are unique. I too might have a difficult time understanding what it means to arrange three objects in a triad according to their "dissimilarity" so I am more than willing to let their own interpretation stand.

CORRELATION WITH THE PRIOR
GOITER AND CRETINISM WORK

The ability to analyze critically is a measure of intelligence. A willingness and aptitude to discriminate among objects may have an adaptive value. The goiter and cretinism work was presented in Philadelphia's Benjamin Franklin Institute at the *Damaged Brain of Iodine Deficiency Symposium* in 1994. A discussant questioned the impact of the original work in eliminating cretinism and improving goiter. We showed that we had made changes in the endocrinologic numbers and in the size of goiters and in a number of physiologic variables that changed before and after the Lipiodal. We could not show that these people were better off, other than being greater consumers of calories, which, I contend, is a disadvantage in the marginal resource environment of Assa. This adverse effect might be offset by cultural adaptability, if their increased metabolic activity allowed them to react more adaptively to the changes in their environment. Perhaps their improved analytical skills would give them more options to choose from, empowering a broader and therefore beneficial choice of responses.

I could not conduct a color interview on a severely affected cretin because they are deaf-mute. The people who volunteered here as informants are perceptive and responsive adults, all of whom are mature males (to further limit variables) who have been treated during the goiter study and returned toward normal thyroid status and normal metabolism. The study tests the hypothesis that the treatment makes it possible for them to respond to the subtle differences they see in their environment and make it possible to choose among their perceptions and carry out a more adaptive course of action. This improvement might empower them to resolve some of their own problems, which they can discriminate more acutely than I, largely through the local use of their own cognition and their cultural expression of that perception and cognition in language.

The Sapir-Whorf hypothesis deals with the effect of language on thought. The hard-line school is that language *determines* thought, and the softer line is that language *influences* thought. Here is a model in which we can study discrimination in a universal modality, color perception, and compare it with shape and object comparisons, in such a way to see if these people have achieved a human benefit and an adaptive advantage when freed of their hypothyroidism. Color discrimination is a noncultural test of intelligence in an environment where the "Stanford-Benet" type of IQ testing would be inappropriate. From whatever obtunded state they had at the time they were hypothyroid, current testing reveals an ability to discriminate and name subtle differences. Improved analytical ability furnishes a means for a greater variety of adaptive responses in the circumstances of a changing environment with significant resource constraints. Options among which such discriminating choices are made might be critical for survival and thriving.

If hypothyroidism is adaptive in environments of severe resource constraints, possibly freeing the population of the burden of hypothyroidism's loss of potential could make possible cultural adaptations to these resource-constrained environments. This anthropologic study may demonstrate the humanitarian benefit to our medical relief effort (Geelhoed, 1999b).

25 RIVER OF MYSTERY

THE ASSA RIVER: "RIVER OF MYSTERY, "
WHICH *MUST* BE EXPLORED WHEN IT IS PEACEFUL.
FOR NOW, I WILL MAKE DO WITH A GPS FIX

July 17, 1998

Nothing was going to stop the ARRC this morning! Or at least not this member thereof. I went to bed at the ludicrous hour of 7:30 PM last night. There could be no mistake that *night* it was. I could neither see nor do anything in the blackness. The waning moon had vanished under rain clouds. There is only so much that can be done in the dark, even with the flickering help of candlelight. I had already done my dictating with the backdrop of the cistern full of bellowing frogs, so I went to bed.

Not to sleep, however, for I thought of the many things I have yet to accomplish here in Assa and beyond, having got more than a good start despite very trying circumstances. Furthermore, there is now a *river* on my mind.

We talked last night about the Assa River, the "River of Mystery," which I had run to on Sunday, and am now determined to explore. Almost as if a red cape were thrown in front of a bull pawing the ground, Inikpio said repeatedly, and the others confirmed, that the Assa River has *never* been explored. It is *right here* waiting for me to explore it. This bull is a member of the National Geographic Society, The American Geographical Society, and the Royal Geographic Society, and has explored unknown jungles before, e.g., with the Terramar Foundation on the Venezuelan tepuys of the Gran Sabana.

Here is the mystery of the Assa River. Hippos and crocodiles find their way up as far as the crude log bridge to which we ran this Sunday morning on our longest run to date. They come up from the Bomu River, a very long river that starts about 150 km east of Assa, near where the Sudan, the CAR, and the DRC share a common border. The Assa River flows from here toward the Bomu River, and around the area of Ebale the Assa River *disappears*. I helicoptered

173

into Ebale in 1992 as part of my goiter work. On take-off, our helicopter had a serious mechanical failure that required a three-day stay while we awaited airdrop of spare parts.

The disappearance of the Assa River is not a total mystery, since it is known that it flows from a grotto into a cave under the *mungas*. But, then the Assa River follows a *subterranean course* for a distance of several kilometers, around one of the other "goiter villages" in the original study, Lumu. About 10 km from Lumu, the underground Assa River joins the Bomu River somewhere *while still underground*! The crocodiles manage to navigate this mysterious passage up river underground and emerge to threaten the fisherman in the Assa River where it surfaces again around the village of Ebale. I had been served catfish caught from the nearby river by Ebale fishermen while stranded in Ebale by the grounding of the helicopter. They reported seeing both crocodiles and hippos more frequently during the rainy season than in the dry season.

The lower stretch of the Assa River presents a challenge. I would want to be coming back to run the river to its mysterious disappearance and reappearance, and "ride the tagged crocodiles" back up to the re-emergence into the light of the rainy season, some day.

Natural coffee "plantations" occupy the course of where the Assa River would have flowed had it not sunk out of sight. In the former flood plain of the river there are collections of wild coffee bushes, according to the young men who made their way into school through the bush craft of knowing a *Rauwolfia* bush from others in the scrub of the bush. These areas seem to be known only to the locals. Many of them are superstitious about this area and avoid it. Several would be willing to guide me there, and together we might explore some of the "Mysteries of the Assa River." Alas, like many other things I would like to do here, that adventure requires a period of relative peace and stability in the Assa area without interference from marauders in or out of uniform.

For now, I will try to roust the ARRC, and despite a good deal of rain last night, head out in the lead on a good morning run, directly toward the Assa River, GPS in hand.

THE ARRC IS ON THE RUN!

It was a good morning for a run, without too many bugs, and although the puddles were bigger, these were no more than we had run around before. I will give you the morning's score in fresh wildlife encounters: I smelled, before I spotted the tracks—an African civet had run down the path ahead of us. To get ahead of this story to the turnaround point in the run, this is an example where we completed the loop on this animal. We smelled it, then spotted tracks, and finally saw the beast itself, casting back and forth across the path on our return.

I was in the lead, and nothing was going to stop me short of the Assa River. André had a sore knee but he gutted it out. He was my only fellow runner this morning and a somewhat reluctant one at that. He taped up his knee in anticipation of the run when he saw me sitting in running gear as he walked out of his room this morning. The last kilometer of the downhill slope to the river was the only point where the red volcanic cinders turned to sticky clay, forcing us to kick off the gumbo clods that accumulated under foot. We arrived at the log bridge, and noted that the river had come up considerably since we were here five mornings earlier.

I stood on the bridge, with booming bullfrogs echoing around me, and waved the GPS in the air trying to expose its antenna to whatever satellites it might find. It took 10 minutes to raise three satellites and start tracking for me to punch in the "RIVE" mark. This "exposure time" meant more to certain little trolls who were keepers of this bridge than it did to me at first.

Among the first wee creatures I became reacquainted with in Assa were the red army ants. Ten years ago, I took a walk around Assa with Tim Harrison, a fellow volunteer physician. In the bucolic setting of a thatched mud hut, we sat on a log outside the fire circle and "communed happily with the natives." The family, delighted, if not overwhelmed, by the visit of a delegation of such distinguished visitors, sent a small boy up the tree growing next to their hut and he banged off a half dozen oranges. Now, those oranges had been there for some time and were within easy reach, so I felt guilty about consuming their "banked stock" but they were saving them for a special occasion and nothing more special would be happening here any time soon.

So, we sat and peeled back the green but delicious oranges gratefully, and began to eat the segments with appreciative gestures while making the universally understood "Ummmmm" noises to indicate approbation.

I was abruptly uncomfortable in this otherwise cozy transcultural exchange. Perhaps I was sitting on a sliver of the log, and had got stuck. No, there was another one, this time at my ankles, nowhere near the log. At first I tried to make my scratching motions coincide with some other gesture, but then I threw the civility of subterfuge to the wind, and began flailing my arms and legs in a St. Vitus dance. Earlier, Tim Harrison had been taken aback by my performance but now he began stamping his feet in such a way as to signal that we had come from a long way away. We were greeting them with this small ceremonial Apache War Dance which was a tradition among Americans extending hands, and feet, across the ocean.

We had discovered fire ants. These little red devils look a lot like ordinary ants, and have the habit of crawling up your leg to some place suited to their convenience, and latching on with a very effective mandibular pincer maneuver. This seems invariably to be a noticeable diversion to the visitor otherwise engaged, but our hosts were nonplussed and looked at us in some wonderment. Well, it has been some time since we have entertained two American Professors of Surgery from otherwise distinguished institutions, and we may have forgotten just how eccentric they can be!

Without so much as a "By your leave," we split, spilling orange peels as we left. I explained that we would be back with some form of interpreter who could give a reason for our abrupt departure, but I hope they were not of the opinion that we rebuffed their generous hospitality. The little buggers had latched on tightly and a slap could sweep away the back two-thirds of the trisegmented corpus, but the head was fixed in position by a vise of its own making.

Descendents of these creatures rediscovered me while I was standing on the log bridge over the Assa River waiting for the stubby little antenna of the GPS to find and hold three satellites. The GPS had trouble holding more than two even though it seemed to have been able to locate quite a few, but lose them on a second glance into that celestial quadrant. Meanwhile, it turned out that what I thought were the hurtful cinders that had caught in my shoes were not sharp little stones, but red fire ants. I jumped off the log bridge onto the muddy path, and tried pulling off the critters, most of which remained as grinning heads still holding on tightly. In some African venues, people allow live ants to clamp the mandibles on either side of a wound and then twist off the body, leaving the stubborn mandibles remaining in a line like the disposable clips used for wound apposition in my part of the surgical world.

The short story is that I got my GPS fix on the Assa River at the bridge both for calculating our running distance and for reference for future exploration. We were running the two legs of a right triangle, whose hypotenuse (not to be confused by the more frequent hippopotamuses around here) was 3.53 miles from our front door. That means our round trip was greater than eight miles or just under 12 km in 70 minutes, a very good run for the morning.

The Assa River at this accessible point, before it turns "mysterious" is 4° 34.03′ N 25° 49.31′ E. **Appendix IV** contains many other GPS marks that will be useful for future reference. You now have the coordinates to know where to look for me later, when I and the "River of Mystery" fall down the rabbit hole to see what wonderland can be discovered.

On returning, I ran across tracks of a large bird and then saw the bird itself. The Secretary Bird (*Sagittarius serpentarius*) is a real prize for birders but quite commonly seen on my treks through the bush in these parts. It is a large, pearly gray and black, long-legged bird with presumed taxonomic affinity to raptors. It uses its long legs to flush and subdue snakes to feed on. Its name is derived from black-tipped crown feathers that project from its head much like the quill pens secretaries of yore must have stuck into the topknot of their hairdos. On a previous Assa visit, I followed and observed an adult Secretary Bird holding a writhing snake in its beak. It flew to treetop level several times, looking awkward in its crane-like flight, and then dropped the snake on the *munga*. After the last fall, the snake was still. Then, the bird pulled it apart with its beak while pinning it with its large feet and ate the snake. When I reported these observations to my fellow hunters back at the encampment, they confirmed my observations, but expressed disappointment that I had not brought this one back for the pot. Neki said, "Secretary Bird — very good!" He was not referring to the behavioral vignette I had observed with fascination. On our return run there were also lots of giant land snails sliding along our course, at a decidedly slower pace than ours.

A RIVER RUNS THROUGH IT

There are two major river systems draining the area around Assa. making for two drainage basins. These two rivers are the Rangu and the Epi Rivers. The Rangu River is just beyond the *Zala* waterhole where I had been hunting so often until recently when soldiers with guns prefer to have all the fun to themselves. The Rangu turns to join the Assa River and they both go out, via the mysterious underground drainage, to the Bomu and then to the Ubangi which drains into the mighty Congo. We are going to do our next run to the Rangu River so that I can get a fix on that as well. Some day, I will come back to this riverine terrain when peace returns. Then I can explore and hunt in the bush without the interference of armed thugs, *avec* or *sans* uniforms.

The Epi River basin drains into the Uele River. The Epi and Bomu are the two watersheds of this area therefore contributing to the Congo at two points. The Bomu joins the Uele at the border with the CAR, and at that junction they form the Ubangi River, a name you have all heard and now know that it means "juncture." At Bangui, the capital of the CAR, the Ubangi River turns south. After about 600 km as the crow flies, it joins with the Congo River.

❦ OUT OF ASSA: HEART OF THE CONGO

A REUNION OF THE LOST ELEPHANT HUNTERS
FROM THE STORY OF ANDRÉ'S ORDEAL IN BEING
LOST IN THE BUSH BETWEEN THE
EPI AND BOMU RIVERS

In earlier chapters, I related a story about André's elephant hunting adventure. André's insight into where they were was based on his knowledge that they had to be between the Epi and Bomu Rivers, and if they only followed any stream to a larger one, he would be able to recognize which river it was by the color of the water. The older hunters had disparaged the would-be schoolboy (recall that the desire for money for school fees had propelled André to set out on this long and hazardous hunt for the "white gold" of Central Africa) but ultimately, whether due to the prayer, or the ritual act of cutting the elephant meat and seeing which way it fell, or possibly the native savvy of having been born in the middle of the riverine orientation of this area of Zandeland, all of the men survived, and André went on to school.

Today those elephant hunters came to see the schoolboy made good. I went to see this event when called by André who was at the time pulling a tooth with a delegation of on-lookers staring in through the window, the light source at which he was working. There were two of them, and they paid me a compliment that comes rather high around here. Through Pazande interpretation they said, "We hear that you are a very good hunter, too!"

I took pictures of this unlikely reunion ceremony. This reunion was probably a lot more meaningful than the one I will be attending in September for the thirtieth anniversary of my graduation from University of Michigan School of Medicine, with a lot of colleagues I have not seen much during those three decades. André was sporting his dental apron and powdered hands from the gloves he had stripped off to greet these long-lost (in several senses of the term) colleagues in rags and bark cloth, as I took their pictures. There may be quite a few of my former running mates who would fit the same divergent pattern of life's "two roads diverged in a snowy (in this case 'muddy') wood: having followed one that seems to have made all the difference." The road to Assa is definitely *not* "the road not taken."

I asked, through translation, if they were doing any hunting now. They said, "We would like to but we cannot, because there are too many soldiers around with guns that would get us."

I replied, "When those soldiers are gone at last, I will be happy to go hunting with you!" First they laughed at the especially good joke. Then they realized that I was serious, and they responded that it would be a great honor, as it would be for me as well.

178

THE FLOWING TOGETHER OF THE DETAILS OF THE RIVERS
AND THE DETAILS OF ANDRÉ'S LIFE AND
PRESENT PLANS TO COMMEMORATE HIS FATHER
IN ASSA IN THE AZANDE TRADITION

The source of the Bomu, near where the borders of the CAR, the Sudan, and the Congo meet, is marked by a large pyramid of stones dug out of a great hole in the Bomu River. A small town there, called Nebaipai, is a market for people of all three nations. They cross freely from one country to another without much concern for national frontiers. It happens that this is the place where André was born, and he got into the school at Dorima 50 km away. He is a son of Zandeland here, and was in Banda and around Assa much of his life. Papa Dix met André at Banda and identified him as someone with promise. Papa Dix worked with André to get him into school and kept pushing him to work hard to be someone who would make a difference in Zandeland, much as he had done with Inikpio, with Bunio, and several others that I had met. This is the second generation of the developmental push that started with Papa Dix at Banda station. We had planned to return there as our next stop after Assa. Since André has family all around there, it would be good to have the death ritual for his father performed at Banda, but that is far away from here and there will not be enough time, if any at all, in our hurried visit to carry out any ceremony there. We will only have time to see patients in consultation, and operate on those who need it before we fly out after our overnight stop there, as long as we can retain the MAF pilot, making his first trip into this area, on the ground.

PREPARATIONS IN PROGRESS
FOR A SPECIAL AZANDE DEATH CEREMONY
IN WHICH I AM A PARTICIPANT WHO HAS KNOWN
EACH OF THOSE INVOLVED

The death ceremony for André's father will be a special event for me in the Azande Culture. Preparations are now being made to hold the ceremony for André's father here in Assa. André's sister and several paternal uncles are here. We are well-known to the whole community for the work we have done with them while here. We have to push to complete the color linguistic study here, since there would be no time to pack any of it into the Banda visit. Any informants that we did manage to round up would have to end interviews with incomplete studies.

The ceremony for André's father's death will be a special one for me. I have known each of the major participants in the event, including the decedent,

179

whom I treated, and whom I recorded in text and pictures at Banda during my 1996 visit there. The poignant generosity of native son and father passing along their pills to an unknown young girl with Burkitt's lymphoma was ultimately frustrated by further cultural customs of the Azande. That diminishes neither the gift from father and son nor the meaningfulness of the final "parting shots" I took of them together.

So, from a running start this morning, you have followed me throughout Zandeland where rivers flowed and traditions of culture have come to reunion. There will be more to recognize as shared ground between us, all those many miles and bearings away, with many rivers removed in space and time but little in life that is important not fully shared and confluent. And, a river runs through it.

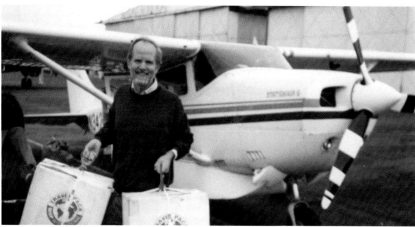

Figure 1. Packing donated medical supplies through Nairobi's Wilson Field.

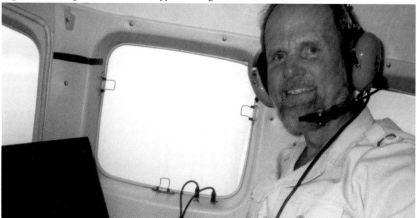

Figure 2. Over the Great Rift Valley, writing in transit.

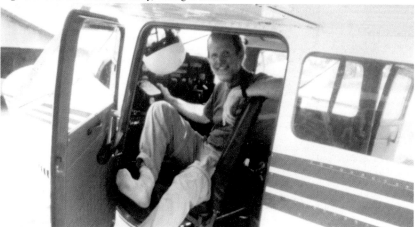

Figure 3. Out of Assa, barefoot again.

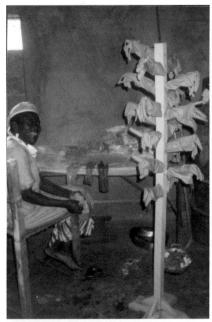

Figure 4. Assa OR recycling: Kinale and "glove-drying tree."

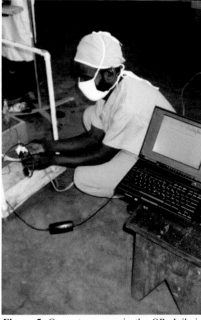

Figure 5. Computer power in the OR: Inikpio jury-rigs connection to battery.

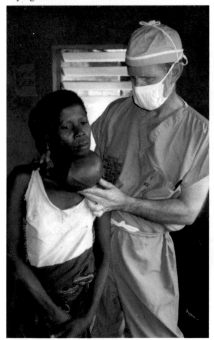

Figure 6. Preoperative evaluation of a massive goiter with airway obstruction.

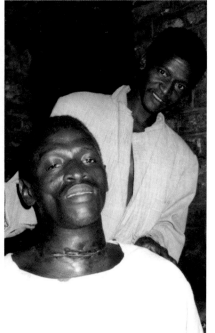

Figure 7. Postoperative recovery after thyroidectomy with patient's brother providing nursing care.

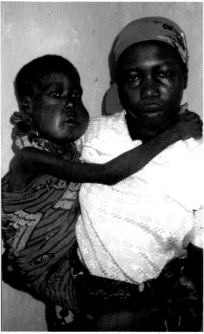

Figure 8. Mother and young girl with Burkitt's lymphoma.

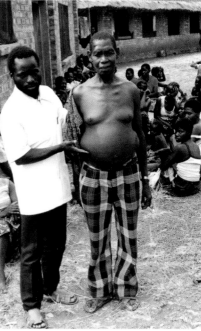

Figure 9. Inikpio diagnoses hepatoma in the outpatient queue.

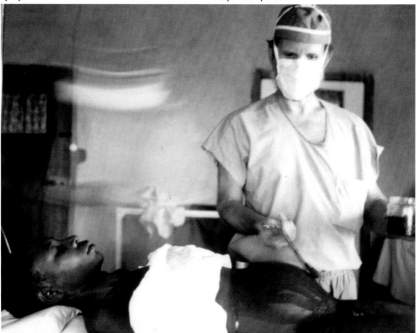

Figure 10. Preparing patient for abdominal hysterectomy.

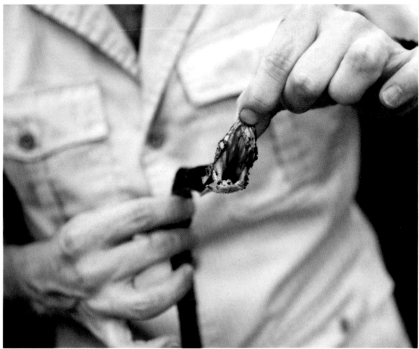

Figure 11. Assa hazards: Black Mamba killed at garden hut.

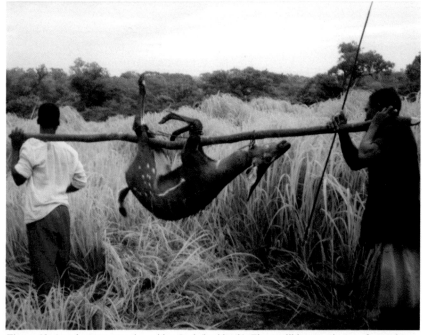

Figure 12. Assa hunters returning with a *Bodi* (bushbuck). There will be meat in Assa for weeks.

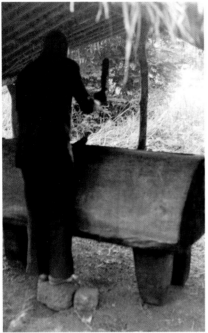

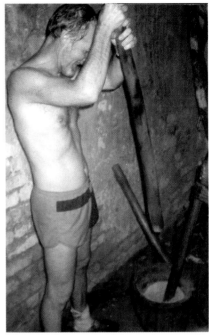

Figure 13. Master drum carver turns musician: Bule beats out a message from Assa.

Figure 14. I try my hand at pounding rice after a run.

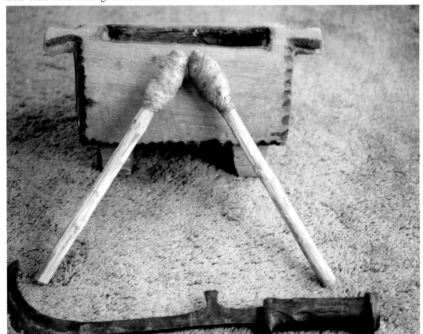

Figure 15. Bule's resonating miniature gift drum and the ancient Azande blade.

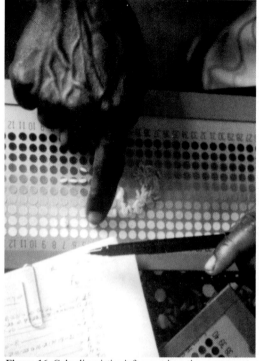

Figure 16. Color linguistics informant in action.

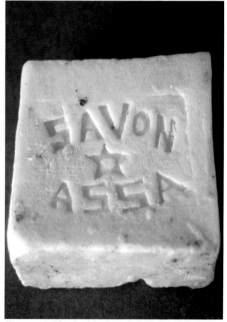

Figure 17. Jean Marco making soap.

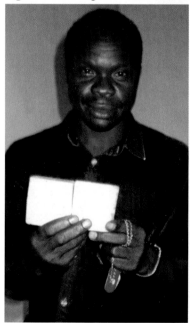

Figure 18. Jean Marco, the proud entrepreneur.

Figure 19. The finsished product: Savon Assa.

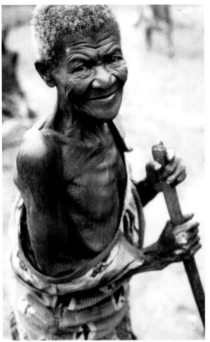

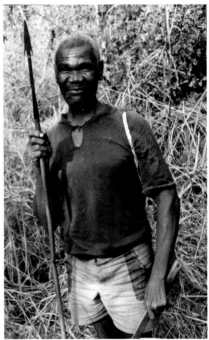

Figure 20. Dignity and grace despite poverty and disease: elderly Assa woman with leprosy and endemic Kaposi's sarcoma.

Figure 21. A hunter-gatherer in the bush.

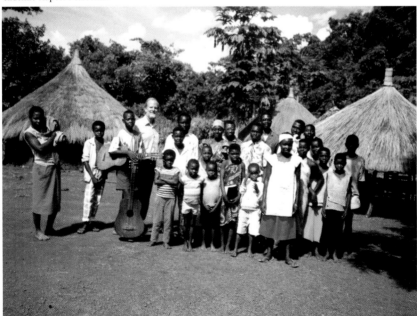

Figure 22. A guest for dinner: a formal reception at Jean Marco's compound.

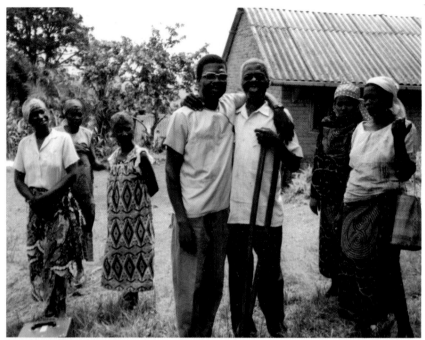

Figure 23. The meeting at Banda: André and his father reunited just before father's death from African melanoma.

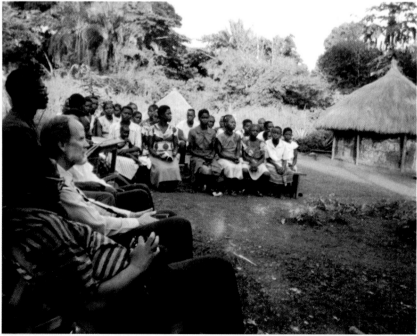

Figure 24. The Azande death ceremony commemorating two fathers: André's and mine.

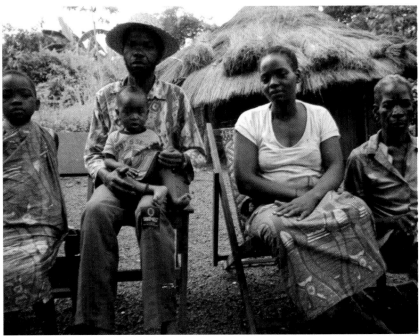

Figure 25. African gothic, an Assa family portrait.

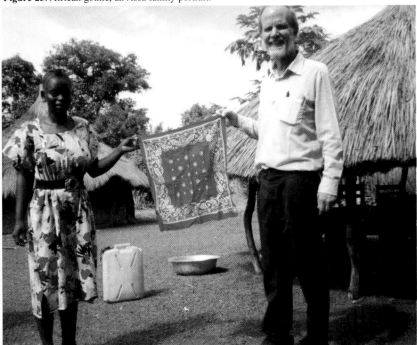

Figure 26. Trend-setting fashion statement: my red bandanna fulfills Siaduwe's wish for a scarf.

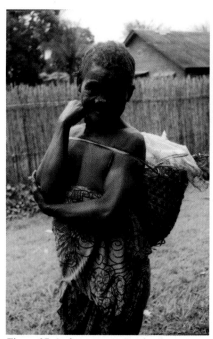

Figure 27. Atobo, a pygmy "cooker."

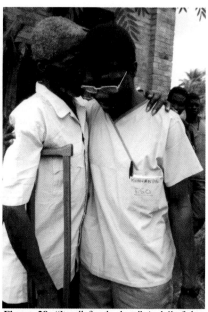

Figure 28. "Its all for the best." André's father passes him the medicine that might have saved the Burkitt's lymphoma girl's life.

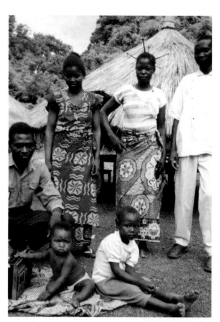

Figure 29. An Assa family in formal portrait poses.

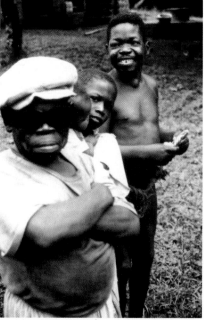

Figure 30. Cool dude Sasa: His dreams fulfilled, Sasa (foreground) sports my shades to the admiration of his fellow cretin Bodo (background).

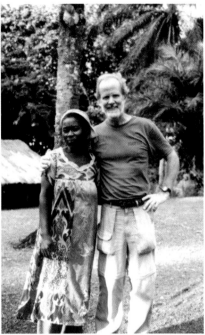

Figure 31. A bashful farewell: OR nurse Ginale says goodbye before my departure from Assa.

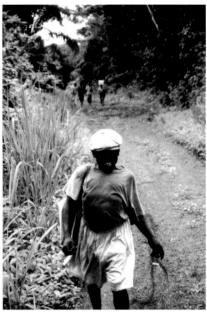

Figure 32. Sasa leads the parade to the Assa airstrip, carrying ThinkPad, camera, and tape recorder. In background, Yuni balances linguistic reports on her head.

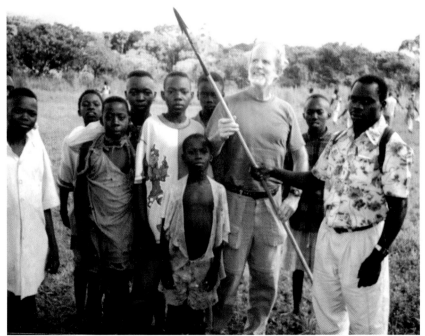

Figure 33. Waiting for the plane, Jean Marco and I examine an Azande spear with onlookers.

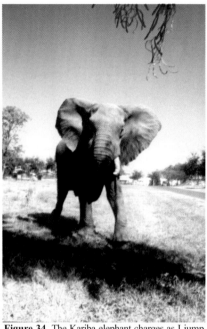

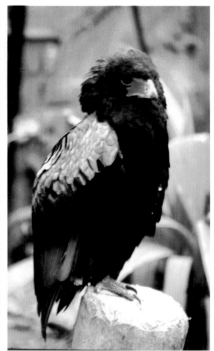

Figure 34. The Kariba elephant charges as I jump behind a small tree and photograph him. My story might have ended here!

Figure 35. The graceful aerialist: the Bateleur.

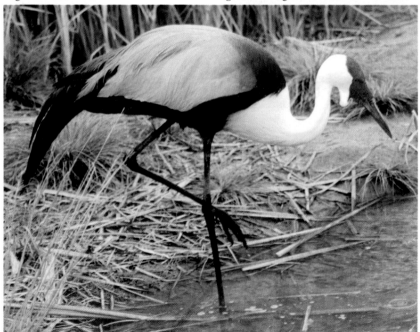

Figure 36. The Wattled Crane at Chisamba Pan, part of the "Garden of Eden" epiphany.

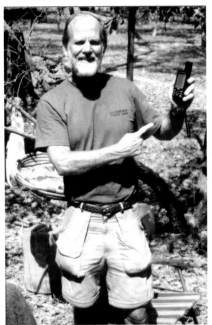

Figure 37. Go ahead, ask me where I am: Marking a GPS reading in Kasanka National Park, Zambia.

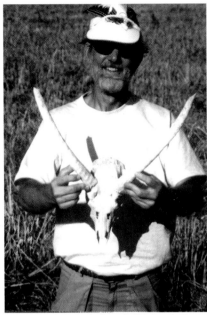

Figure 38. A Kafue lechwe skull in hand, *Kanga* feathers in cap, a happy camper on vacation in Zambia's Lochinvar National Park.

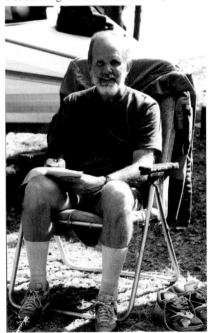

Figure 39. "I'm on vacation!" Author making notes in Wasa Camp, Kasanka National Park, Zambia.

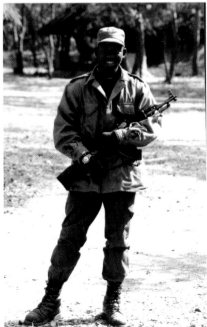

Figure 40. The game warden at Kasanka National Park, Zambia.

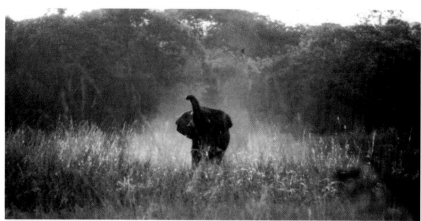

Figure 41. A bluffing charge by a bull elephant near Sitatunga Hide, Kasanka National Park, Zambia.

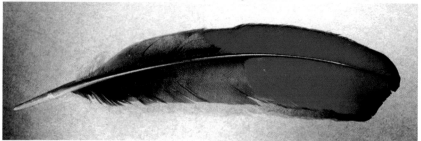

Figure 42. The beauty prize: turacin-stained wing feather from Ross's Turaco, flushed by a Crowned Eagle in the forest near Kapabi Swamp in Kasanka National Park, Zambia.

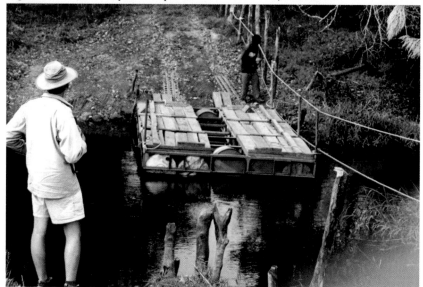

Figure 43. Peter Tetlow summons the pontoon ferry for crossing the Kasanka River, Kasanka National Park, Zambia.

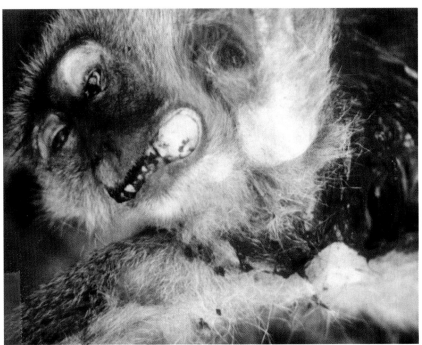

Figure 44. Young yellow baboon killed by Crowned Eagle, still clenching mbola plum in his teeth.

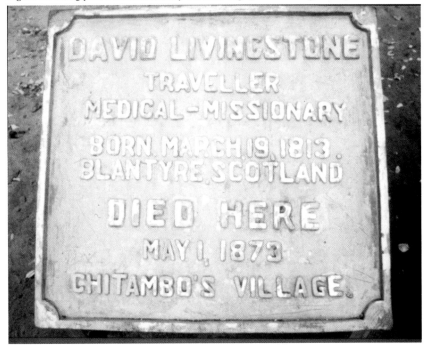

Figure 45. "Dr. Livingston, I presume." Chitambo's village, Zambia.

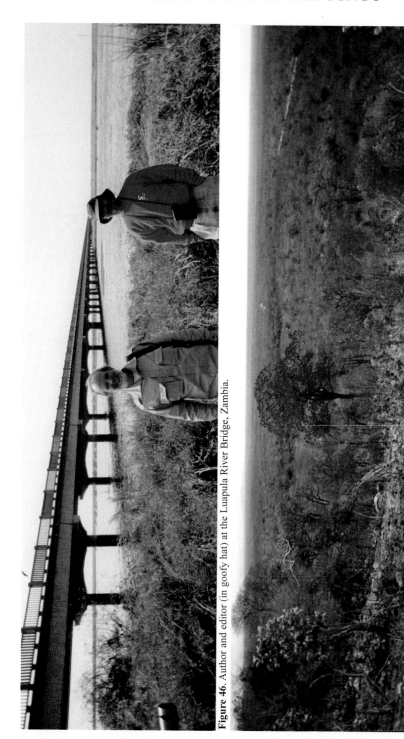

Figure 46. Author and editor (in goofy hat) at the Luapula River Bridge, Zambia.

Figure 47. "All Africa" from the Zambezi escarpment, watching a lone bull elephant tromping through "miles and miles of bloody Africa."

26 THAT'S AFRICA BABY!

THE COMPUTERIZED THEATRE IN ASSA

July 17, 1998

Who said we are primitive here? We have the only computerized theatre for may hundreds of miles in any direction. We have the latest in equipment, tools and toys. Why, here is a GPS, there is a Nikon N 8008, and we have an IBM ThinkPad running off the battery-powered OR lamp. While a hernia operation is in progress, the Author in Africa is using the same energy source to continue his tales of the bush. I am surgeon, anthropologist, and author, all in one-stop shopping! As long as Inikpio continues to play nursemaid to the two copper wires cross-linking my D/C auto cigarette lighter plug-in, you will continue to hear from us.

This narrative has taken extraordinary effort, and if it is to be forwarded to you as soon as I get to the first e-mail connection, which might be the MAF server at Nyankunde, it might add up to astronomic expense as well. On my way in, I had been delighted to find a way to send you the message of arrival and passage through the entrepôt at Bunia that included even the "airborne" message I had typed up from the copilot's seat, plugged into the Cessna's cigarette lighter. I even cheerfully paid for the messages sent at $1.00 per kb. If I might guess that by now I have likely generated 50 kb chapters at least 30 times over, the e-mail transmission fee would probably come to more than the cash allotment I had dropped as "import duty" on freely donated medicines.

But, I will continue as long as the electric charge trickles. When I stop in Banda, possibly at this time next week, it will mark the shift from these chapters of entry into Congo through the Assa experiences, the high point of the whole of these African excursions. Subsequent chapters will take us to Banda, en route through Nyankunde and Bunia, to return to Nairobi. The next section of the book will take us through Zimbabwe to a birding expedition in Zambia. The final chapters will detail my return to South Africa, on a visit to Umtata in the Transkei, and then the homeward bound journey. Now that you have the outline of the book, come along and see the movie.

THE NEW AND SHINY SHOES FOR ASSA

When I left the theatre to go back over for lunch, I passed an interesting sight that made me stir into my bag and pull out the camera. There behind the cistern was one of the kitchen men who had just lowered the leaky, weighted plastic pail into the cistern to draw water. He was using the water to scrub two sets of shoes: the Nikes and the Red Ball Jets that had just made the roundtrip this morning to the Assa River. They have not been so clean and sparkling in a long time. He is apparently unaware that he is shining his own shoes. I do not intend to carry them back with me.

When I came to lunch, I am aware that, as in most other matters of precedence here, I am supposed to be the first to wash hands while the basin is clean and unsoaped. Until I scoop up the rice and serve myself a heaping plateful, no one else eats. I am expected to take the first helping of the *zigba*, which must be running low by now, with no one out hunting to replenish the stock, but that I should go without, or have less than a lot is not part of the expectation. I would have thought that by now, I would have become a commoner, rather than royalty.

SETTING UP A FUND TO SUPPORT PARTIALLY SOME OF THE MANY ASSA REQUESTS

I went over with André my interest in having him administer a fund that I will leave with him in Nyankunde for the support of various projects we had discussed, without taking on the sole support of any individual applicants. I told him not to count on it any time soon, but that I was meeting on my return to the US with the attorney who would officially make them a part of my residual estate in the Geelhoed Private Foundation. This charity can do a lot more with a little in this area of the world, where there are many of the "least of these my children."

One of the least of the least is Sasa, the cretin adult brother of the late chief Sasa, who greets me with great dignity each time I enter or leave the house, with a handshake and a request. He makes the cretinous grunts (he is deaf-mute and stunted) and motions with his fingers putting hooks around his eyes and his ears saying as clearly as an announcement could make it, that he desperately wants sunglasses to make him look more distinguished. The last set he had were ingenious home-made contraptions with latex lens and vine-like frames. He would peer over the top of them like some banker with his half-glasses perched low on his nose studying your accounts.

Jean Marco stopped by and I learned the name of his 18-year-old daughter whom I am partly supporting. André is opening his home to her on the basis that JM is going to carry her on his bicycle as close to Nyankunde as the rainy season will allow. Her name is *Kulungbu Zangatunga* (Rachel). The first name means "little wooden basin" the kind of carved chalice that I see here often being the equivalent of a server, wash basin, collector of things, tray for eating. The second means "seedless," or "no seed." She was named after her aunt who had no children. The third is biblical, Rachel, searching for her children, which I suspect you would do too if you turned out to be infertile.

ANOTHER KIND OF DIP IN THE POOL

Rachel turns out to be named after her aunt, Pastor Bule's sister. So now I know who it is when someone asks after the welfare of another goddaughter. Our conversation was interrupted by yet another example of "*Sic transit gloria mundi*" happening behind the room where I am staying. I looked out, and there were two fellows nonchalantly prying up the boards from the "deck" of what would have been the "Downing swimming pool." This was an inspired project of David's after I had sponsored their travel to Namibia in 1992 for the hunt with Suaro Albertini. Outside the guest cottages, there in the Namibian desert environment, we luxuriated in a swimming pool supplied by a windmill-powered water pump. David, a nonswimmer, believed that one of these would make a nice improvement outside his bedroom at Assa, so that he could walk out in a robe on a sunny morning and take a bit of a dip before breakfast.

Pool construction shifted into high gear on their return from Namibia, even as he was troubled by a letter he tucked into his Bible announcing that the mission had heard and confirmed some unfortunate news about his behavior in Assa. He had to leave the mission. So, the pool liner was smooth and the beveled treated lumber was laid out on a bias for the deck, and all was in readiness for the luxury of the Assa swimming pool. Then the trapdoor fell out from under the whole Downing family and their future in the field, and David's part in it. He made only one final trip to Assa with one of the mission staff to liquidate what could be carried or sold, and neither Diane nor the rest of the family whose lives were centered here for quite a long time have ever returned, nor do they seem likely to. So the never-used pool has, like Assa, fallen upon hard times. Here, almost casually, are two fellows who recognize prize firewood just ready for the prying up—in the treated but now decaying lumber of the rotting pool deck. To quote Robert Burns, "The best laid plans of mice and men gang aft agley."

PLANS FOR AN EXTENSIVE RUN IN THE MORNING
RUN AFOUL BY BEING CLEANED—
A GOOD EXAMPLE OF "TAB"—"THAT'S AFRICA, BABY!"

OK, what would you like first, the good news or the bad? You recall two facts from my description of earlier intents and events. First I had intended to do a long morning run away from the Assa River to see the Rangu River, and GPS mark it for a better understanding of the riverine orientation around Assa. Second, that I had seen Red Ball Jets and Nikes being scrubbed clean from the morning run to the Assa River. Saturday morning is usually a prime time for a run. It would be if I were in Maryland on the Rock Creek Park running trail for the morning run with the MCRRC. The ARRC is a legitimate daughter organization sharing in the spirit and membership of at least one of the members of the W (for worldwide) RRC. This Saturday morning run would be the last chance I would have for a long and focused run here at Assa with the running shoes and other gear that is going to remain behind. This would be the last time I could expect to use them. So, here I am, ready to roll!

Not quite, remember this is Africa. The best intentions in this continent seem predestined to be frustrated by even better interpretations of those intentions. Count on "TAB" coming through far more often than a plan carried out as it was intended. The bad news is that, sure enough, both sets of running shoes are clean and bright enough (and also wet, but that is a small matter), but they have been taken all apart in order to do a thorough job of cleaning them. That is, the sole inserts, arch supports and all the components have been stripped out, and they are lying next to the clean carcasses of the shoes, but the laces are missing. Now, no African would regard that as a particularly worrisome absence, since, after all can you not still pull these open sheaves of clean Nikes and RBJ's onto your feet? So what if they flap around a bit, that will just draw attention to their freshly cleaned and shiny status. Why they are now perfectly good for running, in fact, better than new, since they are now so much easier to get on and off.

So my candlelight inspection of the remaining carcasses of the running shoes shows them to be totally useless for the primary function for which they were brought out here on their one-way trip for their big run tomorrow. There does not appear to be a very good reason to be going to bed just now, other than that there is nothing else that can be done. Going to bed at 8:00 PM or before just because you cannot see or do anything at least had the redeeming feature that I would be up before dawn and could use that precious first light to run out into the dawn. There will be no run, long, short or indifferent tomorrow, and I may have done my last run with the fledgling ARRC.

These plans are just all another shrug and a "TAB." So what if these running shoes are totally functionless now, they *do* look better, now, don't they? So, I have done my job, and deserve thanks and praise for my part well-played in your plans to further explore the mysterious rivers of the Assa area. My intentions were nothing but the best, and if they have frustrated your intents, well, "TAB."

And you thought that just the underground confluence of two African rivers here was a baffling mystery!

27 WATCHING SOAPS IN THE CONGO

ENTERING THE HOME STRETCH

July 18, 1998

I spent most of the day writing letters to people far and wide, and I addressed them for posting when I get to the nearest reliable postbox in Nairobi. My serial letters from Assa will number about a dozen. The postcards will be also a dozen, largely to people who have contributed surgical instruments or medicines. My book *Out of Assa: Heart of the Congo* is getting near the end of the longest part about Assa. In the next two days, I want to complete the linguistic study and medical consultations. I also need the last battery recharges that have kept me writing to you through the disc that will be carried out upon my person. I hope that the computer carrying these precious chapters also escapes to the outside world to continue the narrative during the rest of my trip.

Getting everything out of Assa is not a sure thing even in the relative security of Assa. Last night as André was preparing his own report of this dental experience in the predawn, he heard voices, and found out what others had just discovered that a window was broken in the pharmacy. A thief attempted to steal what I had brought in, since, now there is something worth stealing following my efforts at resupply. All of my stuff is at the same risk, I presume, since they would want to have anything that looked foreign and modern and, more importantly, could be bartered for something really valuable, like salt, soap or matches.

But the value I have tried to secure and plan to carry if I have to smuggle it, is not just in film, tape and notes of my past adventures. This time, I will be packing out the book-length narrative on the disc of hard-won, typed-up communication. I will have written the bulk of *Out of Assa*.

Another communication has come by runner and drummer from the CAR. This message could not come to us directly nor can we interact through a nonfunctional "phonie." We discover that we may be here only until July 21 when the MAF pilot will come to make a quick in-and-out pick-up but will *not* be carrying us on to Banda. He wishes to return directly to Nyankunde to get out of harm's way.

A quick inventory of what remains to be done is necessary since no communication can be sent back. I still aim to complete interviews for five informants, four of these to begin from the ground up. I interviewed four young men whom I worked with all morning. I was already frustrated by my difficult earlier interview of Pastor Bule, who could neither see (without his glasses, nor very well when he got them two hours later) nor write. He has bilateral carpal tunnel syndrome and scars from their releases. Further he was sweating profusely when he got here and had a chill. I treated him with Tylenol and then dosed him with mefloquine. I finally shepherded him through the completion of the objects/colors triads when he felt better.

The young men's interviews were nearly useless. One of them is Lazunga's son who is constantly lying in wait to speak to me urgently and privately, and that has distracted him from doing the job on the study properly. I am sure that the reason he wants to see me and wants no one else to hear is that he wishes to give me large sums of money for the benefit of all the citizens of Assa and he would want to be an anonymous donor. The informants kept asking for repeats of nearly every color disc I showed, they tried to cheat off each other's pages, not recognizing that I had staggered them for Pazande/Bangala, and the only ones who did it quickly did so by leaving most of the answer sheet blank. One had filled it in all right, with about a half-dozen Bangala terms and all the rest in French.

So, once again, in chorus, it has not been easy. But, I am getting close to completion with an allowance for the kind of chicanery I had expected and seen today. All of them are eager to be sprung from the second half of the study (the opposite language) for the big ceremony tonight in honor of André's deceased father, and that means I will have to go through this same drill tomorrow. At least I found the laundered shoe laces and the Nikes are ready to roll in the morning before taking on the further frustrations of the informant pack!

THE VERY DEFINITION OF A "COTTAGE INDUSTRY"

There are two big celebratory get-togethers this "weekend" (a term that I doubt is used or useful here). The first is the Azande death ceremony in tribute to André's father. I am much involved as a treating physician of André's father, and friend of André. The next is a dinner celebration thrown in my honor by Jean Marco, as much like the *fête du chasseurs* from the last time as possible even without the *chasse*. "*La prochaine fois!*" says Jean Marco and all the others who know how much I love the hunt with them. Kazima went out last night despite the ban on hunting, and got a *bodi* (bushbuck).

I asked him, "Was it near Mambasa?" He immediately knew that I knew just where he was and what might be there.

"Yes, and while I was out there, I saw the bongos!" quoth he. "*La prochaine fois*, indeed!" Next time! Next time! I have waited for the better part of two decades now anyway!

Jean Marco asked me to come over today for a special look at his soap-making operation. I had expressed interest since I have now seen it in three parts of the Congo. JM has the best product going. It only needs work on color, scent and pH. He had led me over to the clearing around his compound. His daughter Rachel was there with his other kids, well-behaved and polite. The compound was all raked and swept in my honor with all the grass cut back into the bush, and a chair placed for me in the shade. The master chemist went to work, even wearing long-sleeved rubber gloves and titrating the chemical ingredients reading the specific gravity with a float (**Figure 17**).

Meanwhile, one of the kids turned the crank on a hand-powered tape that played some gospel music, including a few Christmas carols in English. The most touching one was "Great is thy faithfulness—o'er all the earth." I wonder if they understood just how appropriate the song was to my visit of their demonstration of this cottage industry?

I watched the whole careful process, which had been rehearsed with an assistant in anticipation of my inspection. Chickens scratched around in the shade of the tree under which I sat. Community members stopped by "to greet," as the South African expression I learned in KwaZulu/Natal would have it. I took pictures of each carefully controlled step in making soap. It is the very picture of what would be called an "Operation Bootstraps" cottage industry that uses the local initiative and materials to produce something with value added.

The palm tree produces nuts from which useful oil can be extracted. That is the (saturated, I fear) stuff in which all my dinners have been cooked. The sugary sap of the palm tree can be fermented and distilled to make palm wine. I have seen a few Assa irregulars staggering around under its influence. It is usually a luxury item for a people who are otherwise marginally nourished and could get the nonfermented calories more directly and efficiently than through alcohol. Palm oil can also be made into soap if it is specially treated with a few primitive instruments, and enough gumption to have a go at trial-and-error production. JM made two big cakes of soap that will be sliced and stamped tomorrow with his unimaginative logo, "*Savon*," the French word for soap.

Beneath Savon is a star and the word "*Assa*." This is probably the first industrial product of this village (**Figure 18**).

JM's soap is way ahead of the competition, looking like a bar of soap instead of the green, vaguely vegetative blobs of flotsam that I saw for sale on a banana leaf in the Wednesday market. This primitive green soap worked well on my Nikes but can't compare to JM's soap. Mind you, JM's soap needs packaging, a color, and a scent to turn it into a personal-care product, and a bit less residual lye to turn it into a good laundry product. The "color fast" colors of my old running shirts are now fast disappearing from too much lye. With 10 liters of palm oil from the overhead palm trees, JM turned a product of the forest from a low value raw material that does not pay its freight to the distant commodity markets, to the most highly sought commodity out in this neck of the bush. There are no *magasins* here. Store-bought soap, salt, matches and batteries are the hot commodities on the local market. Soap-making is a winner of a cottage industry.

GO "TO GREET" AND TO CHECK OUT THE PREPARATIONS FOR TONIGHT'S CELEBRATION OF ANDRÉ'S FATHER'S LIFE

I felt guilty about having delegated the color interviews to André and Kazima so that I could watch soap-making. I told JM that I should get back to them. He pointed out that "No, I was needed where someone had died and they wanted a picture."

I thought this was macabre, but said, "Lead on." I am glad I did. I was carrying both camera and tape recorder as we made our way through the village from hut to hut "to greet." I watched people change into their better clothes if they had any other, and the young women getting their hair plaited into the "electrified four-poster effect" for the ceremony tonight (**Figure 29**).

I was taken over to the common ground of the community center where an enormous pot of rice was boiling, and saw colorfully dressed groups of women cooking the *pondu*, and the palm oil sauce that will go over the rice in the feast of the celebration. The food will be served in waves over the course of the evening from dusk to dawn. The young girls were busily pounding the rice in a ceremony of shared labor at the mortar and pestle.

Everyone knows that I would be part of this "*Dernier Adieu*" for André's father. I was asked by JM to stay with his family in their hut tonight. It is only a little way along the path, and I could find my way back, but a 12-hour ceremony may be a bit over my limit now, although I promise to be there early as guest of honor. This time they know I will be taping and taking pictures following André's direct requests. I don't need to worry about intruding on their ceremony. After all, the last pictures of his father's life, and the only ones of them together before his death at Banda, are those I had surreptitiously taken. These remain André's most prized possessions.

As I mentioned earlier, the decision to have the Azande death ceremony here in Assa was a good one. Here, we will have enough time and family present, even though André's father died in Banda. The reason became even clearer this morning. We have no "phonie" that functions here at Assa, but Nyankunde called the CAR post in Zemio, and they bounced a message back here this morning saying that the gun-shy MAF pilot would come directly on Tuesday morning, July 21, without going on to Banda at all. We abandoned the plans for dividing the supply of medical goods to leave some at Banda, as devastated as Assa, and will no longer be able to do cases there. On our last visit to Banda, we made an overnight stay and kept the pilot with us. Without the plan to do this ceremony here at Assa, André's father would have been buried without the memorial service, a disgrace in the Azande culture.

It is the rainy season, so that extensive plans are made with tentative reservations. We decided to hold the ceremony under the thatched roof of the community meeting hut, covering ourselves for the likelihood that the rainy season would serve up a serious, gully-washing cloudburst in the rainforest. Moving under shelter will not disappoint them since all the preparations are as much a part of the community ceremony as the "*manifestation*" (Sonny Mwembo's term). What may come as a surprise to those who are reading these pages is that the celebration is not simply with me as anthropologic participant/observer, but much more direct than that. They knew that my father had also died at nearly the same time as André's father through a tribute to my father I had written and sent to André at the time of my condolences on the loss of his father. To my surprise as well, my father and I would figure prominently in the planning and performance of this memorial service. This unusual link came through a tribute to my dead father that I had written and given to André. This tribute reached half a world away and touched down in the Congo on the subject of traditions of never-changing importance. This will be explained in the following "joint tribute" to both fathers being commemorated here in the "Heart of the Congo."

SWAPPING FATHERS
TRADING TRIBUTES

André pointed to the chair next to him at the table for me, and said, "I feel now in this *Dernier Adieu* that I have gained you as my father." He was very interested in my written tribute to my own father. I sent the tribute to my father to André and enclosed the pictures that I took of André and his father, just before the father's death from melanoma. To my amazement, André has carried that tribute with him here to Assa. It turns out that all the others from Nyankunde had read it as well. My tribute struck a responsive chord with them, since it seemed very impressive how both fathers were not simply marching to the same drummer, but that they both "walked with God." Despite very different circumstances a world away from each other, both had the same priorities and faith they had wanted to pass on to their children.

So, this celebration is of both fathers' lives, and is sung in a thousand tongues in the place to which they have gone together. These voices do not need linguistic or cultural translation, although here we still do. I will have to carry with me some of the interpretations that André will whisper to me as we go now to celebrate the lives of our fathers in an Azande tradition similar to that of my own *with the same songs sung in the same heavenly tune.*

**A BIG SUNDAY FULL OF CELEBRATIONS IN ASSA
BEGINS WITH MY WALKING OVER FRESH CARNIVORE TRACKS
TO WATCH THE SLICING OF SOAP, THE FIRST PRODUCT TO
BEAR THE PROUD LABEL"MADE IN ASSA"**

July 19, 1998

Last night's celebration was preceded by the news that soldiers might be coming through Assa on their way to Gwane, the *Chef du Collectivité*'s seat for this area, where Chief Sasa's successor, Emmanuel, was before fleeing for his life. This visit was part of the investigation by the administrator of the district newly appointed to replace Buta, who had fled into the bush after the military occupation. This news was passed by word of mouth. It dominated the early buzz around the compound. We went forward to sit in the honored spots where we were to wait until all the preparations were ready for the Azande celebration of the life of André's father, and by incorporation now, my father too.

While we sat and waited, André told me the details of his father's life in English, as he would later in Pazande for those assembled. I was struck by the similarity of the lives of our fathers. Both were simple men of conviction who valued education for their children. Their lives were congruent. Both were men of faith who had never known each other in this life on opposite ends of the earth. These two fathers no doubt have a lot of notes to compare as this celebration in their honor is proceeding with their sons, still alive back here on earth, attending it and reflecting on their father's lives.

This time there was no reticence for pictures to be taken, and in fact, they were quite pleased when I took some and disappointed if they were not in them. It is a good thing that for this one brief shining moment, my Nikon NTT autofocus flash camera worked well since it was its "last hurrah." I took pictures under the Azande torches lighting the areas of cooking and preparation. We were then seated under an overhanging canopy of a roof made of thatched palm fronds with those same Azande torches perilously close to them. We finished the very good feast in the dark, and even had a "calabash of *kawa*," the local coffee, as the final course. The altogether familiar dinner consisted of rice with palm oil gravy and the sacrificed chickens of Assa, which must now be down to a fraction of their former population.

As we ate, an event unfolded over us that would determine much of the evening, although I did not suspect much of it for starters. The golden weavers had been squeaking and carrying fibers stripped from palm fronds to be used for nests being built in the trees. They were hanging upside down on their yellow wings as the last tinge of the sunset disappeared and a few clouds rumbled. By the time of the *kawa*, however, there were a few drops of rain spattering around us. No matter, quoth we, we will just sit under shelter a bit longer…like all night.

A RAIN CHECK FOR THE MAJOR CELEBRATION, CALLED ON ACCOUNT OF RAINY SEASON IN THE RAINFOREST

When it began raining in double earnest to the point that the Azande torches were sputtering, we had to move over into a mud hut under a thatched roof complete with the hurriedly moved chairs on which we were royally enthroned. We moved in on three women with two sleeping babies who never could get over the intrusion and were so embarrassed at our presence they could not raise their eyes when we brought a kerosene lantern into the thick blackness. I thought they were overwhelmed by the presence of such strangers in the only small intimate space to which they could retreat. There is even one fellow taking flash pictures of the sleeping babies and us. André's interpretation is that they were embarrassed, but since we were men, what could they do?

It was an anthropologist's dream, an intimate view of life inside the hut, typically the province of the women's separate world. I rather enjoyed it for the first hour or so of entry into the hut and hearing the soothing sound of the rain on the thatch. It rained hard enough that even Bodo, the cretin in the bark cloth loincloth, came inside. I noticed that he did relatively well with Inikpio's children and seems to eat at Inikpio's back door, doing some minimal chores besides coming over to greet and grin at me. I asked Inikpio, "If you are feeding Bodo, who feeds Sasa?"

"We all do," replied Inikpio. Sasa apparently moves from hut to hut and is fed at various places. He has a fair amount of dignity, dressed in his cap and shorts with a tee shirt that is now soil gray. Every day he asks me with circles of fingers around his eyes for sunglasses. Won't he be surprised before I leave. I noticed that he was often at our backdoor chopping wood into fire-size pieces for our stove and doing a neat job of it. Is he ever going to be the talk of the town!

Monsieur Sasa is about to have his simple lifelong dream realized! Sasa will be the only one in town sporting designer sunglasses. Granted, there is a big scratch on the left lens, but they are no doubt clearer than the surgical gloves he once had for lenses, and a whole world cooler.

I predict that despite jealousy about one of them having such a coveted item, this being the one small thing in his life that would make such a difference, that no one will take Sasa's glasses from him. This society's treatment of cretins is a reasonable indicator of civility and compassion in their "accessibility" and "mainstreaming." Bodo and Sasa appear to lead rather happy lives. They are accommodated well in the village, perhaps a bit like some people with Down's syndrome in the US. I noted several other adult cretins I had not seen before, including two women. They were also accorded respect and not patronized.

Émile fell sleep in his backward chair with his head face down on folded arms. I said to André that he had collapsed the way the *Soko Mutu* had, dying with his head on his arms the day after he had been shot in the chest with a shotgun, and served up as a feast to unwitting humans at Nyankunde. The feasters would not have been sure that it was right to eat something that could "almost be human." This caused a good laugh by all awake which did not disturb Émile's slumber.

Finally, there was a concession about 10:30 PM that this was an all-night rain. The first course in the feasting had gone to the honored guests. Others could now eat from the remaining stock, and the celebration ceremony for which everyone who would contribute had rehearsed would be resumed tomorrow at "*seize heur*," 4:00 PM, with light enough for photography without flash. This is now important, since I tried to take a photo or two inside the hut, and we did manage a few until I ran out of film and reloaded with the fresh roll I had carried for the ceremony itself. The NTT seemed to make little struggling noises, as though it was getting signals to start and stop, and it did not extend its lens when I tried to make it do so. So, with a little coaxing, I got one final photo of the large fire around which these ceremonies are held. Then we went home, with a kerosene lantern leading the way and an umbrella wrestled out of somewhere held by Dr. Sonny Mwembo over the guest of honor as we walked back. He said: "The rainy season is not the best for *manifestations*."

FOLLOWING THE BIRDSONG OF DAWN AFTER A RAINY NIGHT AND A MISTY DAWN, I WALK OVER TO JEAN MARCO'S AS PROMISED

I was up early, although there would be no run this busy day, after a rather wet night. I was alone as I trekked down the road to take the trail to JM's house, which will also be the site of the afternoon reception and dinner, the *fête du chasseurs*, with only the pictures of past hunts, and promises of *la prochaine fois* for the next ones. I walked over the muddy track and stopped. There were big pugs in the mud between my house and JM's. I stopped to look, and spotted the track of a paw with no claws. Along came one of the underemployed secondary school teachers, possibly to get the messages to be relayed by the Azande drum. I pointed and asked, "*Chui*?"

He said "*Mais oui! Chui!*"

As I walked the trail to JM's compound, I saw another track going right past his hut. This one was only slightly smaller, and had toenails. I found JM and his assistant setting up the home-made apparatus for slicing the two large blocks of soap made yesterday. I showed them the closer of the two tracks, confirming the latter as hyena, a stone's throw from JM's door, and the *chui*, which was between his house and mine and a rifle shot from either. This time, the evidence of these dangerous predators was in the living compound.

I watched as the large slabs of soap were sliced into small usable pieces. A brand name was impressed on each with a blow of a hammer on a dye: *SAVON ✴ ASSA* **(Figure 19)**. I had seen the completion of the product of the cottage industry and will carry back a cake of one of Assa's few manufactured products.

RETURN IN TIME FOR FRESH IRONING AND START OUT ON LONG AND DETAILED ASSA CHURCH SERVICE

I thought the problem with the NTT Nikon was that it might need a new battery, although it did not act that way when it went down. Ironically, I had always carried back up cameras in the event of any equipment failure that could not be repaired in the field. The two other NTTs I had are both in the Republic of South Africa, since I loaned them to a friend, Magdelena Botha, but never got them back. I can see what will happen if the appointment I have tried to make on my next pass in two weeks through Jo'burg results in a meeting with her to recover my cameras. She has them both, since she borrowed one for the Kilimanjaro climb, then dropped it the day before the climb. I gave her the back up with a new battery and set her up with my one remaining NTT camera. I lost a third NTT before arrival in South Africa in 1996 to robbers in Mozambique. This time I had both a flash camera that was disposable and the plastic covered Weekender submersible (ideal, I thought for the rainy season) but I loaned JM the flash camera, and told him to use up the film before I leave so that I could carry back the film and arrange for its development.

I watched a woman ironing some of my freshly washed clothes and took her picture with the rehabilitated NTT. This is the way to get this bit of history to come alive. The iron is a flat iron with a hollow box in which glowing embers are placed, and the whole is set down in a cradle to avoid scorching everything around it. These are found either in museums or in Assa's kitchen for the daily use when guests come, infrequently. I had coaxed the NTT to perform this one last time and it went down never to come alive again. A special notice had gone out to one and all that this would be *Bwana*'s last Sunday and he would be taking a picture of everyone next to the church. This is a promise that I aim to fulfill. I will have to fall back on the very big and clumsy N8008 Nikon. With its special lenses and all it is very professional looking, but it does not have a flash attachment. I will take pictures by daylight, avoiding overcast and the perpetual midnight of the inside of huts.

OFF TO ASSA CHURCH FOR A SPECIAL SERVICE
IN WHICH I, AS GUEST OF HONOR,
GET THE CHAIR IN FRONT FACING THE AUDIENCE
FOR A MARATHON SESSION

This church service was one in which you should start off with an empty bladder. Tiny little kids sit and do whatever their uninhibited natures allow, before drifting off to sleep. Siblings who look less than a year older than their charges often mind the youngest children. The children periodically pee into the dust of the floor of the church. Only slightly older sisters shuffle the dust over the wet spot. I rather envied them by the halfway point in this long service.

There were about six or seven special events, including every singing group, a Bible School graduation, and a farewell ceremony for us the visitors, and special performances with two major interruptions. By my watch it lasted four hours. I was able to maintain an interested expression for the Pazande sermon, listening to André's whispered translations. Then they delivered several touching tributes. One was in song, and one was in dance from a very unlikely source.

"*MBOTE, MBOTE*! WE GREET YOU, WE THANK YOU,
WE HAVE NOTHING TO GIVE YOU; BUT WE GIVE YOU THIS
GREETING, SO THAT WHEN YOU RETURN
TO THOSE WHOM YOU HAVE LEFT, YOU WILL HEAR THIS
'*MBOTE*' AS ECHOES OF ANGELS"

This touching song is sung to a shuffling dance beat where alternate feet are shoved forward in the dust. André interpreted the words for me and I taped everything. An older cretinous woman dressed in rags, stood up and tottered forward. Facing the performers and staring at their feet, she shuffled along with them, doing a little bobbing dance step. The congregation at first chuckled and felt embarrassed for my sake. No one restrained her, however, as she came forward to render her tribute in a manner quite dignified, as if saying, "We all do what we can, and this is what I am going to try to do!" She is mute and probably deaf. She was doing her little shuffle credibly well, using visual cues. Despite the ungainliness of her gait and station, she was putting the correct foot forward in time to the beat, with only a few last minute corrections. She was doing a better dance than most good Dutchmen can muster. I thought hers was the most touching tribute of the service, which was especially poignant given her limited physical abilities and her inability to hear the song, even though it was lustily belted out by all the other participants, several with babies on their backs.

I busied myself taping and photographing the celebration, particularly the imposing parade of headloads of peanuts, maize, pineapples, cassava, and rice bowls coming down the aisle at offering time. Then I took pictures of the congregation as they were coming forward. I then had a brilliant idea, which came to me just before the second homily. I went behind the church and photographed first women and children in a "nursery" there, next the congregation from the back, and finally the pastor through the open door with this harvest of produce at the feet of the offering table. I hope the pictures turn out well but the brilliance of the maneuver was my short bush sortie to relieve a distended urinary bladder before re-entering for the second half.

AN ABRUPT, ALTHOUGH NOT UNANTICIPATED, INTERRUPTION

The dreaded visitors arrived during the pastors' special thanks for our services. He had just said, "We do not know if we will ever see him again, that is in God's plans. He alone knows them; so we wish him now well and many thanks for making so much of our lives here at Assa possible in many instances and richer in others." This was probably a response to my earlier statement that I would certainly try to return to them again, as I had so many times before.

"We have nothing to give you." They have given back so much more than I have extended in their direction, and they are far more generous than I am. Such sentiments are a clear re-enforcement of any motivation for my efforts.

"Our lives are so much richer...." If you could see me sitting in front of the first row in which many are dressed in rags, you might understand the phrase "for richer, for poorer." You would recognize how much richer these people are than many of the stuffed shirts in the other world in which I move who are suffering only the ennui of surfeit.

Suddenly, we heard the roar of an engine. A dust-colored, unmuffled, open-backed Land Rover drove up with a uniformed driver. Three soldiers in the back seat were clutching Kalashnikovs as they bounced along the road over the morning's hyena tracks. Many of the people, and all the kids, stood to look out the open sides of the church. The soldiers were in a big hurry, and passed the church despite all the little heads sticking out looking in their direction. They wheeled around at the hospital. Inikpio walked out to see them, wearing his Sunday Best shirt and tie. He had a brief discussion with them. They were still in a hurry and shortly roared off in the other direction without so much as slowing down near the church. Behind them was a trail of black oil leaking from the vehicle, which like everything else in this part of the world, had seen better days. The way the vehicle was being driven, it would have looked broken down even if nearly brand new.

With an impressive show of courage and dignity, despite the fear that clutches at everybody here within sight of any soldiers of any kind, the pastor turned to Inikpio and asked if he would briefly tell us what the circumstances were, and then we could proceed with the service. Inikpio reported that the soldiers came here for water for the car's radiator, and were in a hurry to be away. They had been to the *Collectivité* at Gwane where the administrator is now with an entourage that will be coming by shortly to explain what they had seen and why they went there. With no more to report, there was a loud sigh of relief and nervous babble from the congregation. The service resumed and continued for several more hours.

From the pulpit then came a list of public announcements. A new drinking water source would be opened down this path next month. Lost and found was announced. Public health announcements and health tips were given. Greetings were extended to neighbors, including one to a refugee from Ango, and another to a man who had come from Ebale for dental extractions. There was then the redundant announcement that their special guests who had already been greeted on the previous Sunday and honored at this special service would be going on a very long and hazardous journey this week to return. "What can we say to you, for all you have done?" They all stood and said *"Merci mingi."* If that were not embarrassing enough, they then started thanking us for many patients who had been treated even though they lacked the nominal fees to pay for them, but we had done them anyway. Now those patients will have good health in order to return the payments later. I do not believe this message was directed so much toward me but more to the entire medical staff. *Bwana* will be outside the church after the service and take pictures of all of us to carry back to the people who have helped us so much by giving the lumber and pan roof for our church. We would like to show our thanks to our friends who have helped us. There was more, but you have the idea.

I am not the only one with a camera in the team, but I am the only one with film, so I spread around my remaining film stock. This is probably fortunate now, since I will not have a flash camera from here on, and they will be giving me the film they expose to carry back. I am also the chief source of development as well as all other things photographic. I went so low in my film stock that I started using the Signature special film, which can come back on disc as well as slides and prints for the same exposure. This triple facility is not very useful in this area of the world.

The sermons were finally completed. Each group of the Bible School sang, one song was a special "graduation presentation" sung in Pazande, Bangala, and French with all the motions attached. A painfully nervous young woman was about to give her presentation, when everything came to a screeching halt, and the service was interrupted again.

CHURCH AND STATE IN ASSA: I AM AN EYEWITNESS TO MAJOR EVENTS IN THE VILLAGE'S LIFE

An enclosed Land Rover came roaring up with the same conviction as had the army jeep, turned at the hospital, and immediately came back to the church. Politicians never lose a chance to work the preformed crowd. The driver headed for a shade tree and a parade of officials came in to sit in the church. They looked in my direction eyeing the *Mzungu* nervously. I am conspicuous at Assa.

Several officials marched into the church and raised their hands over their heads and gave a salute. These big shots were: 1) the Commandant of the Army Battalion; 2) the Chief Inspector of the Police; 3) the District President of the ADFL—"*Alliance des Forces Démocratique de la Libération*" for the whole of the Bas-Uele District; 4) the Administrator of this zone based in Ango, Buta's replacement. The Administrator took charge and acted as emcee. He did the introductions and got the crowd to "Hmmmmmmm" back in response to questions put to them. First he had a pocket full of bills, and he paraded them out one at a time with a little explanation that this was the new money in the DRC, and the old money would be in valid circulation for one year to make the conversion. He added them all up and had the congregation repeat back. According to Sonny Mwembo, he was not a bad instructor in the Bangala that he used in rather good form. He kept looking over to me and nodding for approval. I simply smiled and taped the whole event.

His information on currency conversion was cruelly superfluous. There is precious little currency in Assa, either old or new. These unfortunate people scratched out their marginal daily existence on subsistence farming, hunting and gathering, and a barter economy. The gross domestic product of Assa, if measured by World Bank methods, is just a tick over nil.

"THE INCIDENT AT GWANE IT IS TO BE REGRETTED, AND STEPS TAKEN TO SEE THAT SUCH MILITARY ADVENTURISM AGAINST YOUR CHIEF DOES NOT RECUR"

The Commandant gave the following speech: "What the soldiers did at Gwane was bad. It should not have happened. What Chief Emmanuel (Sasa's son) did was bad; that might be, but that is not the way to judge and carry out the punishment for such alleged misdeeds. These must be called to the attention of the administrator, and appropriate investigations will be carried out. I regret it is not possible to get back any of the Assa property that was taken by the soldiers from the chief's compound. We have been present in Gwane at the *Chef du Collectivité* headquarters and made our inspection of the premises and the remains of the evidence of the soldier's presence. We have seen the grave that we believe was dug for the burial of your chief, but we assure you that he is alive and we will be in communication with him. Now, thank you for your attention, we are in a hurry to get back to where we have many urgent matters of state to attend to. *Attention!*" With that the Commandant, raised both his hands in salute to the congregation and shouted —can you believe—"*Vive Democracie!*"

The small group wheeled on their heels, and exited, with a second rush of the mud and dust, and the second major interruption of the service over. Now, can we resume the next hour of the service?

THE NEXT SECTION OF THE SERVICE, SOMEWHAT AN ANTICLIMAX, RELATES TO THE BIBLE SCHOOL GRADUATES AND THEIR THRILLED FAMILIES

So much for the narrow division of church and state in the new DRC. The graduates of the Bible School were to have had the graduation celebration at a separate session. Because of the uncertainty and insecurity of the soldiers in the area, it was postponed until today. Several people in the congregation were wearing ties, not far from some women in bark cloth loincloths nursing babies. Each graduate had a presentation to make, including a fellow with a high-pitched voice who had to explain to the audience that might not have known him that although he "may speak like a woman, he is definitely a man, and has the following things he wants to say." It was no problem for me to figure out that he has a goiter, and he has probably had disruption of both recurrent laryngeal nerves, since on later inquiry, I learned that he had a weak voice until last year when it became a whisper. As the thyroid gland grows into a much-enlarged goiter, it can constrict the larynx (the voice box) or the trachea (the windpipe). In a few instances, the goiter may displace or disrupt the motor (recurrent laryngeal) nerve that goes to the vocal cords. The breathy, high-pitched voice of this speaker lacked the usual modulation of a person with normal control of the larynx and vocal cords. As he spoke, he became tired trying to make himself heard, and, finally, raising his hand to the goiter under his chin, he broke off before he had finished his speech.

Even the grades and final scores on the examinations were reported for the finalists. It was like a scholarship competition, in which family members cheered as they do at GWU Medical School graduations.

One little kid toddled over to carry his sibling who was sound asleep and wet, to a family member on the other side of church, quite a feat when the difference in their weights was about two pounds! One other toddler walked up to the offering table, now loaded with all the produce, looked inside the collection box, and with a loud fart, toddled back to his seat with the other kids and dozed off. There was a general good-humored murmur at his performance.

I was grateful that I had taken my own "photographic leave" earlier, now totally forgotten, since the two interruptions of "church" by the "state," or else I could not have gone the distance either!

CANDID CAMERA
AFTER CHURCH FUNCTIONS

The pastors were unable to organize a group of posers for the photograph of the whole church despite several efforts at herding the group together. I wandered around shooting a lot of film. I was out of print film, so these will have to be converted from slides eventually, but I do not believe they are expecting rapid turnaround, "MotoPhoto" service! There are dozens of requests by everyone to take their family portraits and then a scramble—first to get everyone together, and then second to get every intruder out who wants to jump into every frame any time a camera is raised. My camera is often taking pictures when not raised, a trick that they have not yet caught on to. I was out of film by the time I focused in on the two new adult female cretins whom I was trying to photograph.

I planned on arriving at JM's compound on time for the afternoon festivities. I had to make a quick stop at the house to pick up a couple of tapes from my dwindling stock and film from the slide stock I had not sequestered in Nairobi for the rest of the trip. If you can believe it, I am only one-third through this eventful day, and they say that nothing ever happens around here! For the rest, you will have to read on for the events at JM's feast, the celebration of the two fathers in the Azande death ceremony, the full story about the incident at Gwane, and the final feast of the day, at Émile Zola's family compound.

And, here, none of you ever thought of me as a "social butterfly" in my "native environment."

29 CHURCH AND STATE

**AN EYEWITNESS ACCOUNT OF THE EVENTS IN ASSA
ON A DAY FILLED WITH CEREMONIES, CELEBRATIONS, WIDE
SWINGS OF EMOTION, AND HAPPINESS SHARED IN FAREWELL
DINNERS AT WHICH I AM THE HONORED GUEST**

July 19, 1998

Upon arrival in JM's compound (**Figure 22**), which this morning was a soap factory and now is a dining hall, I gave my first gift to one of the rather persistent requesters. A young woman, Siaduwe, who, like all the others, has approached me saying in primary standard stilted English, "Please, Sir, I must to speak with you." This introduction was followed by a request to take on the support of her continuing education. From this initial starting point, the argument continues that I represent the supplicant's one and only hope. They believe that their prayers are well-placed and confidence in me would not be disappointed. But she had made one request that, at first, I didn't understand. Her head was *découverte*. This was translated through André to mean that she wanted a scarf of some kind. She had none and coveted most this special crowning glory. I would probably be the last one to stand between anyone and their desire for *haute couture*, but do I look like a designer? Still and all, I started thinking of "this one thing I have."

MY ROLE AS A FASHION TREND-SETTER

My wardrobe is reduced to some rather slim pickings, but what I am being begged for I just might have. Sasa's dreams have been fulfilled and his simple life will never be the same since he now has designer shades and the people here will have to respect him. I did not happen to be carrying $50,000 in US hundred dollar bills to scatter around Assa to the mendicants who could not wisely handle as much as a whole dollar put into their hands at one time for the naïveté of their requests. But, I do have what remains of the hunting gear stripped from me since it looked too military. This obviously shows that the customs officials have never seen civilian, bowhunting, "treebark" camouflage pattern on any gear in their lives. I had a red bandanna of the kind farmers or cowboys have worn around their necks or on some particularly sun-struck days, knotted over their heads. The last time I wore mine was en route up the glacial slopes of Mount Rainier as a sun shield to keep the glare off the glaciers from burning me into a red neck. *Voilà*! My farmer's hip pocket bandanna has become the height of fashion in Assa church circles and the envy of all nubile young ladies who wonder how many more there are where that singular item came from.

I presented it to Siaduwe (**Figure 26**), erstwhile primary school teacher and persistent supplicant, who has now achieved her most lasting passion, her very own fashionable scarf, direct from the designer runways of America. The prize has already turned heads. She performed both in the chorale and in the band playing the trumpet dressed up now to the top of her head in a florid red bandanna tied with a flare.

DINNER AT JM'S RECEPTION

We had dinner under JM's thatched roof in the compound where this morning I watched him make soap. For the first time, Tasamu, Inikpio's wife, joined the men being honored. She is *not* serving us, but is dressed in her Sunday Best finery. She is a very competent health care professional in her own right. She is having dinner with us—a very nice idea, I think—but her status would still not allow her, for example, to sit on the men's (right) side of the church.

After our dinner, Bule showed us pictures from a file he had kept very carefully, that includes his fame as the stalker, shooter and killer of the man-eating leopard that had lain in wait for the Assa villagers—killing it with his *fabricacion* muzzle-loader. The most intriguing of these pictures to the group was not photos of me standing over waterbuck trophies, big Cape buffalo, or recent bushbuck, but Mrs. Pierson's fancy casket at her burial at age 101! Later, I found out why they had this fascination with our burial practices.

In 1996, the last time that JM had invited me and the attending group over for the *fête du chasseurs*, we dined on *zigba*. This animal gored him with its enormous tusks. Those massive tusks were given to André and those were discarded in panic at the approach of the soldiers in the fierce fighting and total looting that had engulfed Nyankunde like a wave. Many vehicles were stolen from CME, but a neat trick that saved some of them was simply to remove the wheels and roll them into the bush. They could be destroyed, but not driven away. As for the Bronco here at Assa, the more recent renegade soldiers rolled the wheels away when they found it wouldn't start.

Kati and some clever fellows salvaged the Toyota Land Cruiser with the twin diesel tanks that was Ruth Powell's vehicle by driving it to old Chief Sasa's compound at Gwane. They sequestered it inside his redoubt, where it survived the looting by the retreating, Mobutu-backed, Rwandan Hutus, because they took an end run around the Gwane complex. In the more recent raid on the Gwane compound, the military marauders made the Toyota priority number one as they made off with it as their best prize. The Toyota that carried us back from the Ebale helicopter stranding was the only reliable functional vehicle in the entire *Collectivité*. It had also provided Kati with a full-time job as chauffeur, a title of which he is stripped along with the loss of the irretrievable vehicle. I cautiously asked about further details of the raid on Chief Sasa's compound following JM's dinner. Everyone politely evaded my questions. Nevertheless, these details came later tonight from another source.

We chatted about the time of our last feast here eating the *zigba* that had ripped open JM. We were eating *bodi* today. A couple of small hunting dogs were wandering about which prompted the comment that the Luba in Kasai Province eat dogs, but only on special occasions, and then it must be for men only, a tangential reference to Tasamu's presence with us. But it was given as a compliment to me, since it was said that these people (the next tribe over to the Azande) would be obligated to feed so high-ranking a visitor as their guest for today the dog that certainly this feast would require. I was happy that the small dogs were free to wander along on their way, at least for the purposes of this guest.

We discussed the intrusion of the four high-ranking officials in the church service. The presence of these bureaucrats was a near farce for me, and the residents of Assa certainly had not missed the irony of *"Vive Démocracie!"* The *party* officials, unelected but appointed by the *military dictator* of a rebel band, interrupted a church service with a slogan to inspire the congregation to further fear of the ruling power. The officials attempted to show that they were bigger than their local chief and would dispose of him, as well as any one who came after him, at their own pleasure. None of this threat was lost on the residents of Assa who realized the irony of the cloak of democracy that the unelected military power structure briefly imposed on their very democratic church service today.

Still, just what had happened recently at Gwane to Chief Emmanuel, Sasa's successor, and how they felt about it was off limits to conversation. Discussion would invoke the sadness they were trying to put behind them in the counterbalancing joy they felt at the presence in Assa of their ever-so-welcome current guests.

The moment nearly passed, when JM got up and came back with a photo folder of his own. He produced the *Time* magazine cover portrait of Paul Carlson M.D., a graduate of GWU medical school. Another photo is of me standing in front of the Carlson portrait (that was the basis for the *Time* cover) in the Himmelfarb Medical Library at GWU. Behind the head of Paul Carlson are the blood splotches against the wall at which he was shot during the Simba revolt, which changed the Belgian Congo to become Patrice Lumumba's communist Zaïre. Lumumba's regime was replaced by anticommunist Mobutu who created a government that became the modern model for a kleptocracy. One year ago, Kabila overthrew Mobutu. The message from JM was clear. With all this political weight being thrown about in some other agenda of someone else's struggle, the welfare of the people, and particularly health care, and most especially the good-hearted effective folk like Dr. Carlson, and by the photographic extension, me, were prevented from doing the beneficial work of the world. These self-appointed political power brokers are seeking to be "president-for-life" while spewing out "*Vive Démocracie!*" The very poor are not always very dumb. JM had another portrait of me and my son Michael, taken at a Washington church. JM and André said together "We would very much like to invite you and your son to visit Assa and be our guests together!"

FOLLOWING JM'S FEET THROUGH THE TALL GRASS OVER TOWARD THE CELEBRATION OF "TWO FATHERS"

After our dinner, we walked over to the rain-postponed celebration. The prerehearsed Azande death ceremony and celebration of our father's lives was prepared to teach what others could learn from them. I followed JM's feet as the growth of tall grass narrowed the path, remembering once, over a decade ago, trying to see two sandals through the predawn dim glow of a sometimes required torch focus—his right sandal was red and his left was green. I had remembered the "red right returning" rules of the road for navigation. I then stared at JM's shoes on this visit, and saw the backs of the heels said "Rockports"—my shoes! They appeared to be in better shape than when I had last had them on my feet several years earlier.

We "made rounds" on each hut in the village as we passed, shaking every hand down to the infants who were eager to touch me. The big advantage about the postponement of this ceremony is that it was now going to be held in daylight, and I was now left with a camera only for daytime photography. And, I used it often, taking a very intimate view of Assa from hutside to fireside. Every member of the community contributed something to this celebration of a faithful Azande father's life, extending to my own father who lived in Michigan. They both had lived for the same purposes and died at nearly the same time, and would be joining each other as their sons had in working together earlier.

The death ceremony was superimposed on everyday life at the Azande hearthside. I watched and took unintrusive pictures of cutting hair, picking nits and jiggers, teasing four-poster coiffures, nursing babies, and children cleaning their parents' toe nails. Other homely chores were taking place: these were rice pounding and *pondu* boiling while the choral processional was arriving. I was seated in a chair at the head of the ceremony, with Inikpio on one side and André on the other side (**Figure 24**). André whispered translations of certain events and the meanings they had to the ceremony. I taped André's tribute to his father in the story of his life, and noted he had in his hand the typescript of the e-mailed story I had written about my father. In André's lapel, he wears a "Gideon" pin, and has in his breast pocket, an already well-thumbed and highly-annotated Gideon New Testament Bible I had given him on my last visit. I had almost forgotten this gesture, which was one of the primary reasons André had said I was now his father substitute. He commemorated his own father and mine, and now passed on to others the wisdom that had been conferred to him.

It was a moving celebration, with school exercises on the part of several students. Rachel, JM's daughter and André's "new daughter" at CME, who hopes to study medicine with the support I am leaving for her, marched to the head of the class for the first recitation. Her hard work and ambition reflected André's father's role in stimulating his children to complete their studies.

SPECIAL MUSIC CONCLUDES THE CELEBRATION; THEN COME REUNIONS WITH SEVERAL FRIENDS WITH GOOD NEWS

I turned to see Kongonyesi. He had been called away to go to Digba to attend his daughter's death! In a rare exception to the general rule that when the Azande say they are going to die, or, more ominously, when someone in authority over them declares that they *will* die, they do not have the independence of spirit to disappoint anyone. They do, in fact, go on to die. Usually, with the called-in family standing by as observers of fact, *they go right ahead and die!*

Not in this case! I asked what was the problem in the first place? I got the circular answer that the problem was that Kongonyesi's daughter was going to die, apparently because someone with an interest in this outcome said that she *would* do so. It turned out that she had begun treatment for both schistosomiasis and for ankylostoma, according to Inikpio, and she was doing nicely, thank you!

207

Schistosomiasis is a kind of parasitic disease that affects the liver predominantly (for one species of *Schistosoma*) and the urinary tract (for another species). Both types are present in Assa. Ankylostoma is another kind of parasite, a hookworm, which burrows through the skin of the bare feet and causes anemia. Inikpio had diagnosed both conditions in Kongonyesi's daughter. Kongonyesi has always been one of my most consistent hunting companions during previous visits, and for him to leave Assa during my visit would be highly unusual unless his daughter was truly going to die. She somehow had mustered the strength, along with a little help from Inikpio's treatment, to throw off someone's malignant death sentence

The second surprise was the appearance of Neke, standing under the tree that gives the date-like fruit with the big pip and scarce pulp. I am told that it yields a vegetable oil, but in much smaller quantities than the palm tree. Neke waited until I should recognize him, so as not to force himself on my attention. His reticence was surprising after all the time he and I had spent in the bush. He was one of the regulars in the hunts, and I looked down to find the dress boots I had given to him just before my departure six years ago. They were recently resoled and shined for this special occasion. I had been worried about him, since I had not seen him. He was in the CAR for the past two weeks, probably related to the incident of Chief Emmanuel being in exile, although he never said so directly. He returned with messages from Chief Emmanuel in a UN refugee camp in the CAR.

No one goes to the CAR casually. Crossing the border requires a permit from the Zemio side of $25.00 US (i.e., two and a half *bidons* [25 liters] of palm oil). Travelers must also pay for the passage on the dugout canoe ferry. A permit must be obtained in advance for another $25.00 US from Bangassou, plus a permit from the "Mayor" of Bangassou, at $5.00 US. All of this means that one cannot get there for simple business purposes without climbing an economic gradient that is too steep for most traders. When I had not seen Neke, I had feared the worst; but he simply greeted me and said that we would hunt again *la prochaine fois*!

News came to Inikpio that there was an outbreak of trypanasomiasis, African sleeping sickness, now epidemic at Obo, Zemio, and Mboke in a circle around Assa. There are many cases but few deaths. This may be the "Rhodesian" variety, which is reservoired in the bushbuck and transmitted by the tsetse fly (*Glossina sp.*), both of which live relatively close to man here. The association is like the white-tailed deer reservoir, deer tick vector, and Lyme disease that occurs on the East Coast in the US.

For some of the tropical infectious diseases, there may be animal reservoirs in which the parasite resides without causing the animal's death.

African sleeping sickness is such an example. The parasite can be carried in animals living close to man, such as the bushbuck, and transmitted by the bite of a tsetse fly. If exotic animals such as the horse were introduced, the organisms would parasitize the newcomer and cause death quickly in such a naïve immigrant without previous experience with the disease to confer resistance. Animals and man may experience "ping-pong" transfers of some of these enzootic diseases, and over time, some accommodation is reached, as with the milder "Rhodesian" variant of trypanasomiasis.

AND NOW FOR THE FINAL FEAST OF THE DAY AT ÉMILE ZOLA'S FAMILY'S COMPOUND WITH THE NEWS OF THE INCIDENT AT GWANE, FINALLY, IN ALL THE DETAILS FROM HIS FATHER

The big celebration adjourned at the brief flare of sunset with me taking a final family portrait of André and all those with a claim to kinship to his father. We entered Émile Zola's freshly swept compound. Flowers had been placed on the thatched roofs over the doors. This is the sign of welcome to a special guest. I well remember this from the *fête du chasseurs* at Kongonyesi's compound in 1992. I learned that their highest honor, as I was served first, is for me to take the gizzard from the bowl of *kanga* gravy.

Tables from all over Assa were arranged in a linear array. The hosts placed me at the head. Then, with the precision of a protocol officer, Émile's oldest brother called out from a list he had on a scrap of paper. The honored guests would come forward in a pecking order that was as rigid as it was formal: beside me was the local pastor, who, for this occasion wore a coat and tie, rarely seen in Assa. Next came André, Inikpio, Pastor Bule, JM, and down through a long list that included Kati, Kazima and others of the school and community, with only a few of the regulars not seated, like Ngasyi, who acted as emcee for Émile's father, the host. Of course, I was first for the hand-washing and service. We ate a rather large and tasty dinner in the dark, which probably always improves the appetite when dining in an *al fresco* restaurant without the gold star of the local sanitation department apparent. André was called over for almost 45 minutes to have a long and animated talk with Émile's father, my titular host. I then found out why. As my host, he was obligated to furnish me what I had requested, and I wanted to know what happened at Gwane. So here is that story, from a man who was there. I taped the full story in translation.

The soldiers came through Assa looting and frightening everyone, and were disappointed to see that things had already been picked rather clean. They demanded of one resident whom they caught, "Where were the riches of Assa?"

They had a wish list: vehicles, the *pikipikis*, and firearms. They began a bit of torture with a heavy club on one of the young men from the Bible School. He did the only reasonable thing and blurted out that Ruth Powell's Toyota had been brought to the Chief's compound for safekeeping, as had every movable thing of high value ahead of the last columns of mixed armed plunderers. They then worked over some other residents to ask if the chief had given them anything illegal, especially elephant meat. The answers to any such questions asked under the threat or initiation of torture is always affirmative. The soldiers then went off to Gwane, after picking out all the parts of the Bronco and a few other things they still could use.

They arrived at the "redoubt" originally built by Chief Sasa but now occupied by his son Emmanuel, and overwhelmed his retainers, and began to beat them, after shooting ineffectively at them—ineffective in hitting any of them, but gunfire certainly won their full cooperation. Persuasion by tire iron (this one being the "clapper" from the "bell" at the Bible School) certainly also helped. The commandant of the rebel unit demanded to see Emmanuel, who had no choice but to come out. They announced to him that he was a bad Chief, and a worse human being besides being a scofflaw in the eyes of this unduly constituted board of review—the fellows waving the guns and occasionally touching off salvos, which kept everyone's attention. They asked for an inventory of the valuables they had heard about in Assa, and started collecting them, the Toyota first, which was then loaded up.

As the Commandant was seeing to the deployment of his scavengers, he had them bring him a cigarette—which André said was opium (probably hemp). He smoked a few of these while he waited and when he was finished he would "finish the job" he had come for—and would the Chief Emmanuel be so kind as to begin digging this large ominous looking hole—six feet deep—in the rocky ground. An askari of the Chief's was assigned to help, who spoke to him in Pazande, saying, "Can you not see that this is your grave and that he plans to execute you? Take-off now!"

The Commandant asked "What are you talking about?" and the Chief replied to the effect that he just remembered another rifle that was hidden and could show them where it was. The Commandant ordered his chief Lieutenant to go with him into the house and fetch it. The house has a front and back door.

The Lieutenant went in and cut a quick deal with Emmanuel, asking, "You see what is about to transpire? What is it worth to you if I let you go through this back door right now?" One brand new motor bike was the exchange rate. The Chief ran out of the redoubt while the Lieutenant, sitting on his new motor bike, roared around shooting. Emmanuel fled in a narrow escape from the lieutenant who had no real intent of letting him do so. Each of the "officers' were a little bit obtunded by that time from smoking the hemp they enjoyed during this reign of terror and looting of the little that Assa had.

And that is how it happened that the entire stock of Assa valuables was carted off in the Assa Mission's own Toyota, and how the Chief's grave at Gwane remains empty and he is in a UN refugee camp in the CAR.

30 MASSACRE NEAR ASSA

**RUNNING DOWN THE TRACK OF TWO OLD SPOOR:
ONE RED AND COLD, LEFT BY THE RETREAT OF MOBUTU'S
SOLDIERS, ONE BLACK AND FRESH, LEFT BY
COMMANDANT'S RECENT RENEGADE BAND OF RAIDERS**

July 20, 1998

Our morning run was 10 miles round-trip in 84 minutes. This was our longest run. We went in the opposite direction of our prior runs, and encountered a few more muddy hills. We have run all but the weekend days, the reverse of the situation back home. Our running here was made more difficult by heavy rain, death celebrations, and missing shoelaces, the usual excuses for not running.

We also saw the fresh spoor of giant forest hog, bushbuck, and African civet. We even spotted the African civet, going back and forth in front of us in the mud to leave fresh tracks. This allowed for us to judge the age of the others after a clean slate due to a recent rain.

But that is the usual spoor I have reported from my runs. Now I will tell you about less usual spoor. One was red and old now but still fresh and burning in the memories of everyone in Assa. The other is black and fresh, the spoor of the military with a leak in what appears to be the old Land Rover's oil pan. This is not a high-maintenance environment for vehicles or people. This explains why they were in such a hurry yesterday to get to Assa and to get water as their coolant. They were no doubt overheating when all their oil leaked out. I found the footprints of the military as surely as the Johnnie Walker Red bottle holding my water, since there, near the massacre site and along the tracks of the tread of the Rover and its black oily spoor was a cigarette wrapper—"Stella" brand. No one in Assa smokes. Such a luxury would be beyond these nearly starving people. Smoking is forbidden in much of the culture and religion here, and would require foreign exchange. The cigarette wrap is as good as a "Kilroy was here." The soldiers also left a body count of four whose gravesites I photographed.

RECONSTRUCTION OF THE RAID OF THE RETREATING ARMY OF MIXED UNITS AND LANGUAGES IN DEFEAT

The spoor is not all that cold from 1997, and the memories could not be any fresher for all the details. Yet, the survivors were reluctant to tell me anything associated with this, their darkest hour, and the recurrence in the recent raid that pillaged Assa. The return of hopped-up rogue military units shooting in all directions brought all the memories from that time as well as the past few weeks into altogether too sharp a focus. The details at last are falling into place. I gathered individual stories in pieces from several individuals who were not in on the fact that I should be sheltered from some of the gorier parts of the story. They had spared me hoping that they might move on with constructive thoughts for the future rather than wallowing in the grief of past massacres.

EVENTS OF APRIL 18-20, 1997

It happened as follows, with several of my Assa friends playing key parts or being eyewitnesses to the worst. The first hit was Yuni, my housekeeper during my last visit. Yuni looks much younger than her 33 years. I just treated her adult daughter for the conjunctivitis that seems epidemic here now. I had made small jokes with her as she picked up rudiments of English.

The villagers heard of the advance of mixed bands of troops who were looting and killing, so they made several trips to and from their houses carrying out whatever they had to hide in the bush. On one of the last return trips, Yuni and her sister were the first in Assa to make contact with the retreating "army" of Mobutu's partisans that was in defeated retreat.

The army was a mixed group containing Bangala-speaking Ngwandi (a smaller northern tribe of neighbors to the Azande) and "refugee" Hutus of the Rwandan conflict. This northern origin is why Mobutu's army spoke Bangala. The "refugee" Hutus of the Rwandan conflict were allied with Mobutu's men. This group inflicted scorched earth pillaging and looting their own or any other peoples encountered as they retreated in defeat.

In contrast, Kabila's ethnic origin and cultural background is from the BiLuba language group of Katanga Province in the southeast—distinct from the BiLuba language of the Kasai—and his long drilling in guerrilla camps meant that he and his foreign mercenary bands spoke Kiswahili. So a guerrilla army that was in "hot pursuit" of the Mobutu allies actually spoke a language better understood by one of the factions of their adversaries, the Hutus. The allies of Mobutu's Bangala-speaking Ngwandi and the Kinyarwanda-speaking Hutus did not understand each other. The Hutus didn't understand any of their victims in this area, whom, to them, represented only so much hominid vermin similar to those they had already exterminated with clubs, hoes and axes in their march through the Tutsi regions further south and east. I paint a picture that may not be pretty, but glosses over their inhuman massacres compared to what they really were like.

The first soldiers that Yuni and her sister encountered were the Hutus, who had pushed ahead of their Bangala-speaking Mobutu irregulars. The Assa women did not understand them precisely, but got a too-clear picture about what they wanted. Soon the Bangala speakers arrived to translate, making it clear that Yuni and the others were to quickly assemble all their valuables and give them up. Yuni was ordered to prepare food for them while they waited for the loot to be brought around. She explained to the Ngwandi troops that she and her sister were here alone and they had nothing. They, of course, would hear none of it, and threatened to beat them. Yuni and her sister ran off into the bush and warned others that these monsters were on the loose behind them in a murderous rampage. The troops swept through Assa, picking up whatever could be carried. After they filled their vehicles, they looked around for people to use as porters for what remained. I have a mind's eye picture of *Man with the Golden Helmet* being carried on someone's head as a tray for whatever could be stacked on top of his portrait! A print of Rembrandt van Rijn's *Man with the Golden Helmet* was the only framed picture on the wall at the mission house in Assa during my previous visits. I have a sentimental connection with this portrait because my last name in Dutch translates loosely as "golden helmet." I had once viewed the original, which had just been sold for the highest price paid for any painting in history, before it was enveloped in controversy as "school of Rembrandt." Since then, this portrait keeps springing up in unlikely places in my life. I once went to bed in the dark in South Africa to awaken in the morning looking up at the only picture in the room. You guessed it. My son Michael has a print hanging in his home in San Antonio without ever knowing these other stories. I arrived in Harare, Zimbabwe to take up residence in the Bronte Hotel. There he was again. These are just coincidences, but *weird* coincidences. Here in Assa, he was my totemic portrait. He disappeared at a time everyone knows too well, during the last military pass through. Everything, even things that were nailed down, was looted, including "Geelhoed."

This ragtag army and a much more ragged band of forced porters were staggering ahead down the road I have just been running. This road has some difficult hills and washouts that are not easy to travel without any headloads.

They headed toward Gwane, the *Chef du Collectivité* site, and the place where all the recent action to and through yesterday, has been going on. On the way, they passed two Catholic mission stations that had small churches, basically thatched huts without any surrounding structures. The parishioners live in distant bush sites, far from these isolated roadside "bush chapels" which do not look like they have been used any time recently.

TWO ROADSIDE BUSH CHAPELS
MUTE WITNESSES OF CARNAGE

Nangume is the name of the first chapel. It looks abandoned. Although it is in disrepair, I learned from Inikpio that it is still occasionally used. There is no priest who lives anywhere near here. It sounds like it is open only when a circuit rider comes through on his bicycle and that has been infrequent since the time of the events around the massacre. I marked it on my GPS as "ASS2" at 04° 39.53′ N and 025° 50.28′ E, and photographed what little is here. At Nangume, the army caught up with four men fleeing on bicycles, and commandeered them to load their bicycles and to strain along, pushing them with large loads of "luggage," as André termed it.

Dianganzi is the name of the next point, the focus of today's interest. I marked it as "ASS3" at 04° 40.33′ N and 025° 50.25′ E. This makes it 2.21 miles from "CONG," our Assa airstrip along bearing 164° or 4.09 miles from "ASS1," the Assa station's front door, along bearing 172°. There is more to these numbers than a measurement of how far we ran in which direction, since the four miles is the hypotenuse of our triangle run which means we did over 10 miles on our round-trip run, in muddy and somewhat sticky conditions with one short rain.

The Catholic chapel here is in somewhat better condition than the one at Nangume. It was whitewashed recently and has a small outbuilding. The name is spelled out with 26 July, 1995, the date of its completion. There is nothing around otherwise, except four recent and stark gravesites, in two rows under a tree. These graves have a longer story not buried with them.

THE MASSACRE SITE
AT DIANGANZI ROADSIDE

The four men with bicycles were pushing their loads of booty down the roads as ordered by the men with guns behind them. As they passed the church at Dianganzi, the chain of one of the bicycles broke, and they could not pump the weight along. The man with the disabled bicycle stopped. After brief consultation with the others, he was delegated to bring the bad news to the Hutu soldiers behind them to see if they had any suggestions of how to replace the broken chain to hurry the procession along. He was the unlucky bearer of bad news to a group that could not hear it, and when translators were brought up, they did not want to hear it. The Hutus were angry with these Azande scum. They accused him of shirking and ordered him back to the task. They punctuated their commands with a tire iron stolen from Assa. When the Hutu soldiers came up upon the stalled bicycle group at the front of the booty baggage line, they became angry.

They took the man who had brought the bad news and beat him with the tire iron in front of the others as a deterrent to more complaints. When the other Hutus came up upon this scene they seemed to smell the blood of previous frenzies, and ordered all four of the men to lie down at the roadside. The killing was not quick. They worked over each of the four with the tire iron. This habit of administering a severe but sublethal beating prior to shooting was perfected during the recent Hutu/Tutsi massacres. About the only equivalent I can think of would probably be the medieval "breaking upon the wheel." When none of the four had any bones intact, one of the Mobutu soldiers came forward, drew his handgun, and shot them dead. Their bodies were left at the roadside as a "signature" of the soldier's presence and *modus operandi*. They wanted to move on, but not down the road, lest they meet Chief Emmanuel's men who may have heard of this incident by any messengers fleeing ahead of them. They wanted a detour off the road.

Two young men of Assa were around (two of many eyewitnesses) and the Hutus summoned one of them. A Bangala speaker asked him if he knew the back trails around the huts and could he guide them around the Gwane *Collectivité* and back onto the road beyond it. So much the worse for him, since he could and agreed to do so. The other youngster fled into the bush. He is the chief eyewitness informant of this part of the story. I was able to track him down after a week of trying. When I finally found him, I realized that I had seen him before on one of my runs.

His name is Mueze. He was hanging around with the other young men outside the house at Assa when I learned of his eyewitness status and talked with him. The soldiers first contacted Yuni on April 18, 1997 and spent the night near here stealing all they could from Assa. They then moved on to Nangume where they picked up the four men and the bicycles as porters on April 19. They killed all four of the men later on April 19 at Dianganzi. The other Assa young man, who served as their guide around the houses at Gwane, was killed on April 20 after he had led them around the back trails. His widow is here and has a one-year-old baby boy. She was pregnant at the time of his death. I had met her before as a friend accompanying Yuni, but then did not know the circumstances that Mueze described.

MUEZE'S STORY

What a surprise in retrospect! Mueze turns out to be the fellow whom we met on the road on the way to the Assa River the first time we ran that far. He was pushing the new fat-tired bicycle, and stopped with us to admire the *chui* tracks, even taking our picture over them. He was on the way to the Assa mission to bring some part of the money owed for an operation on a woman done three days earlier. Here are his eyewitness details on the names, the ages, and the times and means of death of each of the four men forced along with the Catholic mission's bicycles, and his colleague, the young student from Assa.

[**Editor's note**: These details were recorded with André's first use of a computer with a little help from the author. This testimony is offered in raw form for authenticity and accuracy.]

Histoire des gens tues par des Rwoindais Hutu 1997

Le velo de la paroisse cathaulique de Dianganzi a' ete' arrete' par ce militaire Rwoindais entre les mains du catechiste en chef Mr ZININGBA ensuiteles quatre autres catechistes ont prefer defendre ce dernier, leur noms sont les suivants:

    1) Mr. LIKITO, Jean Pierre
    2) Mr. KPIO, Froreburt
    3) Mr. BI, Marcelle
    4) ANINYASI, Justine, 17 ans et eleve a l'Institut de ASSA
    5) Mr. NGBALINDIE, EMMANUEL qui ete' arrete' sur le chemin de GWANEE le 20 Avril 1997 et tue' a' 15 heurs parcequ'il ne voulait pas manger avec les autres prisoniers arrtes' pour le transport des bagages. Les quatre autre qui ete' tues' a' Dianganzi etaient elimines de la maniere suivante:

    Mr Aninyasi ete tue' le premier par le coup de pistolet a la nuque puis le deuxieme ete Mr Kpio ensuite venait le tours de MrBi Marcelle. Le quatrieme repondant au nom de LIKITO ete' ligote et apres etre battu ete tue aussi par le coup de pistolet au niveau de la gorge. Tous etaeainet tue a 17 heures.

THE DEATH OF MUEZE'S ASSA COMPANION

The marauding band made the end run around the backsides of the huts when they could see the road ahead. With no more ceremony, and —it is to be suspected, no formal "thank you"—they turned to their guide, and shot him through the head, leaving his body on the trail they had taken to rejoin the road.

Of the five victims, then, one was from Assa, and the other four were Catholics from Nangume, only two miles from Assa station. When I had first asked the name of the Assa victim, they had said, "You know him," and later they even said to me that he was one of the porters during your hunts, but gave no name. I had not seen Neke at the time, and worried about him. Who should appear last night at the death celebration but Neke, still wearing my shoes! He had no idea why I should be greeting him so enthusiastically. He still lives in the same nearby hut. He had been gone for two weeks over the border in CAR and had just returned in the middle of the ceremony and heard that I was there, so he hung out timorously at the back of the event until I spotted him and came to greet.

IF A BODY MEET A BODY COMING THROUGH THE RAIN

André and I had made the turn at the Dianganzi gravesides, where I took a photograph. We were headed back up the road as a light rain started. The moisture was a little harder on his bright white Red Ball Jets than on my equally shiny Nikes. We looked ahead and saw the African civet, and much later, a form coming down the slick path toward us. It was a woman, wearing only a loincloth. She seemed oblivious to the light rain, but looked embarrassed to be encountering two men. She covered her breasts, an interesting and unusual gesture in this society I had not seen before. She had a large goiter, and did not seem to recognize either of us. This is unusual because by now we are well-known around Assa. She became more animated when she could speak in Pazande with André and learn what we were after. She had a lot of further information. As she now gestured and forgot her earlier embarrassment, she exposed both breasts to reveal a completely duplicated nipple areolar complex on the right.

Yes, she knew what we were after and had told André where to find it. It is unlikely that anyone not directed to it would have recognized it as it was—rather like the roadside crosses at the site of a head-on collision. There are four planted banana palms at roadside, with vine entwined cross pieces three quarters up the small slender trunks. This marks the site where each of the four men were beaten and then shot, and the site is commemorated by this set of markers, only to those who would seek them to remind them of the horror of the recent past.

And the fresh spoor I spotted showed that the horror is not all past. At an interval of every few meters was a streak of black engine oil between two tracks of probably the only four-wheeled vehicle that has been on these roads for a long time. That vehicle might probably have been the same as the one that had been sent through Assa two weeks ago bearing some of the same soldiers. They were still plying their trade, snatching the left front Bronco wheel and anything portable as they were on their way to clean out whatever other valuables had escaped earlier plunder by being spirited away to the Chief's "redoubt," as André had described it, at the *Collectivité* at Gwane. Again, I thought how hypocritical was the administrator's expression of *regret* at the church service for the recent theft of valuables from the chief's compound, his banishment, and, again, the irony—"*Vive Démocracie!*"

RECONSTRUCTION INITIATIVES

We passed a classic example of swidden agronomy, or "slash and burn" farming methods. The forest is chopped and set afire when it is dry enough to clear some of the debris. Amid blackened scorched trunks, a few plants were stuck into the ground. There, closer to Assa as we came up hill, we stopped running to walk, and "to greet" one of the older men working in his shamba. I heard André come in past midnight last night, after he finished his familial rounds in the dark after the death ceremony. He had also counseled some of the men about what to plant and, more importantly, *where*.

Since the 1997 events, everyone in Assa built a new house out of sight and farther away from each other, and had to go still farther away to find a small plot to till. They were afraid of marauders, principally animals. André and I had run across a thick patch of forest bush in which a very large crash was heard as of some buffalo-size creature running away from us. Lately they have also become afraid of human marauders. Decentralized plots were designed to evade marauders but André argues that this makes problems worse. He believes that they should build their houses closer together for protection and they should all cultivate adjoining shambas. That way they could share guard duty and warn of an approach of elephants, Cape buffalo, or even soldiers.

"Well, that may be a good idea in urban planning, but where could we build such a place?" asked the elders.

"Take my lands that I am now having cultivated in rice and bananas." said André unhesitatingly. Further, he is trying to institute what would be called in America a "rural co-op." The idea of "banking" is slow to catch on here, since hand-to-mouth existence does not generate a lot of surplus, and when it does it is expended—I fear a good deal of it recently—in royal receptions for honored guests.

André is trying to encourage the idea that each family should contribute something like one half dollar a month to a fund. This would keep the kitty growing for special needs. If one of them had to go to the hospital there would be some funds for that purpose that could be withdrawn. Despite our donated medical supplies and labor, Assa station has to "float on its own unsubsidized bottom" on under $200 per month for the district. In essence, this co-op would be a combination insurance fund and growth and development strategy. I have promised to help get it started.

SOME HELP FOR SELF-STARTERS

André and I talked about what would be required for the commitments we have made thus far. For example, $5.00 per month school fees for Rachel and her airfare from Isiro. For the people of Assa, we decided that there will be no gifts, except for the things I am leaving here. We will fund only sustainable start-up aid for projects that will pay back into the community. When we look at what is required for what we have projected already, that comes to something around $300.00. An additional $ 200.00 could start a long-term revolving loan, gathering ideas and projects to help them help themselves. So, I will ask new mendicants to make application to the fund with a proposal outlining how soon they could pay back their loan with what benefit it would have for the community. Even huge handouts disappear into the bottomless well of African need without a ripple. Only some kind of recycling system of self-help can be effective in doing something that seems to make a difference in their lives.

The crossed sticks at the roadside, and the dripping oil of the leaking truck of their own army are the spoor behind the animals that have savagely been predating these poor people. These relics should not symbolize these people as perpetual victims. The development loan program we discussed and instituted following this morning's run may let them define more about themselves than the roadside crosses.

31 WHAT A ZOO!

LEAVE-TAKING AT ASSA IN A RUSH OF UNFULFILLED PROMISES AND FURTHER PROMISES FOR WHAT WILL COME NEXT TIME.

July 21, 1998

I am leaving. Everyone knows that I am leaving. Therefore the crowd at the door is thicker than ever and the requests for immediate aid are being pitched fervently. Meanwhile, I have experienced Assa's revenge against the vaunted sin of seeming accomplishment. All day yesterday, I waited, going in and out of theatre to keep the ThinkPad charged for my last chapters and to oversee some final cases: bilateral lipomas below each scapula, an ovarian cyst, and several minor cases not requiring close follow-up. I had apportioned all my clothes to be given away, planned a good morning run before the final "bath" and then packed up the completed 20 bilingual protocols. Then, I changed into my "going away costume." No one else in Assa makes such plans so far ahead. Nevertheless, they all plan to see me off, bringing their entire family for the mandatory portraits that seem to be *Bwana*'s full time job.

LEAVE-TAKING FROM ASSA:
THIS IS NOT INTENDED AS A DRESS REHEARSAL

But, now, what about those five additional protocols that had got started with the four young men and one older man on Friday? They all were eager to get close to *Bwana*, especially Lazunga's son Lipay. He managed to make it to the house on at least five occasions to get the *Bwana* alone to speak to him about a highly important matter, after having soaked up 50% of last year's "foreign aid package" with no apparent yield. He found me busy each time, and figured he ought to join in the action. So, to get into my good graces, he was among the four young men on whom we attempted to complete eight color interviews. Immediately, he set about doing the honors in the color interviews. They all

221

performed abominably. Several of them looked like they were going quite fast, never asking, as did a few of them, for a repeat of each color disc. Later I discovered that this speed was due to their leaving most of the 330 entries blank. When they did write down a term it was often in French. At least one did all right on one of the languages, and we gave them a reprieve to go to their gardens and also to attend the celebration of André's father. They promised to come on Saturday. They cannot say we were not here since we did not go out for our run either Saturday or Sunday. In fact, they never showed up again.

So, of the study that would have been complete with their entries, they have sabotaged it by using up the time, the forms, and starting only one fourth of it (badly). They agreed to return but did not, although they were prominent participants in the feasting and celebrations that attended the closure of our stay. These fellows are probably going to be the final mendicants besieging me as I walk to the plane.

HAZARDS AT DUSK ON THE POOL DECK

I have given my last roll of print color film to André who has the last functioning flash camera. I then took the ThinkPad off to what is left of the poolside deck. This may be the only recreational use being made of the deck around the pool since it was built, although there is a smoky haze in the air that probably reflects some use being made of quite a few of the planks at nearby hearthstones. I had to work my way out there very cautiously in the dimness of twilight to catch the last light of day, and to avoid falling through the gaps where rotting wood and pried up planks made booby traps. I turned on the machine and started the drain of the precious energy in the battery, when I began getting buzzed. Like a magnet, this activity at twilight drew people who had never before gone behind the house to come on out and to tell me they wished to write a letter. Very well, do so. Well... I know, I know, you have not so much as a single scrap of paper. That is right. They now get the paper from me, and while I am at it, I will wager that you do not have a pen either. Bingo! So, after the last of the four dozen pens I brought has been distributed, I try to come out and try again in the now jet black dark.

Again I am buzzed. It is too late for people to be coming out to harass me, and yet I get "close passes" by each ear in a kind of "humming" low fly by. Then I get it. I am out in the darkness with the soft glow of the computer screen being the only light and a few insects are hovering and I am attracting passes from low flying bats! So, my one attempt at "lounging at the poolside deck" has come a cropper, from the continuous buzzing of mammals, first humans, and now *die fledermäuse*.

PRECIOUS PAPER

The subject of paper brings up another sponsorship. I didn't carry the reams of paper needed for the linguistic studies across the Atlantic because the shipping costs exceeded the price in Nyankunde. I took all the paper I could find in Nyankunde with me to Assa. By drawing on both sides of the paper, we have conserved some of this stock, which was paid for at Nyankunde prices. We have a full ream of unopened paper, which André asks me if we should carry back to Nyankunde. I said, "Of course not!" I do not want to pay the freight on carrying it back and forth. It is already here where Inikpio will need it. I just gave the paper to Inikpio. Good idea. If I put it on the plane I will pay freight that is greater than the value of the paper. This seems like simple arithmetic, and besides, I am jettisoning everything to lighten the load for the return trip, right? I will be going back very light to Nyankunde. Right?

THE ECONOMICS OF AIR-FREIGHT *OUT* OF ASSA

Guess again! I just tripped over the freight that is stacked up for the return flight—at least twice the tonnage of the freight coming out here! I was congratulating myself on at least not having the two big air-freight boxes of medicines that were delivered here. What's this? Two large air-freight boxes, heavy as lead, or make that rice!

Recall that we had saved out a stock of medicine that we were going to carry on to Banda along with instruments. The pilot is afraid to delay by landing there so we will not be going there now. I suggested to André that we leave it here at Assa with Inikpio, where it will eventually be used well. André is reluctant since he owes a great deal to the Banda community which now has less than Assa does, and by "over-stocking" Assa we make it a bigger target for the kind of pharmacy break-in attempted the other night. I do not think it wise to make a roundtrip with this weight back to Nyankunde with the faint hope that there may be another flight out this far any time before I return. André has packaged up all the stuff for Banda and it will go *by bicycle* at some future time to resupply them. Well that has saved a lot of weight and my freight charges, right? Wrong.

FOREST PRODUCTS AIRLIFTED OUT OF ASSA

Now another "guess again!" I have just rounded the door to find *three* bidons of palm oil for a total of 60 liters—is that all? No, since around the door is the Émile Zola supply in a 50-liter drum. "It is very expensive in Nyankunde,"

223

was the response—which is true—it costs almost *half* the air-freight charges! Ah, but you are neglecting one of the fundamental economic laws that apply here as well as elsewhere. The air-freight charges are *my* expense, and the sale price in Nyankunde is *their* profit! So, it would work the same way as my carrying three boxes of copier paper from Washington to Assa. It is very cheap in Washington. If it were not for the economic pain of surplus luggage charges, it would be cheaper for me to carry the paper from Washington to Assa. This is the very same reverse reasoning that has me paying for the excess ream of paper that I am leaving at my cost to Inikpio, to lighten up the air-freight load to be filled now by 110 kg of "free" palm oil and rice. And do not forget the mango pips to be planted there in Nyankunde, and the unusual medicinal plants that have been gathered here, and the peanut butter, and the gifts of other staple commodities that would otherwise just have to be bought in Nyankunde. These can be carried from Assa at no added carrying charge to the intended beneficiaries.

Foreign aid takes many forms, including the subsidies with which such a trip as this is frequently burdened. Opportunity costs may mean different things to different observers, especially when there is a high profit opportunity. Assa economics makes every bit as much sense as almost all farm subsidy programs and tariffs and other barriers to trade in which the only perspective that matters is whose ox is being gored versus whose is getting fattened!

CHAMPION OF THE *CHAMPIGNONS*
ZUNGALANI LIPAY: SENIOR "COOKER"
FUFIYO DIENDONEE: JUNIOR "COOKER"

One potential calamity *did not* happen! At dinner last night I was surprised and delighted to note one new dish—the first surprise since my being here. With a variety that is lacking, this was a welcome change. I asked, "What is this very good sauce?"

"*Champignons,*" was the response. Mushrooms!

"Where do they come from?" I asked.

"From around here," was the reply from André.

"Who found them?" I asked.

"The cooker!" was the answer.

They were very good. *After* I had eaten more than my share, André, as is his wont, launched into a story about his father. His father went out to string ground nets along the ground so that a hunter (and perhaps some dogs) can use them to drive the *kangas* into them. Guinea-fowl fly infrequently and mainly scoot along on the ground, only taking to the air consistently twice a day coming from or going to their roosting trees. As André's father searched for the right place to set his nets, he came across a large fairy ring of mushrooms. He was delighted, since hunting is a chancy thing, whereas gathering is pretty much a sure thing in such a bonanza. He went back to tell his friends about the find. He came back with them and they gathered all they could carry and feasted well on all the mushrooms they had collected.

That is, until later, when each glutton awoke desperately ill. The critical timing of this story sapped it of some of its humor, as we waited to hear the outcome of the hunters turned gatherers. Some remained sick unto death but there did not seem to be much that could be done for them. I thought about the toxicity of muscarine, a potentially deadly neurotoxin from the common North American mushroom *Amanita muscaria* and phalloidin, a nasty liver toxin produced by *A. phalloides*. I realized that there probably was nothing available out here to help us anyway. If poisoned, we would just bloody well be forced to writhe around, froth at the mouth, hallucinate, and weather it out if possible. I also gave some thought to the idea that this would be an unusual, but less than desirable, way to spend my final night in Assa. Finding the *choo* in the dark among hyenas and various flying things from insects to mammals is something I would want to avoid even if it could be pursued at leisure. The worst case scenario was that the experience would be slow, dreadful and fatal.

I asked, "How much does our cooker know about such things?"

André said, "Oh, I told him about my father's experience, and he told me not to worry!"

I am here to say that we each spent a very normal night and awoke in the morning of a day full of hurry and last minute details without further thought of the very good *dejeuner* by the "Champion of the *Champignons!*" He deserved the present I gave him this morning, the dress shirt he had so carefully ironed and folded with the flair of a professional launderer. His assistant has a pair of shorts that once were red, but now even the patches have patches. Since it is his only set, I surprised him with the khaki Bermuda shorts that have made the back and forth trip to Africa at least four times. They looked brand new after he had washed and pressed them. He also has the fabric belt that once belonged to the khaki safari pants that were left here on my first trip, now more than ten years ago.

FEW LOAVES AND SO MANY FISHES

Not that every mendicant was so well-satisfied. The hospital guard on whom I had operated earlier this past week, came "to greet" early this morning. I gained some spare time when I realized that the press of other activities and the light rain would wash out the planned run. He positioned himself between the door and the *choo* to say "*Mbote*" and present me with his flashlight. I recognized it as a GWU model from many trips ago. He showed me that it had no batteries. I have neither batteries nor flashlight, unfortunately. Rather dumbly, I carried only my tiny Mag-Lite to a lampless land with 12 hours of darkness and expressed that in unmistakable gestures of futility. OK. On his next pass by me, he showed evidence that he had encountered Sasa, and circled his eyes with his fingers. He wanted to look at least half as cool as Sasa. I came with two sets of shades and now I have none for my own onward journey.

Not to be discouraged that this *Bwana's* traveling Goodwill Store is not very well-stocked, he then came around the other door and rubbed all over his naked torso, showing that he was cold and wet in the light rain. He surely could use the clothes I was wearing. What I was wearing was what remained of my wardrobe. The apportionment process had stripped me down to the single versatile outfit of my tee shirt and the khaki pants with the zip off legs to become shorts. That would do nicely, he seemed to say.

When I shook my head, having allocated everything else already, he smiled, as if to say wordlessly, "It never does hurt to give it one last try." Then, not to appear ungrateful, he patted the fresh bandage, (now getting quite dirty) on his abdomen where the ventral hernia was repaired four days ago, as if to add "But, *Bwana* has already given me a pretty good gift from this trip!" Now, at last, the path to the *choo* is left unguarded.

THE LEPER COMES TO CALL

But already, painlessly making his awkward way down the path to me is the old leper who had met me at church to say again through his unblinking eyes as he pointed to my shirt and said, "Mingi, mingi." He said you have very many, an accusation that from him is as true as an arrow. He was wearing the identical repatched rags in which I first encountered him well over a decade ago. Leprosy is a bacterial disease that can destroy sensation in the extremities. This man had no sensation in his hands. Consequently, his hands had been burned repeatedly and he had lost fingers and toes. I really should have taken off my shoes and given them to him, but he now has one of my newly pressed and laundered shirts. I am sure I will see it again on my next visit. At any rate, he will probably wear this shirt for the rest of his life.

A very helpful teacher at the Bible School, whose hyphenated Pazande name includes the suffix "Peter," has a good little son whom I recognize by his single Chicago Bulls "Threepeat" Champs tee shirt. This youngster was a real trooper. The child could sit patiently at his father's side for hours as the father did the boring tabulation of the data on the sheets. Peter got my light brown wool pants, for which he was very grateful. I figured that he saved me 48 hours of digital drudgery and so I felt that the better part of this bargain was on my side.

KONGOYESI COMES "TO GREET" AND TO PROFFER SERVICES IN THE FUTURE EXPLORATION AS GUIDE

Kongonyesi came to say goodbye with apologies that he could not accompany me down to the airstrip since his responsibilities of working his garden would require him to leave directly for the work there. But he wanted to remind me of one request he had made last time and add to it another. He had asked for a harmonica, and I had looked for but never found one. He asked if I could also search for a melodica, since that would complete the series of instruments I have been delivering out here with each trip. This is the little flute-like wind instrument with a keyboard with finger holes. Does anyone have a clue where I might get an instrument that has been as obsolete as the "penny whistle" for kids that have grown up on computer generated bleeps?

Since I had Kongonyesi's wish list he wanted me to know that he understood mine. We will hunt *mingi mingi, la prochaine fois*, of course, if only I can get the rifles and *cartouches* and the permits to try. Well the bongos out there are worth the effort, if only I can get to them. But, that is not all. He said through interpretation that he knew I wanted to explore the River of Mystery. He was prepared to outfit a group of stalwarts to undertake this mission with me and act as guide, especially since I was the one with this marvelous device that they had all been talking about, that told where you were from the artificial stars. They thought that I had planned for this in advance by hanging them right over Assa, rather like the Christmas star. So the River Assa and the "Big Hole" beyond Gwane are on my adventure travel plans. Such a trip would be a first time exploration for me and perhaps for anyone, just like the first ascent of the tepuys of Amazonas. I hope you will be reading about these explorations in the not-too-distant future. Kongonyesi left with new shoes. I still have the shoes I am wearing. I have plans for those. The old leper has lost two more toes from his senseless feet.

Others have already done an inventory on what little remains on my person on this final morning. My "mascot" Sasa is now nearly always at my heels, virtually strutting in my shadow. He is saying "Ba-Bab-Ba" to others to call attention to his elevated status in life as my unofficial aide de camp and wearing his celebrity dark glasses with which better to scan the crowd. When we rounded a *Rauwolfia* bush, he saw that we were alone and there were no others to be a security threat to his charge, or to witness the request he was going to make. He tugged on my sleeve, and started tugging on his tattered tee shirt, then pointed to his feet that have the splayed out station of the cretin's constant stance. He has never had so much as sandals, and has had only this one shirt since I have known him. The shades are the one item he has coveted more than anything in life, but now back to basics. He seemed to say, "You are going back to the land of tee shirts and shoes. Here I am the lowest of the low in the farthest African outpost beyond the end of any supply line. What are you going to do about that?"

The Lipiodal has certainly improved Sasa's ingenuity, industriousness and persistence! Again, I shrug as if to say that there is only so much I have to give. Sasa smiles broadly, and claps his hands. With his perfect cretinous delight, he readjusts his glasses, and bursts out with a chorus of "Ba, Bab, Ba, Ba, Bah!" I am sure that one meant "*Merci mingi!*"

I am called from the theatre, where I am trying to add the last chapters and charge the battery for the last time. Three families requested their portraits, for which everyone gathered to display their kids, best clothes, and anything that looks like it was manufactured somewhere, no matter what it is—like a castoff broken plastic toy (**Figures 25 & 29**). One call is to come to breakfast the final time, prepared by our "cooker" to send us off. As I walk back over, I am besieged. Sasa will not let me carry even so much as the computer D/C adapter cord, but marches proudly holding it high over head. A dozen groups are awaiting their pictures to be taken. The wonders of photography have been well-learned from *Bwana*.

BWANA, CHIEF PORTRAIT ARTIST OF ASSA

With the APB going out to *Bwana* to do his duty as a portrait artist, interrupting the call to breakfast, comes a crisis. At the rate of accumulation of people for their official "sittings," a military airdrop of film bricks would be an inadequate stock for even my usual ample supply. But, worse, I had packed my bags, including the small Denver General Western Regional Trauma Symposium bag, in which I had placed my camera, and all other valuables, and all the mail for which I am the postmaster general of the entire literate population of the Assa region. I was carrying the computer, now charged, to put into this carry-on bag, and to take out the camera for my photographic chores. I returned to my room, to discover that my door was—well, not quite locked—it was jammed. Since I packed, several people must have come to weigh the bag for the flight. If my load weighed little, they could pack the plane with more rice and palm oil—this stuff is expensive in Nyankunde, you know! In leaving my room, they pulled the door—which had never quite shut—and to force it shut, they had pulled it past "true" so it was now warped into a stuck position and would neither open nor close.

The panic from would-be photographic models occasioned the first concerted scramble I had witnessed in Assa since my hunts on previous visits. Once, after we killed a huge Cape buffalo, people seemed to materialize from the bush as if by magic. They volunteered as porters in a long train of moving buffalo parts to Assa to claim a share of the booty from the bush. This morning, a dozen assembled around the door to try to bend it and pry it open. It looked like the door was about to splinter. The senior and junior "cookers" ran around outside with a machete, and within a very short time, had pried out the louvered glass from the window, so they could get in to push from the inside. The heavy random beating on both sides of the door probably neutralized controlled movement in any one direction. This assault certainly stressed the structure of the wood itself. Then, by random chance, one side was pushing while the other side was pulling, and the door burst open, unhinged!

No one seemed interested in the door and its destruction any longer. They did reinsert the glass plates into the louvers, however, to keep any others from noticing how quickly this break-in had been accomplished. They quickly guided me to my carry-on bag to fetch my camera and the one remaining roll of film. I brought it outside, and one after another the subjects tried to jump into everyone else's picture frame and to exclude all the interlopers from their own. For one picture they wanted me surrounded by them, causing a struggle over who would take the picture. The risks and benefits on either side were formidable. They wanted to handle the big Nikon N 8008 and see how it was possible for so many people to get into the wide-angle lens of this very modern looking and expensive device. If someone were the photographer, then he could not be in the picture. Nevertheless, they wanted to do both. Sasa strutted out in front of the group. Then everyone swarmed around me making sure they were next to me, while covering me from view entirely. The black faces swallowed up the white one, a common occurrence in this area of Africa.

I called to Bodo, the other adult cretin, who is much less coordinated than Sasa, but can hear a little, even though mute. He staggered over in his bark cloth loincloth. I said to the others that Bodo and Sasa were also citizens so they should make room for them in the picture. After it had been taken, I gave Bodo a packet containing the socks, toothbrush, toothpaste, and minor toiletries from the kit from my long overnight British Airways flight nearly three weeks ago. He toddled off to cherish his new prize. I used up the last of the film taking a picture of Sasa in his shades, standing proudly upright to his full three-foot height, fiercely holding my carry-on bag with all my valuables, next to Bodo, who was sitting on a rock sporting new blue socks to go with his bark cloth loincloth!

When I first visited Assa, no one understood photography. They denied that the pictures that I distributed showed images of themselves, although they recognized the likenesses of others. There are no "looking glasses" in Assa. At first they were curious about how the "little animal" had crawled into the two dimensions of the paper they were holding and would turn it around and look at the back side. They would laugh uproariously at a picture of a pair of them, saying, "That person looks a lot like Tanda," for example, but would deny that the other person could be they. "No, that cannot be, since I am over here!" Only after later trips, with lots of photographs, had they grown accustomed to the idea of images of themselves and other things on a flat surface. They understood that there was some miracle (hard to explain, either then or now, to them, or to me) which freezes an instant of time to be lived again later in the memory, now burned onto this little piece of paper.

Now they are not only used to it but they have a high demand, now close to insatiable, to throw themselves in front of any lens pointed anywhere. They will pose automatically when they see a camera, since they know that *Bwana* will raise it to his eye, and then the miracle happens. A year or two later we may see the results. For that reason, I took quite a few candid pictures from the hip when they were not posing. This is a little trick they have not yet caught on to. I left disposable cameras with JM on each trip. He gave one to MAF pilot Don in the CAR with a letter for me. I received neither the letter nor the camera to send his pictures back. So JM now has my disposable flash camera, and has carried it for me to return with now.

I am no longer the only one with a camera. André and Émile have simple autofocus cameras. I assure you I am the only one with film. I have exhausted my film supply. I did my best at the morning's photo review and tried to retreat to breakfast. There is one more item of note on the photography issue. Pastor Bule and JM had a folder of photographs (as all of them now seem to after my many trips and deliveries of many different pictures). There is a picture of Mrs. Pierson over age 90 in some Pennsylvania nursing home, very feeble and being propped up in front of a birthday cake. She was the wife of Papa Piesey, and the first European missionary woman in this area. The portrait that interests them most is of a spray of flowers on a shiny bronze funeral casket being carried into a Cadillac hearse, with a date and a note on the back explaining that this was Mrs. Pierson's funeral. The little kids came back to that photo again and again, and each looked longingly at these big and fancy shiny objects—all of them much finer than any things they had seen anywhere in their lives. When it was explained that this was a funeral and that casket was buried in the ground with Mrs. Pierson, they were baffled. "Why would anyone take anything half so fine, and make all this huge expense, just to bury the whole thing in the ground?"

Well. . . ., it is not at all easy to explain!

AN EMOTIONAL MOMENT, TOO BUSY TO BE WALLOWED IN, BUT WITH A TOUCHING SYMBOLIC "RECESSIONAL"

Last night we had a dinner, not at all unlike the breakfast that we had today, i.e. there would be no *petit dejeuner* when the "cookers" had turned out the best of their (only) menu for us—a heaping bowl of rice with a lot of gravy with both *zigba* and the last of Assa's slow-moving chickens. Our visit has put a real selective pressure on the slow runners among the fowl of the area. Half the chickens here when I arrived have been eaten. Over time, we may well improve the speed of the breeders that remain.

As it could be our last supper, we invited Kazima and JM to join us. André made his final rounds in the bush village to gather up intelligence and gifts to be carried to Nyankunde. These gifts included some "bush meat," some unidentifiable smoked "*viandes*" of some species best left unspecified. When we were here alone with JM and Kazima, I asked them if they had anything to add to what André and I had picked up on our own regarding the troubles, both in 1997 and last month. When we arrived, we asked about the news of what has been happening in Assa. They said they would prefer to wait for us to be rested, and they would tell us much later so as not to dilute their joy of that moment. They didn't want to recall the unhappy events to upset either us or them. We are now rested, and I think that I will be comfortable hearing the truth that can be gleaned from those who had so directly suffered these hardships. I felt that sharing the sad stories might help them in knowing they were not alone in their troubles. I had already pursued a fairly rigorous journalistic track in confirming the details as I heard them from multiple sources. Were there any other facts they would want me to know?

The response was interesting. They said, "Some problems have a way of finding us and we do not have to go looking for them, nor recounting these troubles when there may be others ahead that we should be preparing for. We do not want you to worry about that which has already passed, and which, thank God, we have survived to do our duty by the present when we must look forward to a better future."

Our breakfast was held on a similar upbeat note. A large crowd gathered at the door with a thick sheaf of mail to be carried by this postmaster general to the outside world. I was going to foot the freight. There were letters to New Zealand, long shot hopes for pen pals who would spot them their school fees, and large packs of mail to the Downings and distant family members. These missives were to be sent in several directions. Two-thirds of the addresses I do not know. Lazunga had been hounding me for a week for one of the two envelopes I have carried here, and I had put Diane Downing's address on this envelope and stamped it with the one of the two Kenyan stamps I had carried for such mail. I told him three times that this would have to carry all the letters to the Downings so I would put it in the envelope with the others. No, he would take the envelope, and bring it back with the letter. I had him carry the letter to me, and then handed him the envelope reluctantly to have him insert his secretive letter. He hid the letter as he quickly stuffed the envelope, as if I was going to peek at his Bangala requests and know that he is trying to dig the same well in two places. This would not come as a surprise to me, of course. I held the sheaf of letters in my hand to follow his into the same envelope. Nonetheless, he quickly licked and sealed it so as to make his the solitary request that would be carried out in the one envelope and with the one stamp that Assa had which was available for this communal task.

I walked out the door to check on the two items that were my highest priority in this trip. The number one objective you hold in hand—*Out of Assa: Heart of the Congo*—the record of my experiences here that I have not been casual about gathering carefully and reporting to you. The second is the completed set of data forms from the linguistic anthropology study in a white cardboard box. I looked at Yuni. Yuni, who always laughs when she talks to me in her four English phrases, was not laughing, but looked away. I came over and gave her a big hug. Think of all she has been through! She squirmed away, and busied herself in picking up the box and perched it gracefully on the top of her head where it rested until we reached the airstrip. I never saw it being supported by her hands. She walked gracefully and never once did I see it slip or fall, but there were quite a few tears falling, unheeded.

Ginale, the mature, pretty, good-hearted theatre nurse, awaited me, with her hand outstretched when she saw Yuni. She turned away quickly to run. When I caught her, I gave her a hug, which embarrassed her no end, not so much because of this very European and non-African public display of affection, but because I had caught her crying (**Figure 31**).

THE RECESSIONAL:
I AM FOLLOWED BY TWO SPECIAL PORTERS
AS THE PARADE WINDS DOWN TO THE ASSA AIRSTRIP

Without a word spoken, everyone waited for me to begin the walk to the airstrip. This moment would have been a quite emotional scene except for an urgent comedy. The garden tractor with its trailer, like everything else in Assa, starts—if it starts at all—only with a concerted push. Kati was on the seat holding the steering wheel—a twisted vine wrapped in a circle around the steering post. Two youngsters were busy pumping up the right trailer tire, which seems to have a leaky valve. Therefore it only holds air for about the distance we would be going. Travel is interrupted by intervals of pumping. The end of the stem was tightly wrapped with a piece of cut inner tube to hold whatever air could be put in the tire during its "breathing spell." The whole group assembled behind the tractor and trailer and pushed, as Kati popped the clutch, each time bringing the whole group of pushers to a shuddering halt as the engine did not kick over or cough. We came to the little incline down the hill and got a good running start down the slope, but it did not start then either. It was only on the uphill slope that the engine coughed and started. All the pushers, some of whom had knocked their teeth hard against all the tarp-wrapped forest products lashed down on the trailer during the false starts, clambered aboard for the ride to the airstrip. *Bwana* was already ahead of the parade as the engine came to life. André came rushing up 10 minutes after his forty-seventh dental extraction, 10 minutes before leaving. He was wearing his Azande robes, carrying a small cross-bow given to him to defend his garden from marauding antelope, now that he has been stripped of any more effective weaponry.

For the first time since leaving the broken door, I chuckled. I remembered leaving from the Rockies on my October elk hunt when I had gimpily arrived at the pick-up truck in which all the camp gear and elk venison had been packed for the return trip to Denver. There, one of my hunting companions, Gene Moore, had taken all his valuables, including wallet, cellular phone, checkbook, binoculars, camera and GPS—almost an identical cargo as mine now, and had put it in a backpack that was tossed onto the back of the pick-up truck. I drove down to Denver with a left leg found by subsequent x-ray to be fractured by the horse that had reared and kicked me high up in Charity Basin in the deep snow. Somewhere in the night, the backpack had left the pick-up truck to be struck by an 18-wheeler and to be recovered in fragments identified by the police through pieces of the checkbook. The police had called Gene's wife Sarah at home and asked her, "Do you know where your husband is? We found the remains of his backpack and a bloody knife." She was startled and thought for a moment that Gene had been kidnapped or killed. She did not realize that her husband was safe and sound until we arrived at Gene's house with an intact husband for proof. Gene had carefully centralized his valuables for safekeeping. So had I, coincidentally, in the Denver General Trauma Symposium bag, which now was securely held triumphantly in the very dirty hands of an unsteady cretin. He was strutting behind me proudly in his new designer shades, and wobbling on bare feet under the 4-kg load of my most valuable surviving possessions, including this computer, equal to the net worth of the Assa District. Sasa could not be prouder of his importance, and would utter "Ba, BaBa, Ba" if no one had noted his rank and station in this parade for a while.

Yuni followed Sasa with the balanced box of linguistic anthropology data gracefully turning around on her head (**Figure 32**). Neither of them had a clue what was so significant about their burdens, Yuni no more nor less than Sasa, but each knew that their burden was important to me, so they were very deadly earnest about carrying out their roles on this short journey and farewell. Behind them in the long queue of this pied-piper parade was a gathering of people who had come from huts or hospital in a serpentine trailer behind the vanguard. As we passed some who had stayed to work their gardens, they had all stopped to stand at the roadside with their hands outstretched to be shaken in passing, down to the most solemn of the toddlers, each muttering, "*Merci, merci mingi!*"

And then, there were the kids. They were about 30 5- to 10-year-old children. They were squirming with eagerness, since they had obviously been over-rehearsed. We had not yet pulled alongside them yet when they got a drop on the protocol and, altogether now, "*Merci* DOCTOR GLENN!" I was the one looking away this time, as they said it again and again embarrassing me more than I had Ginale.

I hurried down the trail faster than Sasa could keep up. I got to the airstrip ahead of the group behind me, happy to have outrun the crowd since now I could find a nice quiet spot in the bush to pee. Little privacies are highly valued when you have been over-treated to the star reception. I rounded the tall reeds to find—-Oh, no—two hundred people!

How they got there I do not know, but they obviously navigate their trails better than I do with the help of the GPS. They all were simply standing, most in the hot sun, and a few under the shelter, just waiting and looking at me furtively. We arrived well before the expected 11:00 AM arrival of the pilot from Nyankunde. The sky around us was clear. We have no functional "phonie." The mission's radio phone was wrapped up in a box carried by Kazima to go back to get its microphone fixed, and probably some cannibalized wire will have to be replaced before it can be made to work again, whenever it is brought back to Assa.

LA PROCHAINE FOIS:
AWAITING THE NEXT FLIGHT

Why are all these people out here in the hot sun of broad daylight? There were always so many activities for which this precious daylight should be used, gardening, typing or color linguistics studies, for example. Many of these had been called off for lack of all this daylight that was now being squandered wholesale as if we were in northern Finland in the summer. This is just the rare arrival of a flight to take us away. They would waste a lot of time chasing airplanes if they did this regularly. I asked Inikpio, "When was the last flight before my arrival?"

"There was one in early March for a brief stop, but none for a year or more before that."

"When will be the next?" I asked.

"When will you be coming again?" he asked back.

WE WAITED, AND WAITED, AND WAITED

We sat. Jean Marco and I sat silently next to each other, for at least 45 minutes without a sound, just appreciating each other's company for the first time we have been together in the bush this trip. I did not want to disappoint the people by turning to something selfish like pulling out the computer to type up the last chapter, so at first I took pictures until I ran out of film (**Figure 33**). Then I shook hands with each. It is now two hours into the afternoon and no one is making a move to leave. A young girl went away and came back with a plastic jug on her head with water and a cup. André asked her where she had found it. She replied, " I found it in the rock." Somehow she found a spring in the *munga* we are sitting on, and had brought water from it. It tasted like iron.

I had an idea for community entertainment. I popped out the GPS, and showed them where the Assa area landmarks were and how far they were away from many things including my home, and in which direction. The gadget stimulated their wonderment for another hour until I looked for shade. There would be no way we could make a return to Nyankunde in daylight by VFR. Perhaps the pilot had set down in a rainstorm somewhere else, and would be coming to overnight in Assa or in Nebobongo. We had no idea, of course, and did not want to leave in the event that the whole parade had to return to get back down to the airstrip quickly, a long roundtrip considering the porters.

While we waited André and I had a prolonged discussion about the use of the money I would leave for Azande development. I pointed out that the gifts continuously asked for by individuals would not be forthcoming, but there would be aid for sustainable starter projects that would return to the community what was invested in it. Lazunga insisted that there would be a return, all right, he could return the moneys that I gave him on my last trip since they were still in the case that he had buried to keep it from the soldiers. This is almost identical to the buried talents of silver. They could relate to that from their Bible School. They then had what could be called a community planning session, during which I backed away and watched. Later, I pulled out my notepad and wrote a bit of my last Assa-based serial letter. By 4:00 PM, everyone realized we were going to be spending another night in Assa, so we would be going back. Nevertheless, no one moved until I did.

I stood up, feeling some remorse about having fought so hard to conserve and use daylight for the duration of my stay, yet I had frittered away a whole day's worth of the best daylight we had yet seen. We learned later that there were such rainstorms that no flight could leave Nyankunde. Three planes tried to take-off but turned back because of the weather.

SO, NOT YET OUT OF ASSA
WELCOME BACK!

My absence from Assa was certainly brief. "*Karibu*" (Welcome) was hardly necessary. It crossed my mind to wonder if the plane was coming at all. Good thing I had my trusty GPS to find my way back to Nyankunde on a bicycle without tires and a broken chain. Right!

**THE RETURN TO ASSA AND AN ACCOUNTING OF WHAT HAS
TRANSPIRED BEFORE A SECOND "GO" AT DEPARTURE**

July 21-22, 1998

"When we asked how soon you could return, we did not know it would be so soon!" said the first person we encountered on the path as I re-entered the rainy season overgrowth of the path leading back toward Assa station. I was not at all unhappy about the return. I did think that it was somewhat difficult for the Assa residents to sustain the emotional pitch of parting for very long. It might have been better to quietly steal away now that we have had a sustained farewell. We will see how far *that* proposal might take us.

Without the "phonie," now, again, balanced on a head bobbing behind me as I made my way up the path, we had no idea what had happened to the pilot or what plans there were for the next try. I worried that this delay would compromise my future plane connections. "Romans 8:28," said André.

I said, "Now we can finish those last protocols," and told him there are few spots I would rather be stranded. I felt sorry for the remaining chickens that had so brief a reprieve. OK, I had not come "Out of Assa"— I was still in Africa, was I not? And, then it happened. Right in front of me!

**THERE IS ALWAYS SOMETHING NEW
COMING OUT OF AFRICA**

André spotted it first, while I heard a swoosh of wings to our right. Almost as if I were hoping for a sign of some sort, it was dropped in front of me like the Boomslang and the frog I encountered on my solitary walk upstream in Zimbabwe last year. Could it get any better? Here is the next African vignette played out, it seemed, for the benefit of the naturalist of whom the principals were totally oblivious.

A *Gwan* (Pazande) had swooped into a tree just off the path to our right and hit something in the branches. We looked up to see the thing "wonderful to see" as André had called it. This big and beautiful eagle, a large raptor that might have been an immature Crowned Eagle (*Stephanoaetus coronatus*), although I have never seen one previously around Assa, had landed in the tree within our plain view. What was that writhing commotion? The eagle had hit a large green arboreal snake in the equatorial canopy, the deadly Green Mamba.

A magnificent raptor had killed a deadly snake overhead, like the symbol of the serpent and the eagle in the Mexican flag and Teotihuacán mythology. Here was the real thing, not played out for our entertainment, but for lunch! For another of those magic African moments, I was a privileged participant/observer in life as it is without explanations, apologies, or excuses. This event was a passing instant of success for one at the extinguishing of another species competing, not for our attention, but for life.

Each of the others in the queue of those behind me confirmed first the type of snake, of which there was no doubt in translation, but no one could add an English name to the *Gwan* they all agreed it was. I shot another exposure as the eagle lifted up and away with its prize using André's small camera which I had loaded with my last roll of print film. The picture will probably vanish into the distance in the frame of the photo, even when enlarged, but hardly ever from my mind!

The next bit of natural history we encountered along the trail was of immediate use to them and the next thereafter was already being used. We soon spotted a green plant (looking a bit like the Neotropical exotic lantana I had uprooted in the Pilanesberg crater in South Africa) that André identified as one of the two kinds of *Nzawa* that grows in the bush around Assa. We encountered one of the second kind later. It was much less user-friendly than the first since it has fiberglass-like hairs on its leaves that cause irritation if touched. A few steps farther along the trail we encountered a woman walking toward the Assa hospital with a poultice of the *Nzawa* on her left maxilla. She appeared to be suffering from a suppurative sinusitis that had the whole side of her face and orbit swollen up. When she opened her mouth, it seemed to have started from a dental abscess in the left upper molars. It was too swollen to see what was cause and what effect. This time, "bush pharmacy" was applied when needed. We made a few cuttings of the *Nzawa* plant to go back to Nyankunde's greenhouse to track down the identity and the ethnobotany of this *Nzawa*. It is used commonly among the Azande who practice the healing arts around Assa.

AFTERNOON DELIGHTS:
A FREE LAST LOOK AROUND ASSA

What a unique perspective! My chores had been as done as I could make them. This reprieve after all the plans for departure meant that I could use the last of the light of day to wander back and look, almost at leisure, at the things around Assa. I had not time for this leisurely walkabout while I was trying to juggle the three main balls of this book, the linguistic study, and the medical work.

Since I had not been out bush-bashing as I always had on prior visits in the dawn hunts, I had missed some of the pleasures of the natural history of the Assa setting, being confined to base by military maneuvers. I walked back to see a beautiful flower I had passed on the march when I had no film in the camera. It was a flower with a dependent bean, looking a bit like a kind of *Heliconia*, yet the internal color of what I now know to be *"kpe ndunda"* in Pazande. I am told that a cucumber-like fruit grows from this plant. Once, one of the men cut a meter-long section of a vine in a demonstration for me. Then, pouring water as if from a garden hose, he took a drink from the falling stream like hoisting a wine skin. The liquid tasted a bit starchy, but it was clear and potable—if not Perrier, certainly better than thirst, out in the bush.

I tried to hook my computer for the last supply of energy. Inikpio helped me reconnect there. I walked out with him on a bit of an ethnobotanic tour. Since he had been a young boy sent out into the bush at Banda along with André by Papa Dix to go look for *Rauwolfia*, I had him pose by such a bush. He and I then went down the trail to a very large tree, next to a kapok, which I recognized as a kind of *Ficus*—a fig—whose bark had been stripped to as tall a height as a man could reach, even if he got a boost from a friend. "They strip the bark, and use it to make a cure for abdominal pain and diarrhea," explained Inikpio. This is different from the plant that Kongonyesi used as a treatment for David Downing's diarrhea on their road trip to Ndamana—so there are drugs of first and second choice available out here in this pharmacopoeia.

On our morning parade to the airstrip, I noticed a small thatched structure with a fire pit in the center of it that did not look like a cooking place. There was a bicycle wheel with the pedal and sprocket attached. At last light I admired this Bronze Age picture of the blacksmith's art, the metallurgical power to smelt, and deliver the hidden metals buried in the earth. Pastor Bule turns out to be the alchemist. He came out to mimic the maneuvers he makes to get the fire hot enough and the wheel pumping air through the charcoal to superheat it. There, looking for all the world like a very proper anvil, is a piece of the *chemin de fer*, a section of rail with the flange that is spiked to the sleepers serving as the base. "Under the spreading chestnut (kapok, in this case) tree, the village smithy stands."

To view one other bit of Bule's handiwork, and the reason he was brought here by Pastor Piesey, we stopped to look at the master drum. It looked different to me. It was still in its old spot under its own thatched roof, but it had a kind of black paint on it, and it looked lower. Inikpio explained. When they finished the new church building, they had even built a "tower" that could be a "belfry," if only there were a church bell. In Assa, an old steel wheel hangs from a tree out front. When clanged with a tire iron, this wheel serves as the church or school bell. What better place for the drum, than to hoist this early master work of Bule up and into the belfry. You can imagine this daylong project by the whole community. First they had to get the drum out of its thatched building on rollers. Then they cut off the beautifully carved legs from this masterpiece. This huge drum was produced from one original master log, with the slit carved carefully. One side (the parent) had a different thickness, and therefore, pitch, from the other side (the child). It was a Zandeland Stradivarius. I would think it ought to have been treated more kindly. They manhandled it into slings and hauled it up the side of the church to install in its belfry.

The moment arrived. Bule stood like the maestro with his two batons, and with the tympani player's stylized runs and flourishes began to beat out the message for all to hear that the church was complete now with the master drum having been hoisted to its rightful place in the belfry.

But not all heard it. The acoustics were all wrong. It seems the lower register tones of the big drum that always frustrate me in getting the sound on my cassette tape, are resonated by the earth on which it stands, in the rocky *munga* hill, and it lost this amplification by being hoisted up high off the ground. The effort was a failure. What is worse, it modified the drum. The loss of its stout legs changed the tone, and the scratches required a kind of "paint job." The community made a decision. The drum would have to be moved back into its former place of honor on the rocky rise next to the church leaving the belfry of the church empty, once again.

Well, not quite empty. What would you think would be issuing forth out of the belfry tonight as I passed at twilight? To quote a not quite original cliché which, honestly, I do not believe I am making up for the very first time in history—my musings seem to have stirred up the *bats in the belfry!*

I returned to my bare mattress, and the nubbin of candle that had been replaced after it had already been salvaged after our departure, as the inexorable dark had turned out the lights on my last evening in Assa. I had literally eaten them out of house and home, and our supper was light. It was a delightful single dish, sliced fresh and juicy pineapple, otherwise my favorite part of breakfast. I saved out my Nike running shoes where I could find them by feel, for the ceremonial last run of the ARRC before the "colors are retired" and the "company stands down" in the morning.

33 *OUT OF ASSA*

THE LAST DAWN RUN IN ASSA BIRDSONG:
THE TEMPORARY RETIREMENT OF THE ARRC

July 22, 1998

And, so it came to pass. Passing just short of six miles in 39:27 at a very brisk pace in the damp cool dawn, the ARRC, down to its hard corps of two runners, and the faithful, well-broken-in equipment of the Red Ball Jets and "first marathon" Nikes, passed into the history of the annals of *Mazori Wazungu* (the *"white man's madness"* = someone running while no one or thing is chasing). So, the Assa Road Runner's Club, a subsidiary of no other local organization, and quite an exotic import, was decommissioned.

I regret to say that the passing of this institution was not witnessed by anyone other than the two participants. No extensive ceremony accompanied the final run. The run was also recorded in no photographic or GPS-annotated record, and no higher technology than the somewhat obsolete aforementioned footwear was involved. Once more, *sic transit gloria mundi.*

THIS TIME, THE DRILL IS FOR REAL!

How was I to know when I had written in those lines—"This is not a dress rehearsal" that the ceremony we went through with tight throats and averted eyes was just that—a dress rehearsal! This time it was more efficient, less emotional (until the final take-off, perhaps) and also a bit more opportunistic. A flourish of activities at the scale came back with the news that the *Bwana's* nearly empty suitcase is now down to 1.6 kg so there may be room for another *bidon* of palm oil.

242

PARADE #2 TO ASSA AIRSTRIP

Just before parade #2 down to the airstrip, complete with the push-start of the garden tractor, and a repeat of the same drill, let me run through a bare bones set of closing numbers. We accomplished a lot in my brief stay here:

21 major surgical operations under general anesthesia
47 dental extractions under local anesthesia
33 chapters of *Out of Assa*
20 completed linguistic anthropology protocols
80 kg of pharmaceuticals and surgical
instruments delivered
11 medical personnel trained or encouraged
$128 in surgical fees generated from OR
A "Project Zandeland Development Fund" established.

The emotion of the moment was not necessarily one of nostalgic poignancy. As I headed up the parade rerun, I was handed a note from an absentee, once again requesting full-ride scholarship support. It was rather business-like this time, with a few more letters tucked in and some parting details conveyed. We passed under a tree that was dropping the date-like fruits called "Ngbandi" in Pazande, which at one time were used to produce a vegetable cooking oil. This was a tree like the one I had seen at André's sister's house at the ceremony for their father. It was explained to me without my understanding that this was the oil for our dinner rather than the more usual palm oil.

We arrived 15 minutes early. The plane piloted by Brad Weston soon appeared in the sky about six minutes late on his ETA. This was only his second MAF landing in Assa. We loaded up the pod and the plane with the over-abundant forest products (including one black plastic trash bag about which André was quite protective). I got in first, and strapped into the copilot's seat, and opened the side window. The others also said their emotional goodbyes, especially Émile Zola with his big family who had seen him return as "the man" after leaving Assa as "a boy" eight years ago with no clear idea if or when they would see him again—after these fortuitous reunion weeks.

OUT OF ASSA:
HEART OF THE CONGO

I shook several more hands, then waved from the open window. I looked up at the end of the turnaround "taxi" part of the airstrip. There stood the old leper, with his unblinking face staring over at the plane, resplendent in his new shirt, leaning on his stick, barefoot with only a few stubs of toes, standing on the *munga*. It had taken a lot of time and effort for him to hobble down this far, and I had not seen him before during the parade and the aircraft arrival and loading. JM came around as pilot Brad was about to shout "*Attention!* Clear Prop!" to be the last to shake my hand.

I looked away from the open window and down at my feet. I loosened my seat belt and darted down to the floor as JM waited with his hand outstretched.

When I popped back up to retighten my belt, I reached out to JM, and said, "Today, I do not walk; I will fly. I no longer will need these!" And, pointing to the old man, I dropped my shoes in JM's hands. Except for the old man with leprosy, whose facial expression never changes, they were all crying. They were not alone.

And, so, I am now *Out of Assa*, again, barefoot.

PART III

ZIM/ZAM: SAFARI FROM HARARE

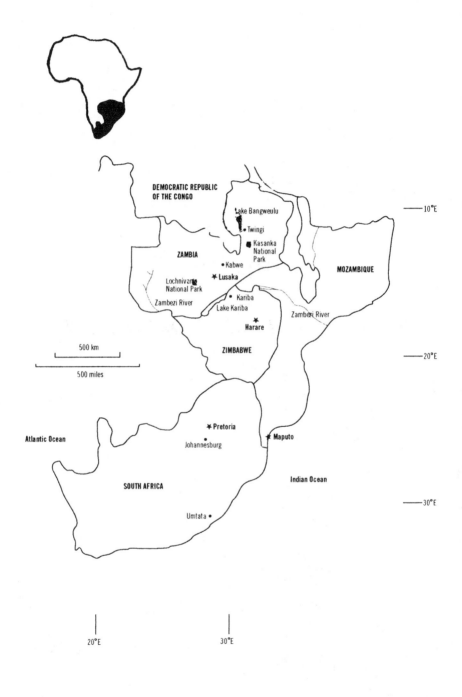

DEMOCRATIC REPUBLIC
OF THE CONGO

Lake Bangweulu

Twingi

ZAMBIA

Kasanka
National
Park

Kabwe

Lochnivar
National Park

Lusaka

MOZAMBIQUE

Zambezi River

Kariba

Lake Kariba

Zambezi River

Harare

500 km

500 miles

ZIMBABWE

10°E

20°E

Pretoria

Maputo

Johannesburg

Atlantic Ocean

Indian Ocean

SOUTH AFRICA

30°E

Umtata

20°E

30°E

34 BACK TO NEBOBONGO

OUT OF ASSA ON A WING AND A PRAYER

July 22, 1998

So what if I am barefoot. "I do not need shoes to fly." Brad Westom bounced us off the Assa strip and we pulled up in a swooping curve over the *Zala* marsh, scattering birds below us. "Would you like a picture?" I would! So we made a sentimental low-level pass over the Assa station and I snapped away as the hospital patients and the staff were still waving at the sky.

As we leveled off, Brad gestured at me with both hands off the yoke, and pointed to the trim tabs. "OK!" I responded eagerly as I took him up on his offer, up to about 9,500 feet. He directed me by saying, "Try for about 150°," and added, "Stay out of clouds, though!" So, he turned around and gestured to the "pax" in back with both palms up. André and Sonny Mwembo applauded and Émile Zola fell asleep. I went swooping along on a cloud-weaving pattern to avoid the big tropical thunderheads I scraped with the starboard wing. They went on up to 20,000 feet. Flying is fun, but is demanding if it is not second nature. In the haze I had to keep my eye on the artificial horizon. I did my best to follow the rules and to *not* use the GPS for navigation, but tried to fly in the right direction off the compass headings and bearings marked on the chart. Airspeed 135 mph meant that we had about 10-mph tailwind advantage on ground speed. Brad did some paper work, as I wiggled my free toes. I planned *not* to get out at Nebobongo to stagger around in the mud on my way to the *choo*.

When we were close to Nebobongo, Brad pointed two fingers toward himself, and took the yoke, putting it into about 5° nose-down for the glide slope. He had changed the trim tabs, which made fighting the yoke a lot less laborious. You could almost fly the plane with the two wheels on the trim tabs without touching the yoke after take-off as long as the aircraft was trimmed correctly. In that sense, it is almost identical to sailing. You can almost let the craft fly itself, and nod off. The only reason to concentrate is to be thinking about landmarks ahead and doing the radio communications and the paper work. What would bug me about the piloting business is the long spell between landings in which you are flying with a finger on the yoke fighting off boredom before phrenetic busyness. When the critical business of landing on approach over treetops in turbulent air is complete, when everyone else thinks your work is done, you become the busiest, weighing freight, refueling, adjusting the loading of cargo, and doing essential ground checks.

ARRIVAL IN NEBOBONGO

As we rolled to the hangar, the fuel barrels were rolled out for us. Brad supervised the adding of 80 liters into each wing tank, through the coffee filter that doubles as a fuel filter. A local pastor requested passage to Nyankunde. To make room for him and his 30-kg of baggage we had to jettison a large amount of the "forest products." I seem to be the local UPS, cash-paying customer/supplier for the rice, salt and palm oil for Nyankunde, to supply a large profit margin for them, at my loss. My passengers were unhappy to have the bulk of their "forest products" left here, although it would be coming to Nyankunde on the next flight on Friday in 48 hours at no cost to them other than what I would already be paying. Émile said he was not sure he had *confiance* in the *pilote*, even though he seemed to have enough in me to sleep through my cloud weaving. That, however, did not involve major economics.

Despite the early return of their prepaid "forest products," they were still whining about their not coming in covered with glory and excess palm oil, the currency of the exploiter of the extractive reserves of the bush. André picked up the black plastic trash bag, and came back to the pod with it and saved that out of the stuff that had been taken out. He would not fly without that, and would rather stay than separate from that bag, so it came along with us.

I could not get out of the plane because of my bare feet. I watched as the delicate negotiations to let the pastor board in place of about 120-kg of valuable raw products. Émile was still worried that he was going to lose the family wealth. With an audience of a lot of little kids waving into the dust cloud caused by the prop wash, we rolled out and with a few bounces cleared the close-in palm trees in taking off from Nebobongo, for Nyankunde, our home base.

I marked some GPS fixes and made notes about the condition of airstrips for future reference. I also marked the Ituri River and the Uele River near Bandada at a fix where there was a road. I heard from Brad Westom about the spectacular Ibina River, tributary of the Ituri River through a deep and spectacular gorge, and also looked up on the maps at the junction of the Assa River and the Bomu, which is rather sketchy, for good reason.

RETURN TO NYANKUNDE, THE "BUSH MEAT" BUST, GREET ERIC SARIN, AND PLAN THE TOUR OF THE SCHOOL OF PUBLIC HEALTH AND TROPICAL MEDICINE, LIVERPOOL CONNECTION

We took off from Nebobongo uneventfully. I settled back on the flight to Nyankunde while Brad and I talked about the navigation. The MAF pilots have always been good to me, letting me extend my hours of airtime with their dependable Cessnas. These planes are both sensitive and quite forgiving to my manipulation. As a return favor I promised to line them all up and do their FAA-required medical exams. We talked about the vast Ituri Forest beneath us as we came over Akokora—one of the pygmy sites near the Newli River. We flew over Epulu where the Okapi Study is opening an airstrip. I would have gone to Epulu this trip if I had insisted on getting more of the pygmy languages for the study that I began in the 1996 series on Kibili and Kilhese at Lolwa. I would also have gone to Mambasa. This town is near the Lolwa Station. I had seen it on the map and got close to it when we took the Dutch-donated Pygmy Project diesel 4X4 driving over rainy season roads over the Ituri River to get back to Nyankunde last time I was here.

I had marked a number of these sites with my GPS with the hope of returning some day. I saw gorgeous narrow canyons with series of waterfalls not that far from Nyankunde. I know that it is harder to get to them on the ground through nearly impenetrable jungle, than by flying a nearly straight course at 118 mph airspeed with a tail wind. We talked about the dead-stick glide slope this aircraft would have if there were a power loss or fuel problem. This entails how much altitude you have and how far that will take you to someplace outside the "endless broccoli" of the great forest which would dismember anything that flew into the canopy. The GPS can give you the quickest regional airstrips to chose from with a push of the button in an emergency, but this region does not have the high density of airfields as you might in Connecticut.

There might be a few roads that have already been marked near villages as possibly wide enough to take a chance at landing. I asked, "How about the river?"

Brad said, "I would prefer the tops of the trees and take my chances with them to any of these rivers. After all, I would not want to make a perfect landing and then get eaten by a croc!"

He had made one trial run at the road they have marked which is a tricky approach and landing so they always check out such unknown spots with someone who has landed there before. He went with one of the other pilots and did accomplish the landing on the road, but upon revving up again, he was on the roll when he had to abort the take-off. Three large bushbuck bolted right out in front of the aircraft and ran toward the plane *down the road.* Another time at one of these strips, he had to wait for over an hour because a pack of chacma baboons just would not take the hint. They stayed out on the strip shrieking to give a warning and threaten off the vintage Cessna Stationair. Collision with them would have sliced up the baboons and damaged the plane.

The recent civil wars interrupted the pilots' plans for their terms on the field because they were all evacuated from Nyankunde. Each family was allowed to carry 40 kg of valuables—the only things they still have—before the army came through on its looting and rampage of killing in the intense fighting in its retreat ahead of the rebels. They lost everything looted from the houses, with a lot of damage to vehicles. All the motorbikes were stolen, which is the usual mode of the pilot's ground transport. There are a few of the Toyota four wheel drive vehicles from "up on the hill" where I stay at the CME Guest House, which were salvaged by a rather clever technique. The wheels were taken off and rolled out into the bush so the vehicle could not be driven, but could only be ransacked.

Most of the MAF families took their photo albums and their other precious keepsakes. I added that this would amount to a bit more than the 40 kg for me. First they went north toward Rethy where the dependants had already been evacuated. They then spirited out the planes ahead of the army. The wretched "customs" bastards in Bunia, even our *bête noire* Umro, had fled to the bush. They were identified with the prior government. They came back after lying low in deep cover, sure they would be killed. When they found out that the new group was every bit as corrupt as the old one, they came back in force to cash in on the newly raised upper limits of what they could skim.

All of the MAF folk who could get out flew to Nairobi where they spent three months, and then many of them took an additional three months of home leave. But the Nyankunde medical personnel had to stay, and the last one out was Ahuka. You will have to hand it to him, since he stayed with the patients in the hospital until the bullets were flying through the wards. Then André, Ahuka and several others scattered over the hills behind the Guest House through about 15 km of bush. André took his stuff and my precious linguistic data kit and hid it in the bush near his shamba. The household possessions that identified him as a hunter, the leopard skin, the *zigba* teeth, and assorted animal skins were all thrown into the latrine along with the elephant ivory. His treasured pump .22 rifle with a scope was tossed from a bridge into the river near Nyankunde as he fled in sheer terror.

Some members of the group escaped by hiring a fishing boat on the lake, formerly Lake Sese Mobutu, but now renamed Lake Albert as it had been in Victoria's time. They actually rowed across to Uganda as storm-tossed refugees right ahead of the gunfire. The MAF hangar was stripped clean, except for the getaway gas in the airplanes they had reserved to escape to Zambia to get them out of harm's way.

ARRIVAL AT NYANKUNDE AMID TWO MAJOR CELEBRATIONS AND "ENTRY FORMALITIES" WHICH ARE THERE TO REMIND US THAT ALL THE GOOD OLD DAYS OF GRAFT AND CORRUPTION ARE NOT ALL IN THE PAST!

We could see the Nyankunde airstrip grass just ahead of the aircraft as we crossed the Ituri River. We circled once around the town to let the group know of our arrival and to clear the strip. As we came in low, there was a large group of people gathered in a field near the airstrip. It was a large funeral, which we buzzed as a distraction to the little kids who could not keep concentrated on the solemnities as we rolled past them on the grass within a few meters. As soon as we pulled up to the hangar, we saw there was a religious meeting going on there as well, with singing and the prayers interrupted by the roar of the engine. But this group would understand. This was the assembled MAF brass since the president of MAF-International was making his first stop on his first African tour hosted by the head of MAF-Africa.

I met both of these gentlemen during a moment when they weren't busy. They were occupied by two further unusual events and the end of their service. They had been talking about me as the kind of support that MAF was designed to give. They were proud of having us roll up just in time to be exhibit A for the president of MAF-International. I could not come out immediately and stayed strapped in until they brought over the dolly for the luggage including André's precious black plastic trash bag. I could then get out and rummage around while standing on the trolley. I was still barefoot and trying to protect my socks from the muddy ground in front of the hangar (**Figure 3**). The word spread around as they saw me coming out in stocking feet that I had done it again, having given away all my shoes. I would have to make an immediate trip to the market in the mud to get something to wear on my feet.

Not surprisingly, there were new "formalities" just instituted this week by a new "government customs official" at Nyankunde. Now why there should be an internal immigration and customs is a little hard to understand, since everything had already been shaken down and extorted at Bunia. But this fellow was excited to see a *Mzungu* getting off the plane, shoes or not. He was contemplating early retirement. His first request was for me to open my suitcase. It got a lot of laughs. At 1.6 kg, all I had left was exposed rolls of film, audiotapes, and a bar of Jean Marco's soap. Everything else that had not been stolen in Bunia had been given away in Assa.

Well, he was not through. The new regulations state that permanent residents of Nyankunde owed $750.00 US paid in cash in US dollars on the spot, and I did not have a visa. Oh, yes I did, and I have been down this route before, you bastards! At this point the good Dr. Mwembo started screaming in French and showing him my perfectly valid visa good for three months through September, but he could already taste $750.00 US dollars crawling up from his pocket onto his taste buds, and he insisted I was a permanent resident. "I am in transit" I explained—my French getting worse as my colleagues' got louder. I am en route to Bunia and out to Nairobi tomorrow.

"Oh but you are staying the night!"

That was his last effort at making a permanent resident out of me. He was shouted down by what was now a large throng of onlookers who were telling us that he was being searched for by the army within the first few days of his appearance here in Nyankunde. He was wanted both for them to discipline and to see if they could not get a piece of this action. He had gone around to each of the missionaries and MAF pilots yesterday, and asked them if they had submitted their census forms. Yes, as it turns out, they had. "No, the short forms!" he said. They had undoubtedly submitted the invalid long forms. Although they cost $200 to submit, they really needed the short form which cost $500 for every household and fortunately, he was the only one who had the short forms. He would be collecting the currency tomorrow or else they would all have to clear out immediately.

I BAIL OUT ANDRÉ, THROUGH BRIBERY
KEEPING HIM OUT OF JAIL, AS HE HELPS ME TO BUY SHOES
WITH WHICH TO EXIT THE CONGO

The newly self-appointed "official" around the back corner of Nyankunde's own MAF hangar was not about to let his prize catch of the day off the hook. He then insisted that he examine the forest products being carried in by my subsidized colleagues. The first thing he wanted to see was the precious black trash bag of André's, the one item he would not leave behind in Nebobongo to arrive on the regular flight on Friday. AHAH!

This is serious! Inside the trash bag was "bush meat." This is the blackened smoked meat from some kill at Assa that was given to André, he says, to be presented to Ahuka as a gift from the families at Assa. I recognized one chunk as a *bodi* haunch, and another as a chunk of what André referred to vaguely as "bush cow." Now I recognize *nyati* (Cape buffalo) on close and personal terms. The chief baggage inspector for this internal flight had determined that the bush meat was from an elephant! MAF pilots said later that he is strictly forbidden to make inspections of the internally cleared baggage. He is doing this inspection only to find what he can plunder and make up infractions that will run up the ticker.

It is obvious to anyone who can see that André has been out poaching elephants, and will go straight to jail. There will be an immediate arrest! But since he cannot arrest him, we will have to get a vehicle to carry him to Bunia— a four-hour trip by road under the best of circumstances. In any event, André is in deep DooDoo!

The Inspector said, "But, in the interest of compassion, for the good works of the *Dentiste*, perhaps if he could just come up with a sum of $750.00 US currency (sounds familiar), all of this could be forgotten right here and now."

André asked, "Where on earth would I come up with that kind of money?"

His tormentor replied, "Well, if you don't come up with it now, you will have to come up with three times as much since the group at Bunia will hit you up for a lot more than I will!"

André asked again, with the earnest serious expression he uses for every one of life's troubles that he has collided with head on, "Oh, sorry! Where do I come up with that kind of money which is more than twice my annual salary?"

"Why, for whatever reason had he not thought about it before?" asked the grafty little bastard—and pointed to the *Mzungu* standing right next to him— who must surely be dripping with US currency. After all, had he not narrowly escaped the payment of the permanent residence visa fee that was the due payment to his humble civil servant? He may have slithered out of forking over the cash before, but now his friend is going to jail in Bunia amid vultures that are even more rapacious than this emissary is! "Ah, that should loosen up those purse strings and return what was due!"

André came over to me after I had already met the MAF officials, hobbling barefoot still and relayed to me that "He says I have to go to Bunia and things there will be very bad for me."

"Ask him if he takes American Express!" I said, and then added quickly "And I need notarized receipts on every transaction that I must report to his superiors at Bunia!"

André relayed a translation of what the official said: "No, he does not know anything about such kinds of transactions, and needs only US cash in untorn and new bills."

I said, "That may limit his take since I do not have much that the scum of Bunia had not already collected."

"He asks how much you have and he will take it!" replied André. I gave him what I had sequestered away in three places. It came to $ 250.00. So, with a receipt written down in the big book at Nyankunde which no doubt lasted about ten milliseconds after he pocketed the cash, our slimy bastard in Nyankunde exerted his Congo-given right to extort at least as much as he could carry away. André was not carted off to do battle from the Bunia jail for three times his annual income.

Now, I had to get some shoes. I hobbled down to the market in Nyankunde on the muddy street, and we stopped at the first stall and asked for shoes. They had two pairs in a plastic bag. One actually looked quite reasonable, probably Chinese made, the most up-market thing in the shop. André had a bunch of NZ in his wallet, not quite enough it turns out to do business, but his credit is good. I tried on the shoes but they were just a little bit tight. No problem, a fellow went across the street to get another pair. They fit. The total of thousands of NZ that André had were handed over for a grand total of $13.00 US, on which he owed the balance and would be back later, since he would not have to be making a trip to Bunia tonight.

A FUND FOR THE PRIVATE FOUNDATION
FOR ZANDELAND DEVELOPMENT SET UP AT CME

I might be out of cash, but I am still not out of obligations! I left funds to support the development plans that André and I had discussed at the airstrip, and to support JM's daughter when she comes to Nyankunde to be fed at André's table and partially supported by my donation for her school fees. All of the earlier restrictions apply. There will be no gifts, but funds may be used for start up of sustainable community benefit that is repaid with interest back into the fund. Payments can be made in soap, palm oil, rice or whatever the currency is that will keep it growing for the benefit of the community. The idea was to create a small endowment useful in resolving human needs in the Assa environment and around Zandeland.

Not a bad exchange for a new pair of shoes!

A BRIEF AND BUSY STAY AT THE CME GUEST HOUSE
AT NYANKUNDE SURROUNDED BY FRIENDS AND SUPPLICANTS

I went to chat with Gary Bishop, the president of MAF-International, and Brent Rapp, the president of MAF-Africa as I came back sporting my new shoes. I thanked them for the help MAF had been to me, and they will be using some of my writings from Assa in their support. As I walked up to the Guest House, I met Ahuka's wife as I was accompanied by a very greatly relieved André. I told her I had one thing to say to her and to Ahuka when he returns from the Durban conference of the Pan-African Association of Christian Surgeons during my visit. When he returns and you and he sit down to a special dinner—I wish you *"Bon appetit!"* She looked puzzled, but I suppose André will tell her later some part of the story, after they have their dinner of the bush meat—from whatever species it is derived!

As I got to the Guest House, the queue of people who wanted to see me had already formed. A Congolese doctor named Hubert Kakalo had come back with an interpreter to ask again when he could hear about a residency in obstetrics and gynecology in US or UK. Apparently he missed the entire conversation I had had with him the previous visit on the way in, and did not have the entire document I sent to him that explained it all. The gist of this is that it is not just difficult, it is impossible. We will await the Pan-African Association of Christian Surgeons to work out the possibility of advanced training in Africa. Then several sequences of students came to me with notes they passed to me, with their name and a number printed right beneath it. The name was followed by the year they were in school, which would be their last unless I came up with the number that was printed right below it—their school fees for this year which were already in arrears. Most of these people I had not met and do not know, but they all seemed to find me.

THE RAPID COMPUTER WORK THAT WOULD ALLOW ME TO COPY THE ASSA STORY FOR THOSE WHO WERE REQUESTING THE FIRST HAND REPORT, EVEN IF INCOMPLETE

A lot of people are very interested in what I saw and did in Assa, and I promised them a report, if I could copy even the incomplete parts of it. I worked late into the night at The CME Guest House to copy onto the disc provided me by Gary Bishop. He wanted it e-mailed but this would be cumbersome at best so I decided to try to copy the disc despite the distractions of lots of people coming to see me at the Guest House.

I was not at all sure that my prior messages from here made it out and particularly whether my recently graduated medical student, Eric Sarin had got the earlier message to come on to Nyankunde as planned. I entered the copy command on my ThinkPad. As I was bent over this effort, I heard a voice behind me in probably one of the best uses of the line to date, "Doctor Geelhoed, I presume." I do look like a sight fresh out of the deep bush, and there stood Eric Sarin, M.D. Not only did he get the message, but he also took off for Nyankunde as soon as he got it. I found out that he will be staying here until September when he will leave Africa and go to India to join me in an upcoming Himalayan medical adventure.

I greeted him and outlined what he could expect when things were back to full speed when Ahuka returned in two weeks. He then introduced me to Dr. Gilbert Krakenbuhl, a Swiss surgeon who has been here for several months already, and who has been shepherding Eric around. We shook hands all around and chatted, making plans for a departure breakfast.

So, with a lot still to be done at dawn, I retired. Tomorrow will be a very busy day. I will repack and get organized for leaving. I promised to do AME physical exams on all the MAF pilots. I also need to evaluate the Public Health School here at CME for my own purposes at GWU and for the London School of Hygeine and Tropical Medicine with which I have been associated. The situation here appears to be burgeoning and is nearly ideal for student electives in international health. Finally, I should take the cutting of the *Nzawa* plant over to the greenhouse for Dr. Mwoembe. He is interested in investigating its uses as a medicinal plant. Five other mendicants solemnly promised me that they would be coming by this final morning. I have forty other things to do but they will want to remind me that I am their last and only hope for staying in school. All of them lost everything when the army ripped through Nyankunde. I came along just in time to save them from the doom they were praying to be relieved from by some miracle. *Voilà!* Who knoweth but that I have come into the kingdom for such a time as this?

[Editor's Note: Within a week after Glenn's departure from Nyankunde, the civil war overtook the area again. All expatriates were evacuated. Eric Sarin escaped overland through Uganda and joined Glenn in September in Delhi to begin their medical mission to Himachal Pradesh in Himalayan India.]

PILOT PHYSICAL EXAMS, TOUR OF THE PUBLIC HEALTH
SCHOOL, FINAL SHAKEDOWN IN BUNIA,
AND LAUNCH TOWARD ZIMBABWE

July 23, 1998

My last morning in Nyankunde was hectic even though I got up as early as possible to carry out the final packing, to help André sort the linguistic data, and to complete some last minute computer work. I did not even ask about the possibility of sending an e-mail, since the manuscript has grown enormously. I planned to make copies of the discs and mail them from Nairobi's US Embassy before I disappear once more into the bush. Unfortunately, right here and now I have to get a dozen things done before leaving.

I had promises to keep. Lary Strietzel, our pilot into Assa, picked me up on the motorbike. He drove me down to the hangar where I had scheduled physicals with the other pilots. I was carrying a loaned, Dutch, battery-powered automatic blood pressure device. It is a better sphygmomanometer than I have in my Washington office. I zipped through my physicals, keeping the records on a yellow note pad until they can be transcribed on the official FAA forms later at GWU. I examined everyone who was within reach. I stacked up the half-dozen forms on the completed exams. I had forgotten how quick and easy these exams are to do. I have gone to a lot of fuss and expense to keep my FAA medical examiner credentials. I wanted to use this credential to do a favor for these MAF pilots. My effort means that none of the MAF pilots will have to leave the country to get their exam, sparing them one hassle that allows them to stay current on their pilot's licenses and thus have more time for their more important missionary work.

OUT OF ASSA: HEART OF THE CONGO

CAN YOU BELIEVE—A SHOWER—
AND EVEN HOT WATER TO GO ALONG WITH IT!

Ah, the little under-rated joys of life! I may have reached for my last soapy bucket for my bath at Assa, although I miss the people and the setting already. A warm shower is a convenience that is awfully nice to have. On the other hand, there is something else about being without these basics where one's skills are desperately needed although being needed gets cloyingly dependent-heavy sometimes. I realized this as I was pampered myself in Nyankunde with a hot shower. I had depended on someone unknown to me to stoke the wood fire under the water heater at night.

I was finishing the last paperwork on the pilot exams, when Pat Nickson came over on an all-terrain vehicle (the kind I would like to use while hunting in the North American bush.) She was riding with her small black adopted son. She was surprised to hear that among the other things I had going for me that interested her was my degree in tropical medicine and hygiene. We bantered a bit about not being on speaking terms since her appointment is with the School of Hygiene and Tropical Medicine at Liverpool, the arch-rival of my alma mater in London. We played "Who do you know?" and we hit all the right chords immediately since David Morley, a pediatrician from London, is her sponsor and chief encourager. He and I are faculty at the East African Post-Graduate Program for teaching appropriate technology at Brackenhurst in Tigoni, Kenya. My name kept coming up in the African landscape. These stories communicated my accomplishments that were of interest to her. She put all the data together and figured out that I was not just an itinerant surgeon but also an M.P.H. with an interest in epidemiology, ethnobotany and anthropology. She pleaded with me to come back as a volunteer lecturer. I may get a volunteer appointment from the University of Liverpool to facilitate this.

I was brought over to meet Kaswera Vulere, a rising star here in maternal and child health. She has more energy and is busier than about any five African health care workers put together. Her husband is off in Canada getting his Ph.D. degree. This would mark him as the first African from Nyankunde with a doctorate. Their efforts give one hope for the indigenization of this whole project.

Kaswera leads a dozen initiatives on safe motherhood and family planning which were hot buttons on the public health planning and funding scene, as I saw recently in the Global Health Council Conference I attended in June before leaving the US. The tour of the facilities at Nyankunde introduced me to people and facilities that bode well for long-term sustainable projects here. I was particularly interested in the ethnobotanic gardens. This kind of initiative could be important for attracting development funds from drug companies. I made a mental note to send them a copy of my book *Natural Health Secrets from Around the World* (Keats Publishing, New Canaan, CT, 1997). Kaswera's programs would be a gold mine affiliation for GWU's new School of Public Health, if they do not politicize them into a policy management process. Some "experts" collect *per diem* and consultant fees while talking policy about public health rather than doing something to move it forward. They make certain that their hands are as little soiled as possible in the real work of the world. Not knowing or practicing health care is hardly a credential for managing it. The hard-working collections of public health students here and in Bunia are real-world, indigenous health care providers and are now part of the first degree-granting piece of the CME program. They are most appropriate as managers here, since they have the credibility of having delivered health care first.

TAKE-OFF FROM NYANKUNDE TO ARRIVE AMID A RUSSIAN FLOTILLA OF ANTONOVS PILOTED BY ESTONIANS, AS THEY FLOG THEIR WARES IN AFRICAN TROUBLE SPOTS

I scrambled aboard a second MAF flight to Bunia, and landed amid what could only be called a Russian Air Show. There were two large four engine Antonov 32's complete with turret guns in the nose bubble underneath the aircraft. They are massive flying fortresses left over from World War II. There was even someone hanging in the bubble as the big plane lumbered out streaming four dirty streaks into the sky, using the entire runway for take-off. The Estonian pilots were hauling cargo, probably to some Congolese destination as independent contractors, delivering low-level flight hardware to some warring factions. While they were at it, they were flogging these used airplanes as exactly the kind of technology that the new Democratic Republic of the Congo badly needs. That's it, all right, fifty-year-old, obsolete, fuel-inefficient aircraft technology. I would be hard pressed to think of anything more important than old warplanes to spread democracy.

Then standing on the taxiway, after this impressive display of aerial pollution, were two AN-2's, big biplanes. The Estonians were doing a "wing walk" to be sure that fuel was being put in and not substituted with something else. The fuel was poured through a felt filter over a coffee can. The AN-2's looked like they belonged in a flying circus, and I would have loved to shoot a picture, but for the fact that the last place to pull out and display a camera like the N 8008 is in the Bunia Airport. Not that this is a highly sensitive military establishment, but it has the highest concentration of official thieves of anyplace I know. I am sure there would be some regulation that requires hanging by the neck until dead—but, for you, our good friend, we will call it all square if you just turn over everything we have not already cleaned you of on the first pass. This, after all, was their last chance at me for this trip and so they did me the honor of coming out on the tarmac to look me over. I saw my *bête noire*, the grand larcenist Umro, walking around at the terminal, but he did not see me. Maybe he was "honoring the point" as his other henchmen came out to see me.

I owed them $20.00 departure tax, and there is one fellow who is not all that bad and even speaks a few words of English who said he would take it for me with the passport. I gave him my only $ 20.00 bill among the three US bills I still had. The others were ones. The $ 20.00 had a minute tear in the corner of the bill, so it was "no good." I explained to them that the bill was the only one I had, and they simply motioned to the AIM Air pilot who was also standing there for the "formalities." They ordered me, "Get it from him!" So, I walked over and asked if he had any US currency and he did. He got me a new $20.00 bill and I delivered that. In order to trade I went over to reclaim my "damaged currency." No go, they had kept the money. This bill was no good for official purposes but that did not make it unfit for private transactions.

There is one bit of good news from the Bunia customs officials. On surrendering my officially stamped and sealed document, I got the plastic bag with my camouflage shorts, shirt and hat back. This gear was too military-looking to take into peace-loving Democratic Republic of Congo!

Out came another fellow with no uniform, but this time he was sporting a cellophane wrapped tag that identified him as Bunia customs agent for the new Democratic Republic of Congo. He came to me and asked, "Estonian?"

I said, "No," and as my passport returned with the twice-bought departure tax, I pointed to it, and said "American."

"Oh! Good!" he said, licking his lips. He continued with, "Let me see your particulars!" going through every page of the passport, holding it up to the light at several pages to see the pretty stamps in it. It is a very long process to go through my passport, and this is even a relatively new one. He took his time asking the kinds of questions that are, of course, in the vital interest of state security of the DRC. "How much currency are you carrying, and let me see it."

"Thanks to your administrative ministrations, I have $ 2.00 US left." I said with more than a touch of sarcasm.

He did not understand my humor. He asked, "What have you been doing here?"

"I have been a medical volunteer, helping your people," I responded.

"Ah, yes, but just what is it that you are doing for me? I like your pen," he added as no particular point except perhaps aesthetically.

It is not that it was a Mont Blanc, but it was my last one, so I said, "It is almost out, so you should get a new one instead."

"That is OK, I will take your 'agenda' instead," he replied. Here in my pocket is the Smythson Wafer Diary that records my life. It has many important phone numbers, laboriously copied over at every year's end when all the changes are edited in. He wants this diary, filled in through more than half the year, that is good to no one else on earth but me, representing several hundred man-hours.

"No, you won't," I said simply. His great disappointment was assuaged with the last two bills the US government had printed to distribute to such larcenous places as this one, our foreign aid in action.

He added ominously "When you return next time, do not forget what you can bring for me, since I will not forget you!" You can bet he won't.

OVER THE FABLED ORIGIN OF THE NILE

Right behind the AN-2, with its crackle of Russian over the intercom, we rolled off the Bunia strip and looked down on the town of Bunia, then over Lake Albert. I was preparing both my ThinkPad and GPS for a little work en route in the copilot's seat. I was intent on flying over the origin of the White Nile, or "Victoria Nile," the one of the two sources of this river that had defied understanding for at least two millennia of speculation by many authorities. The source of the life-giving Nile, cradle of Egyptian civilization, had brought out many people to search, including my hero David Livingstone, who never did find it although he had the right idea. He was headed toward Lake Bangweulu when he died at Chitambo in Zambia. He was at least two lakes short of the origin, but he was right in his assumption that the source of the Nile was somewhere in this Great Rift.

Later explorers, such as Burton and Speke, had been right in saying that the great Lake Victoria was the origin. There was an ancient civilization at the source of the White Nile as it exits from the Lake east of where we reach Entebbe in Uganda. The town is *Jinja* where a flooded-out, prehistoric civilization lies under water. I marked this site on the GPS and recorded it for later exploration of the White Nile, along with my great interest in exploring the Blue Nile, as it come from Lake Tana in Ethiopia. The great gorges that drain Lake Tana are the Blue Nile's source. Together these rivers flow toward Khartoum where they join but don't mix. The waters of the Blue Nile and the White Nile flow side by side for another 25 km down toward Ondurman, scene of General Gordon's last stand, where the two Niles eventually mix and become one.

So, we flew over Lake Kyoga next. This is a lagoon-like diverticulum rather than a dammed impoundment of the Victoria Nile, like the great sudd in the Sudan, which is chock full of the Nile cabbages that the hippos like to eat. Rivers of size in this part of the world that are not flowing fast through rainforest cataracts appear green, not blue or white, since they clog up with vegetation. Maybe the run off would be faster in the sudd if there were more hippos, but that would not make it a more user-friendly place.

My AIM Air pilot was Steve, from Bellingham Washington, who grew up as a mission kid (MK) in a SIL family with Wycliffe Bible Translators in Bolivia. I asked him if he knew about JAARS—"Jungle Aviation and Radio Service" that is the SIL branch in South America that does what MAF and AIM do here. He was too young when he left there to have participated, but JAARS was the inspiration, along with the Moody Bible Institute, that got him started here.

One of our passengers who had come into Bunia on the earlier flight while I was doing flight physicals in Nyankunde was an English internist named Nigel Pearson. He lives in the area of Virunga Park, in the Similiki Valley, DRC. I would get to know him better at Mayfield and when we arrived at Nairobi, since he was traveling back to England by way of France for a month of holiday and to pick up books that he planned to donate upon his return. Since he had no Kenyan currency and had not been through Nairobi recently, he would ride with me over to Mayfield. We agreed to rendezvous later, when he discovered that I had an adventuresome streak and wanted to go out into the Kenyan countryside. Stay tuned, and we will see just how far into the Kenya hills we can get.

36 NGONG

**RETURN TO MY MAYFIELD STAGING AREA, DEBRIEFING BY
ASSA SUPPORTERS, EDITING DISCS FOR *OUT OF ASSA*, AND
CLIMBING THE NGONG HILLS**

July 23-24, 1998

We deplaned at Wilson Field, where I often meet someone I may faintly recognize, but either I know their name or they know mine. On the way outbound to the Congo through the multiple tries we made to thread out through the weather front, I had met Rob McKee. I might not have known him, but I soon found out that we shared interests in linguistic anthropology of the Congolese people as I described in Chapter 4. As I waited to leave Nairobi, there was another fellow with Rob, also with SIL who was in Nairobi. I had later met him at Nyankunde with his wife's parents. The family was about to disappear into the northeast of the jungle for a long period. Her parents were playing grandpa and grandma. I had envied them as I saw them throwing a ball to a grandson, who would be about the same age as Andrew William Geelhoed, my first grandchild, and videotaping around the CME Guest House.

This time, as I deplaned in Nairobi from the Congo, the same grandparents were seeing off their other son and daughter-in-law, both of whom seemed to know me. They were with MAF and just returning to the field after the disruptions. I guess, by now, I am accepted as one of the "regulars" here, since I am hearing legends about me from others, and find I have to explain less about what it is that I am doing. There is a fascination with Assa, as the "back of beyond." There are a number of people who want to sit with me and "debrief" everything I can tell them about Assa, which they may have wanted to visit once or at least were fascinated with the place about which they had heard stories.

♦ OUT OF ASSA: HEART OF THE CONGO

I AM THE LIONIZED EXPLORER OF THE INTERIOR HOLDING LATE DEBRIEFING SESSIONS AT MAYFIELD

I arrived at Mayfield in the taxi with Nigel Pearson, who asked me about Assa. I promised to provide as much information as they wanted after dinner. We were just in time for dinner. I carried my pitifully small luggage and picked up the small amount of "left luggage" I had stored in Mayfield. I thought I had been rather clever in leaving behind the computer carrying case, so that I would have a "stealth device" to smuggle in with me. But there are disconcerting rattles that sound like loose nuts and bolts floating around inside the ThinkPad, which has not been handled gently, by either cretins or euthyroids. I had left one complete set of safari clothes at Mayfield, and, now, with the new Chinese shoes I had bought in Nyankunde, I look like some ersatz Abercrombie and Fitch advertisement, absurdly over-dressed for most bush environments, and completely out of place in most civilized cities.

As soon as I sat down to dinner, people came clustering around. These included Steve and Debbie Wolcott, who have been very interested in my experiences in Assa, as was a fellow named Jim Pinkerton. Jim works now in Emole, Congo. He is a former MK and worked for Baker Oil Company putting out wildfires in oil fields before retiring and coming back to the Congo as a missionary to pygmies. He is a hunter, and we exchanged stories and promises to return. I also met a couple named David and Joan Sercombe. They turn out to be missionaries assigned to Assa after the Downings left. He is a Welshman and she is a long-time missionary companion of his. They developed a deep affection for Assa. They were reluctant to leave when the last hostilities shut down the station. I did not know it at dinner, but the lounge had been set up for the debriefing session that went on with a large audience until nearly midnight.

Nigel Pearson and I had made plans for the next afternoon after I finished several chores. I had to go to the AIM office to pay for the flights and the excess baggage fees for the medical supplies. Combined with that business trip, I hoped to visit the US Embassy, and relay the messages from *Out of Assa*. I worked on editing them far into the night at Mayfield after the debriefing. So, I worked hard to get all of *Out of Assa* reduced to a single disc full of transmissible data.

FELLOW ASSA FANS FILL ME IN ON THEIR STORIES AND I MAKE DISC COPIES FOR ALL

Nigel Pearson had his own chores to do in Nairobi. We reserved the taxi we had hired to take us back from the Wilson Field to return around noon to take us on an excursion. I wanted to climb the Ngong Hills in "Karen," named for the author Karen Blixen (who wrote *Out of Africa* under the pen name Isak Dinesen). I gathered together all the letters for deposit in the embassy postbox, and as I still worked on getting the disc ready, David Sercombe took a taxi to get a box of discs for me to copy my manuscript for him and others. By now, lunch was served at Mayfield. This worked out ideally, since we could eat at Mayfield, and did not need to carry the mangoes and other goodies we had planned to picnic with in the Ngong Hills. We planned to have the taxi driver wait with us. We were his only sure thing as far as business, so he was happy to stand by. I finished copying the discs. My hard-working IBM ThinkPad can work its magic while I have electricity to keep it going.

I learned a lot from the others at lunch about events in the Congo. There is a big but under-reported war going on in the Ruwenzori Mountains. I aspire to a climb in this fantastic place. Richard Burton explored and descibed these "Mountains of the Moon." I had once programmed a climb up these mountains from Zaïre and down in Uganda. Unfortunately, there always seems to be a nasty war breaking out in this very remote area every time I get good and ready to make the climb. Nigel tells me that there is an army of 200,000 troops called the National Army of Liberation of Uganda (NALU) which is a Moslem group fighting for the overthrow of the Ugandan government. They are well-equipped and well-supplied. One might ask from whom? It seems the Moslem connection would be weak as a link, until I learned further that the hostilities are right over the top of potentially huge petroleum reserves. Apparently, the limited exploration that has gone on when there has not been active shooting over it suggests that these reserves may even be larger than the oil fields of the Middle East. This is in the estimate of the Baker Oil Company for which Jim Pinkerton worked, but more importantly, according to Jim, the Chinese. The Chinese are counting on this reserve to fuel their development through the next half-century, with the target of full exploitation by the mid-2000's.

Big time power groups are interested in the oil, but the squabbling of several groups over the area has kept all deals off. Aramco/ELF proposed a 64-inch pipeline to carry off the high volume yield that was expected from this potentially rich oil pool. This was to be a deal cut between Mobutu and these US interests, tilted to the West to get it away from the Chinese. This deal collapsed with the ouster and death of Mobutu. So, this massive wealth is up for grabs again.

With massive wealth sitting under the fringe of the new Congolese state, and some bills to pay to allies in Tanzania and Uganda, Kabila wants to get this area explored and exploited. Where is President Kabila this week? Up north, in Libya, with Muammar al-Qaddafi!

There is a Croesus-like fortune at stake here with important global dimensions. Terrorism is a tool that Qaddafi knows well. Perhaps Kabila will learn to use it as effectively. Look for a big blow in this area of the world to raise the cost of doing business to dampen the enthusiasm of the West, and tilt it into the Chinese influence already primed.

There is an enormous road construction effort right now funded by the Chinese, not necessarily altruistic, going on right around the disputed area of the potential oil field. Kabila has definitely "tilted" away from the West (who are putting him up for the War Crimes tribunal for his role in killing hordes of Tutsi in paying debts to his Hutu allies) and toward the Chinese. He has suggested that the Africans should solve their problems, without relying on Western leadership, and a huge source of wealth is under his eastern border, under Lake Albert—where from ancient times to the present, there have been natural oil slicks on the surface. With limited seismography, it seems that the entire area of the Rift Valley is a treasure trove beyond calculation, right under the beautiful Similiki Valley. Environmentalists can be expected to protest, but they don't stand a chance to defend Virunga Park, gorillas in the mist and all. The most promising prospect is at the border of Congo and Uganda. What this major geopolitical struggle does—at the very least—is postpone for at least another two years my attempt to climb the Ruwenzori Mountains. By the time this part of the world is safe for me, I may no longer be quite ready to leap tall mountains in the mist at a single bound.

Where are all the arms coming from that fuel these large-scale conflicts? Could it be the Saudis? They have a hegemonic grip on the biggest oil reserves currently exploited. They might find it appropriate to support their NALU Islamic brethren in carrying out a massive campaign of destabilization on the African continent. This would discourage any further exploitation of a wild card oil source in their OPEC world.

I would say there will be a big token threat against the Western friendly governments nearby to teach a lesson to everyone about how to play oil-dirty pool. Look for something nasty to happen, for example, to the US Embassy in Nairobi where I have just dropped off my letters and the precious disc.

[Editor's Note: This material was written before the terrorist attacks on the US Embassies in East Africa, which followed within three days the author's visit to the US Embassy in Nairobi.]

I MEET ENTHUSIASTIC INTEREST IN MY LINGUISTIC DATA EVERYWHERE EXCEPT IN MY DISSERTATION COMMITTEE

Jim Pinkerton and I are enthusiastic about our common interests. He is studying with the pygmies in a remote area of the Congo deep in the Ituri Forest. He is working in SIL with the Lhese, and I have Kilhese data from my interviews with pygmies in Lolwa. We both hunt and fish, and have talked about going up the smaller Congo River tributaries in the Ituri Forest in dugout canoes to catch trophy tigerfish. The disincentive is that we expect the sudden startling of dangerous Nile crocodiles on the banks in a stream narrower than the length of the canoe. They do not take kindly to being surprised. They can and do overturn canoes with a single sweep of their tails and then dine at leisure on the toothsome former occupants.

I told him I was interested in shooting a bongo, and that ironically during my Assa stay when I could not hunt, there were regular bongo sightings all around where I hunted previously, including a magnificent bull along with a group of five reported on my second to last day. He told me that deep in the Ituri Forest, there are herds of bongos. They have minimal encounters with human hunters and thus show very little fear. The pygmies call the area the Nandas after the big tall trees that are so dense that they block all sun from penetrance below the canopy. One can travel very easily through the dark understorey of the *nandas*. One of the pygmies had counted sixty bongos in a single group. When asked where that was, the reply is "Eleven sleeps under the *nandas*." That means *eleven days travel* in a straight line in the clear understorey of this immense rainforest. He says—and I echo—that "We have got to do it!" I hope for a future pygmy hunting party when I join with them in exploring the *nandas*, perhaps all the way to the Ndoki Swamp—-one of the least explored places on earth, where there is supposed to be the *Mokélé mbembé*—a surviving dinosaur. Redmond O'Hanlon's disturbing and hilarious book, *No Mercy: A Journey to the Heart of the Congo* (Knopf, 1997) describes an expedition to Lake Télé in The People's Republic of the Congo. I highly recommend it to those with an interest in the remote parts of the "other" Congo.

One of the pygmies tried to describe to Jim a very large bird-like reptile. "Right!" he said. They insisted, and drew a crude picture of it in the sand. It looked so startlingly like a picture Jim had of a pterodactyl that he got a book on furlough and carried it out and showed it to these pygmies. They had never seen a book before.

"Oh, you know him, then!" they said. "That's him all right." When asked how long it has been since they had seen this animal, they responded, "Two moons ago."

"Where?" Jim asked.

Once more, "Eight sleeps under the *nandas*." Count me in! I'm there. These people must need some medical attention.

One of the pygmies had come upon a very large herd of forest buffalo that were startled by some other predator than he. They stampeded past him as he took refuge in a tree. He is an acculturated pygmy, one of Pinkerton's informants, and even wears a watch. When asked how many buffalo there were, he replied, "I do not know, *Bwana*, but it took them two and one-half hours to pass on the run!"

Jim Pinkerton supervises the construction of a new airstrip at Emola, the SIL outpost to reach these pygmies. When it is completed he will let me know and I will program that region as part of my next visit, for both medical and linguistic investigations. Then, of course, for purely food-gathering reasons, I will have to take my GPS and whatever firearm the hoped-for forthcoming calm will allow, and go many sleeps under the *nandas*.

Jim Pinkerton is missing a distal phalanx of his right thumb. I asked him, "How did that happen?"

He replied, "A very interesting looking snake, which I got too close to." He got close enough to identify it very well, a viper *Altractaspis congonensis*, the Black Burrowing Asp. When hit, he went down and tried to compose himself as he faded away, with what felt like a high voltage shock that went up his arm, paralyzing him. The amputation saved him from more serious poisoning. The digit was necrotic anyway. The surgeon who treated him said that if he were not such a big man, he would not have survived the envenomation. *Ex Africa semper aliquid novi*!

We compared notes, such as the Pazande meanings of some personal names, thought to be beautiful when conferred by the grandparents. Kati's wife, Sendekpio, means "She who is torn asunder by death." This is hardly a lyrical name, but it fits perhaps as well as that of Assa's chief medical officer whom I call "Doctor Inikpio," much to this good man's embarrassment, since he is very careful and exercises very conservative judgment as the chief medical officer of the entire district. Inikpio means "He who walks hand in hand with death!"

THE NGONG HILLS NEAR NAIROBI

Since I will neither be climbing the Ruwenzori Mountains nor sleeping under the *nandas*, I am on my way to the Ngong Hills. Once I visited the "I had a farm in Africa…" house of Karen Blixen which is in the area of the Ngong Hills where she tried to raise coffee. The elevation is just a little too high for good coffee to be grown. But she liked the area, now named after her—and now made famous in a movie based on her book *Out of Africa.* "Ngong" means "knuckles" since the Masai legend has it that a very large giant was buried there, and all that sticks up out of the ground now are his knuckles. There are seven of them, and I climbed and scrambled over five of the seven.

Nigel Pearson and I took our patient taxi driver and went on errands to mail letters and disc. Then we went on to Wilson Field to the AIM hangar to pay my bill for transportation to and from Bunia. We then drove on to the entry to a Forest Preserve, where there were two young white women and a single black man. They had picked him up at the base of the hill, as a "guide," but were rejected from entering the reserve because of a "security risk" according to the armed guards at the gate.

Nigel spoke with them in Kiswahili, and would speak with me in French, when we were trying to decide how long to keep the driver and how much we would negotiate for payment. This was a perfectly good system until we discovered that one of the women was French. The other was German, and they had just met each other. They were eager to go somewhere for a strenuous bit of African exercise. What was not calculated into that plan after they had had a taxi drop them off here, is the reputation that the Ngong Hills have of harboring dacoits, the thieves that make a good living by robbing tourists in this isolated place. Two white women would be ludicrously easy pickings.

Some part of the rumors of the inevitability of mugging, or worse, may actually be promoted by the guards. Exaggeration of hazards to personal safety decreases their work load, and also creates a demand for their services if the unintimidated are still intent on "hill-walking" as the British would say. The guard said, "Anyone who sees a white person immediately thinks of their money," present company included. There is a fee for entry into the park. The entry fee includes an armed escort. But here we were, an African, an American, and Europeans, a serendipitous group in the form of a UN entourage. I said we would all go together. That took a while to negotiate, since combining into one group knocked out a fee for some armed escort's services. It seemed redundant to have a guard when what we had was a whole UN delegation. Each of us had our own language, culture and nation. All were interested in scrambling up and over the hills to gaze over the Great Rift Valley spread out at our feet.

SERENDIPITY MAKES FOR UNUSUAL FELLOW CLIMBERS

Here we are. Nigel Pearson is a British generalist physician who has lived in Eastern Congo under the shadow of the dangerous Ruwenzori Mountains. He speaks French and Kiswahili more than his native English. He is en route to France tonight on Air France, from which he will look down on this beacon for air navigation on the top of the first of the Ngong Hills.

Suzanne Kustner is a German woman who has volunteered at a project in Tanzania, who will next be working as an au pair girl in London.

Sylvana Doblier is a French woman on holiday in Africa. She met Suzanne at a hostel where they each stayed last night and they decided to come out to the Ngong Hills. They hired a "guide" from among the loiterers in the bush at the gate of the Forest Preserve. He was a single man who might lead them into a trap of his friends, so they paid him off and now were our dependents for the duration.

Henry Osmaston is our Kenyan taxi driver. He seems to enjoy this break from his usual routine of sitting long hours each day behind his steering wheel. Now, only because of this chance encounter with the crazy *Wazungu*, he is going to look down from the top of the Ngong Hills instead of only up at them as he has all his life. He reported that he could not wait to tell his wife what he was paid to do today.

C'est moi, an American Africanist vagabond, who murmurs French in Kenya—where Kiswahili is the rule, and stammers Spanish in francophone Africa, and who carries a GPS with which he is making frequent marks. This hybrid freak has two cameras, one of which is nonfunctional, one roll of extra film, a tape recorder, and a safari jacket in a Steamboat Springs Marathon bag from Denver General Trauma Service, while walking over and accurately identifying the hoof prints of the large "Kafir bull" Cape buffalo.   He also carried a telephoto lens which was too much work to take out of his bag when Augur Buzzards (*Buteo augur*) were floating overhead at close range. Due to this sloth, he missed the shot at a beautiful prize any other birder would envy, the Lammergeier (*Gypaetus barbatus*).

Not one of these hill-walkers came from the same country. Each had a primary home language that was common for only two of them with an ocean between giving a different accent and meaning to much of what they would have said was a common language. This motley crew shrugged off the danger of hostilities and plunged ahead over the hillsides to see what lay on the other side of the Ngong Hills.

WE ARE ALL PILGRIMS IN TRANSIT
OVER THE NGONG HILLS IN REVERIE AND REALITY

There was also an interesting series of single men going up to the top of the Ngong Hills to set up their blankets, and spend the night, alone, under the moon and communing in prayer and fasting. These were pilgrims. They had fasted all day, and were contemplating their future and their place in life and eternity with the attempt to get closer to their God on the top of this mountain. I punched in "NGON" and located us at 01° 23.29′ S and 036° 38.27′ E at 8,850 feet elevation. This is a good halfway point to be suspended between heaven and earth, and to contemplate our various roles and futures in each.

I rather liked the idea of the pilgrimage and our own peregrine status. So did Nigel, who said he would look out of his Air France window tonight at midnight down on his fellow pilgrims, and say a prayer to the same God—even though he would be having a fine French wine (denied to him in the field by the Church Mission Society of the Anglican Church) while the remaining pilgrims were shivering in their blankets after a long day of fasting and the exertion of the climb. I, too, will wish them well as I look down at the Ngong Hills from over the Great Rift Valley in the morning as I wing my way over them heading south to begin the "Safari from Harare."

At present, we were looking over the vast sweep of the same Great Rift, and thinking our own thoughts as the wonderful vision of the Lammergeier came over me. The Lammergeier is a large vulture-like bird. Its name is based on the allegation that it would carry away lambs as prey. In fact, it feeds mostly on carrion. It eats the marrow and the bones of the dead, in essence, recycling carcasses. This unusual bird gets at the marrow and breaks the bones into digestible fragments by dropping them on rocks from great altitude. These ossuaries are probably used for centuries and typically consist of thousands of bone fragments, bleached white in the intense sun in the clear mountain air.

I was in some degree of reverie until I suddenly started crazy contortions—while rapt with the wonder of it all, I had stood in a large colony of the fierce biting red ants! I tried swiping them away, and when I did that brushing action, all I did was separate their bodies from the solidly clenched mandibles, that held on tightly with a grin as they drew blood with their last bite before decapitation.

Africa is always ready to temper any reverie with reality!

37 ON SAFARI THROUGH HARARE

July 25, 1998

I am up very early for a flight that is taking off for Harare at 10:00 AM. It is not for an early arrival at the Jomo Kenyatta International Airport that I am up even before the muezzin sings out his call to prayers, and a good two hours before the Hadeda Ibis (*Bostrychia hagedash*) announces his shift in position for the day. I am joining a family for an "early breakfast" (a bowl of Weetabix). They are the Shales from Bakersfield, California. He is a radiologist, and she is a family practitioner. They have just done a six-week stint in Tenwek, a Kenyan mission hospital I know well. Coincidentally, we are all heading to Zimbabwe. She grew up as a child of Free Methodist missionaries in Mashonaland. They are taking their three small kids on a holiday for three weeks. I am guiding them a bit, since this is their first time at doing anything like this. They have taken two months off from private group practice.

But, it was for the reader's sake and not the early arrangements for take-off that I have been up early and in bed late in my Mayfield staging area. I finished the writing of serial letters and editing and copying of *Out of Assa* to mail here in Nairobi. The potpourri of stamps I used to airmail a letter and the disc to the US made a colorful package.

HEADING SOUTH OVER THE GREAT RIFT

I boarded the Kenya Airways flight to Harare with the Shale family spread out in the row behind me. I have my charged-up ThinkPad on the seatback tray in this 737-300. On this trip, I had written often while propping it up on the copilot's yoke on the flights in and out of the Congo over the Rift. It is difficult to explain to the Shales while we are flying on such a civilized flight as this scheduled airliner, that I am often hopping over large jungles or bodies of water, intermittently typing or steering my way around thunderheads in cloud-weaving on VFR.

The experiences of the past three weeks are going to be hard to explain on the next entry into the bush, since, after all, we are voluntarily entering the *bundu* (Kiswahili for the forbidding, hostile unknown). In doing so, we are giving up basic necessities as on a camping trip where one voluntarily foregoes the absolute luxuries of plumbing and power. In much of Africa, these luxuries are simply not available and can't be had just by coming in from the bush, having finished a camping experience to the point you would like to leave it behind, when it is convenient.

I am currently twiddling with both GPS and tape recorder. I might try to get a disposable flash camera to replace my broken one, but my otherwise minimalist kit is quite compact and versatile for moving between the highly developed and primitive worlds. This portable computer is especially important to me. I am using it as I write over Zambian airspace.

ARRIVAL IN HARARE CHECK-IN AT THE EXPANDING BRONTE HOTEL, MY "ZIM" STAGING AREA

I talked with the Shales, whom I helped through the blessedly routine arrival formalities in Harare. It is high, dry, clear and cool, winter in the highveld. The climate resembles that of a mountain resort in the Western US. They were met by a local evangelical who also took me along in the overloaded vehicle. We had stopped at the Baptist Conference Center near the airport. Sarah Shales told me that they were going to take a dilapidated VW combi and drive to Victoria Falls, a trip that may be risky for someone with three young kids. Fortunately, her husband rebuilds engines for recreation, a skill that may be useful along the way. They wanted to know where to eat, and I recommended the Manchurian, where you can pick your own combinations of ostrich, antelope, chicken, beef, pork, and assorted vegetables. The chefs stir-fry everything on a flat table. I said I would try to meet them there, depending on when Kurt Johnson arrived.

Kurt is my friend and colleague at GWU where he is a Professor of Anatomy and Cell Biology. He is also my publisher and editor and a keen birder. He dreams of identifying and "listing" half of the 10,000 or so bird species currently extant. He would be joining me in the Bronte Hotel by prearrangement. The Bronte is our rendezvous point with Gary Douglas, one of our two African professional guides who would be taking us off on our safari to Zambia early next morning.

I walked into the new marble foyer of the lobby, with new rooms being built along the way. The Bronte has grown larger every time I have checked in from the first time I lived here in 1996. It was a great "discovery" of mine, a garden hotel in close proximity to the Parirenyatwa Hospital of the University of

Zimbabwe. It has expanded its capacity to double the original number of rooms, but it still remained overbooked, and at a rate that doubles every other month. In 1996, I had a room that was up-market from my Courtney Hotel ($11.00 per day) to the Bronte ($15.00 per day with breakfast). My discovery seemed to have been noted by others. Last year the same room was about $ 50.00. This year it is $90.00. The room remains the same but for the price increase. All these are the rates in US dollars, since the inflation rate keeps them from even listing the Zim dollar rates. The Zim dollar exchange rate is currently between 17 and 19 to the US dollar, depending on whether one is buying or selling.

The economy of Zimbabwe is on the skids. It seems "Comrade Robert Mugabe, President-for-Life," whose house several blocks over from the Bronte means that all the surrounding streets are closed off after dark, has made more strident efforts to get approval from his sycophant population as the inflation rate passes 40%. He has found a real political crowd-pleaser. Increasing intolerance of the minority white population has been continuing. There are 80,000 whites in Zimbabwe among 12 million blacks, or less than 1% of the population although they made up nearly 100% of the population I saw in the shops and in restaurants like Fat Momma's.

There is an ongoing economic nosedive in Zimbabwe. Somehow the good Mr. Mugabe has managed to squirrel away one of the world's great fortunes. He has a mansion in the UK and about every other place on earth where there are few questions asked after the size of the payroll is discussed. So, at more than $ 4 billion US, Mugabe ranks among the richest men in the world, the typical story of the African President-for-Life.

A porter wheeled my bag to my room, passing the lounge where the *Man with the Golden Helmet* hangs, scowling at me, his namesake. I repacked my large bag and filled it with things to be left behind for my August 1 return to Harare. I am back to one small carry-on and the computer bag with the D/C charger cord, hoping to get a "toke" of energy out of the cigarette lighter of the Toyota safari vehicle to keep typing my adventures into the ThinkPad. Having mailed off the disc of the experience that ended in Assa, I am ready for *vacation* with guide-catered services. For a change, I will be the recipient, rather than provider, of direction through the unknowns of the Dark Continent and its wonders hard ahead.

I had just finished the consolidation, when there was a knock on the door. The porter opened it, and I heard Kurt say, "Doctor Geelhoed, I presume." This is the same greeting that, although unoriginal, served to alert me in Nyankunde that my former medical student, now Eric Sarin, M.D. was standing behind me. Kurt and I had arranged months ago in my GW office to meet out here in Africa and then go on our Zambian birding safari. This is the place for Livingstonian comparisons, and Zambia (his last stop) even more! Kurt Johnson said he was glad to see me alive, having received the cards from South Africa and Nairobi and the last e-mail out of Nyankunde. He brought me the clothes I had given him before departing the US to replace the stuff I had peeled off and left in Assa. Gary Douglas ("Golfie," from his pilot call letters) called and said he was running around Harare renting vehicles and trailers, and buying supplies. Our other guide, Peter Tetlow would fly to Kariba, where we would be headed by early morning for rendezvous. Helga Patrikios is going to pick us up for dinner at Fat Momma's, the restaurant in the nearby Russell Hotel at which we had dined before with her niece and boyfriend. Helga is the Medical Librarian at the University of Zimbabwe. I had met her in 1996 as I staggered around her library, seeking help to e-mail something back from my Fulbright assignment in Zimbabwe. She is a charming and witty woman and has been a helpful source of perspective as a "Rhodie insider/outsider." She is quite liberal politically and was a forceful critic of white minority rule when Zimbabwe was Southern Rhodesia. Nevertheless, now that there is majority rule and she is white, she is subjected to quite a few indignities.

So, all the pieces are in place, and I am ready to roll—on the way from "Zim" to "Zam."

"MILES AND MILES OF BLOODY AFRICA" PUNCTUATED
BY ONE BLOOD-CURDLING INSTANT

July 26, 1998

It happened like this.

A VERY LONG DAY FROM ZIM TO ZAM

It is now evening and my ThinkPad is plugged into the cigarette lighter of our Toyota Hi-Lux in the remote Zambian Lochinvar National Park, 1000 km from Harare. The full day included one unique, potentially lethal, experience at the shores of the big lake Kariba along the dammed Zambezi River.

Gary Douglas, bird-guide extraordinaire, came by the Bronte as we were eating breakfast. He sat down and we offered him the already poured cup of coffee and piece of toast we were not planning to eat. This caused the waiter to have a real problem, since Gary was not registered in our hotel. So after an investigation through multiple levels he rendered a new bill for 10 Zim dollars (about US $0.50). I paid for Kurt's phone call home to reassure his wife that he had arrived safely and Gary's "extra" breakfast and we checked out. With a final pack up of the Venter trailer and a securing of our camping gear with a cargo net in the back of the Toyota 4X4, we were on our way out of Harare for a long road trip into Zambia, ultimately destined for Lochinvar National Park about 200 km southwest of Lusaka, Zambia's capital city.

Gary Douglas is a highly qualified professional guide, licensed in Zimbabwe. In years past, he directed a paramilitary organization dedicated to saving the black rhinoceros. Their horns became so valuable (as a source for aphrodisiac powder as well as hilts and sheaths for ritual knives called khanjars in Oman and Yemen) that eventually Gary had been involved in virtual wars with poachers. His units had orders to shoot on sight anyone found in restricted preserves designed to protect the rapidly dwindling wild populations of black rhinos. He and his troops had even been involved in fire-fights with regulars from the Zimbabwean army. Later he worked as a guide and guide-trainer for Zimbabwe Sun Hotels at several locations in Zimbabwe. Kurt met him in 1996 at Chikwenya Lodge in Mana Pools National Park and was so impressed with his birding skills that he hired him to guide a birding safari to the Eastern Highlands of Zimbabwe in August, 1997. Kurt invited me along as a payback for some help I had given him with his medical publishing business. Peter Tetlow, Gary's friend and colleague at Zimbabwe Sun Hotels also came along on this expedition. We all had so much enjoyment that we decided on a new adventure in Zambia.

Gary now works at Malilangwe Wildlife Reserve, a new conservation trust and tourist facility set up by a 40-year-old American, who made a lot of money in the stock market. The benefactor now leads a lifestyle that includes establishing a nature preserve and jetting his friends and paying customers out into the Zimbabwean bush. The guests are put up in private accommodation filled with original art and serious luxury in the African bush. The Trust also runs two twelve-bed camps in an intact Big Five ecosystem and is working hard at reintroducing native game. The camps and staff can be rented out for $400 and up per night. This organization is competing with the up-market camps at Saba Saba and other insulated communities along Kruger Park's borders, where there are private luxury accommodations for hire.

KARIBA: A MORE CHILLING THAN THRILLING INTERLUDE WHILE AWAITING THE REST OF OUR TEAM AT THE ZIM/ZAM BORDER

We arrived in the mopane woodland on a long and winding course throughout the large national parks that line the upper and lower Kariba area. The Kariba Dam blocks the Zambezi River. The floodwaters behind the dam backed up in 1962 to create the large Lake Kariba. This reservoir harbors the tigerfish that make for good sportfishing, Lake Kariba is home to many enormous Nile crocodiles and herds of elephants who cling around the edge of the lake, sometimes causing trouble for boaters or passers-by.

Mopane woodlands are collections of scattered, stunted trees, a brushy understorey, and sparse grass. The mopane tree (*Colophospermum mopane*) dominates mopane woodlands. Mopane wood weighs 1.2 tons/m^3. It is one of the densest and therefore hardest woods in Africa, like the ironwood I had burned in one of my first South African safari camps. Lake Kariba has many skeletons of dead mopane trees. The resins in these trees as well as their hardness make them as solid now as the day they were killed in the flood that backed up in 1962 behind Kariba Dam.

The treetops could rip the bottom out of any passing boat that might consider them rotten. Drowned mopane trees are still pulled out and used as very acceptable solid wood today despite the 36 years since the lake was created for power, recreation, flood control, and irrigation. In flooding the rich Zambezi Escarpment, the submerged trees increased the surface of the lake by ten-fold, providing a substrate for aquatic life like sponges and jellyfish, making it somewhat like an inland sea. The rising Lake Kariba marooned animals on islands like Fothergill Island, named after the game ranger who launched the Noah's Ark-like rescue operation to salvage the stranded animals. Fothergill Island is the base from which Peter Tetlow, our other guide, would be arriving by air at the Kariba airstrip. This airstrip is in the middle of a remote wilderness. Its proximity to a major tourist attraction, Victoria Falls, means that modern jet aircraft can land here.

Peter manages safari operations for the Zimbabwe Sun Hotels. Although Gary now works for a separate firm, they were close professional colleagues and remain close friends. This trip brings them together for the first time since Gary began his new job. They were on a bit of a busman's holiday while being paid by us for the birding safari. It was a good deal all around. They can holiday and explore a new habitat for their favorite outdoor activity, birding. Gary had never been to Zambia. Peter was born there but had not returned since his family left when he was a child. His father was a mining engineer in the Zambian copper belt. The trip would be a bit of a homecoming for him. Kurt is a totally urban person who was being deposited in wild African bush for only his third time. He was being looked after by guides with years of experience in wild Africa, so he felt secure. I could do some uninhibited bush-bashing. Everyone was happy and in high spirits in anticipation of our adventure.

We stopped at Kariba airstrip to pick up Peter. His wife and two children were going on holiday to his wife's native Germany. We would be having our "boys night out" for a week bird-spotting, bush-bashing, learning more about ecological relationships from them, and telling lies around camp fires. Last summer, Kurt and I had hooked up with them for a similar adventure to the Eastern Highlands in Zimbabwe near the Mozambican border. We had such a good time that we decided to do it again in a different venue in Zambia. Originally, we had planned to hit Zambia, Botswana, and Namibia but limited time and various difficulties with getting permits and camping reservations forced truncation of our expedition. We would "only" be able to cover a few spots in remote Zambia.

The Zambezi Escarpment is a branch of the Great Rift along which runs the 2,760-km long Zambezi River, Africa's third longest river. The surface of Kariba Lake is now 5,000 km^2 filling what was the Gwembe Valley. Not too many years ago, there were thousands of black rhinos in the Gwembe Valley. Gary had to patrol constantly against poachers who pursued the dwindling rhinos. There are now less than a dozen remaining from this population. They are all kept in a guarded compound. Plans are underway for captive breeding and release of this magnificent creature back into the wild world. There is an odd habit difference between the two species of rhino. The white rhinos become much more irritable and dangerously unapproachable when in confinement. The black rhinos are typically very shy and aggressive in the wild bush but become tamer in confinement. They also become easier to poach in nature preserves. I have a story to tell about aggressive animals that become accustomed to humans.

THE ROGUE BULL ELEPHANT
AT KARIBA AIRSTRIP

When we arrived at Kariba, Peter Tetlow and his family had not yet arrived. The pilot who was going to carry them on the brief flight from nearby Fothergill Island was still at the airstrip. Gary pulled away from the airstrip to a roadside filling station to fill up the truck and our auxiliary tanks with diesel fuel at about $4.50 US per gallon. We picked up one of bachelor Gary's ideas of *haute cuisine*, warm Polly's chicken pies at Polly's Ice Cream. These local specialties were classic road food. They tasted good because we were famished. Several local birds including Lilian's Lovebirds (*Agapornis lilianae*), lovely little green parrots with reddish-orange heads, were in a large cage outside Polly's place. One had escaped the cage and was pecking at the seed from the outside in, a position in which it was legitimate, Kurt figured, to list it as a wild bird spotted. We packed up the drinks and chicken pies and returned to Kariba airstrip to await Peter's arrival, and to list our valuables for the Zambia customs before crossing the border. On the way back to the airstrip, I spotted a bull elephant we had seen and photographed earlier.

AND, NOW, COMES THE STORY--
THAT MIGHT HAVE BEEN THE LAST OF THE
"SAFARI FROM HARARE"

As we pulled out of the gas station and headed back toward the airstrip, we were passed by a caravan of Afrikaners on holiday. Like us, they had an extensive kit pulled behind 4X4 vehicles in a Venter trailer. These utilitarian camping trailers have a supported cover that can be raised secured for loading and then closed and locked to keep gear dry and safe from thieves. I waved as we passed them to go on to park under one of the few trees available for shade to open the camp kit and have our Polly's Chicken Pie lunch.

I walked over to see the unusual sight of a one-tusked bull elephant encroaching on the airstrip. The elephant threatened a group of people who were walking down the road, by advancing on them with flapping ears and trunk held high. They scrambled to the fence along the airstrip, and I walked the road in the direction opposite them as the bull stood up to tear branches from a lone tree on the other side of the road. A worrisome comment had been passed along later when we found out that a "problem elephant" had crushed and killed a schoolboy awaiting a lift to school at the turnoff to the Kariba airstrip. Could that killer have been *this* elephant? I thought of this possibility later.

I walked down the road, away from both the airstrip and the elephant, to get the wide-angle view of this bull acting up in front of our camp kit. Golfie had gone to get his camera from the trailer. He was fussing over it since it seemed to be giving him some trouble. He was within shouting distance of me. I was about 150 m from the elephant and about 300 m from the trailer. I was walking down the tarred road toward the intersection away from the airport. When I turned around to look back, I saw a very startling sight. The elephant was in a full charge, bearing down on me!

I saw the open-mouthed but speechless look of horror on Golfie's face and the dust kicked up by the fast-shuffling elephant who was silent and had his ears pinned back flat. His eyes were locked on me, and the most dangerous sign was that he had curled his trunk under his mouth, and he had pulled his head down for the collision. This was no bluffing threat display! His intent was obvious, and he was closing fast!

Golfie finally found his voice as the killer elephant closed. I was aware of the slender single tree on my side of the road, I was backing toward it, not turning and not running away from the beast who could obviously outrun me at the speed he was closing. "The *tree*!" yelled Golfie.

I made one jump when the bull was two meters from me—one body length. I got behind the six-inch trunk of this puny tree, half the size of the one the bull had been tearing apart at the time I had passed by him off the roadside. He screeched to a dusty halt and raised his trunk and blasted a trumpeting scream!

Everyone at the airstrip stood at the fence watching what was happening. Several shouted advice, most of which involved getting someplace else. I was eyeball to eyeball with an extremely annoyed five-ton beast as he crab-walked around the base of the tree. I reciprocated on the opposite side, keeping the tree trunk between us, even if he would not find that a very big impediment if he charged again. I played little white Sambo with a large gray pachyderm chasing circles around the base of the tree, an adrenaline surge focusing my concentration to avoid being reduced to bloody grease as I circled the tree. He sidled away with ears flapping and head and trunk held high, periodically turning around to see that I was duly impressed—and I was.

When Golfie pulled down the flip top of the trailer, he drove the vehicle over to get me, while the bull was still 15 m away. I backed up to enter the Toyota from the side opposite the trumpeting elephant. "Are you all right?" Kurt was freaked—he was a witness to the near flattening of the African explorer who had talked him into coming to Africa despite his abundant worries about safety. Gary said it was the closest call he had ever seen in eight years of professional guiding to losing a colleague or a client, and paid me the compliment of saying that I was one of the former rather than the latter. "Weren't you terribly scared out of your wits?" they asked.

Well, I probably might have been, had there been enough time to think rather than to act reflexly. My reflexive actions included shooting a dozen shots on full wide-angle manual focus of the rogue bull in full serious charge, the last of which exposures are from a lens-filling range of two meters (**Figure 34**).

"Great final photos!" was the comment at the airstrip after everyone had retold the story as Peter and family arrived with a good deal of laughter to break the tension. It is not good advertising to have an experienced Africanist greased by an elephant at the tourist take-off point into Kariba. I recounted the story earlier of my respectful dance in the marshes near Assa with a big bull elephant who had silently come up behind me. He crab-walked around me with his trunk high before he trumpeted and backed away after his threat (see Endpiece). I had unknowingly got between him and the cows of the herd I had spotted while stalking the Cape buffalo bull that had driven them off—and which eventually became the final bull of my 1990 hunts, this one even captured on videotape.

This elephantine episode was not taped. Fear paralyzed the camera holders behind me in the bush as they were hanging from trees when they saw the big bull emerge between them and me. I was holding a .375 H & H Weatherby Magnum at that time, although I never raised it from waist level, since the elephant bull and I treated each other with the utmost respect.

Somehow I knew that the big bull at Assa was bluffing and reminding me that I was in his turf and he was entitled to do jolly well whatever he wanted to do in it. I agreed.

This Kariba elephant was more used to seeing people and that familiarity made him much more dangerous. I also knew, even before Gary characterized it completely, that this was no mock charge as a bluff or threat display, but this rogue bull was intent on deadly mayhem. I am grateful there was a friendly thorn tree nearby, however flimsy it looked in retrospect. It is also a good idea that I did not run, both for the futility of it and the further enragement of this unpredictable "problem elephant" who is altogether too close to people and the airstrip, causing havoc not only to the arboreal vegetation but also to people. Golfie said he had already made his bluff to the workers he had scared off earlier. Therefore he would not threaten a second time. Now the elephant would have to run down his target to make good his threat with the same witnesses still looking on. The game rangers at Mana Pools National Park were already on their way to shoot this big brute, particularly since he is the same one that killed the boy the previous week. I am glad that the same outcome was not the case for the sake of this narrative, and a whole lot more.

This set off a couple of hours of banter from Peter and the airport personnel and Gary. They then put the incident behind them and turned to the next things. Not so with Kurt, who was not just upset but obsessed with the event, and spent a restless and sleepless night, contemplating the "Great Void" ahead. When asked later by Gary if this event had scared him, he responded, "Yes, but additionally, I scared myself!"

THE REST OF THE DAY'S ANTICLIMACTIC EVENTS INCLUDED A LONG RIDE LOST THROUGH ENDLESS BUSH TO FINALLY ARRIVE NEAR MIDNIGHT AT LOCHINVAR WHERE WE PITCHED CAMP

I could tell of the various events of the rest of the day—the crossing of the Kariba Dam, the exit from Zimbabwe and the entry to Zambia, or the scrounging of a few kwachas for incidental purchases. The exchange rate was 2200 Zambian kwachas to the US dollar. We passed through customs uneventfully but respectfully under the photo of Mr. Frederick J. T. Chiluba, the boyish-looking fellow who is the Zambian head of state, displacing the founder and major party political power, Kenneth Kuanda. We would be traveling through Gwembeland of the Batooku Valley among the Bembe people. The drive was long.

Gary had explicit directions to Lochinvar National Park. Darkness fell before we began searching in earnest for the sign indicating the entrance to the park. On the first try, we drove right past it. This was not altogether due to inattentiveness on the part of Peter, the navigator. We asked directions several times. One man was riding a bicycle and when we stopped to ask directions, he looked at us with terror and pitched off into the bush on foot, leaving his bicycle in the road. He was probably terrified by Kurt's goofy hat, a dark green affair with a huge front visor and absurd flaps to protect his neck and ears from the ferocious sun. The hat even had a short cord with an alligator clip on the end to secure it to one's clothing. The hat was functional but goofy-looking (**Figure 46**). Other pedestrians we questioned reported variously that it was 40 km in one direction or 10 km in the opposite direction. We stopped at a small lighted encampment that was occupied by several men who worked as a road repair crew, judging from the road grader parked nearby. They were watching a video recording of a kung fu movie. They didn't have much of a clue where the park was.

We thrashed around in the dark for what seemed like hours without finding the sign for the entrance to the park. It should be noted that my GPS gave me regular marks concerning our location. Too bad I didn't have a GPS mark for our *destination*. The effort was not totally wasted since we saw several Giant Eagle Owls (*Bubo lacteus*), a Spotted Eagle Owl (*Bubo africanus*) (as they flushed from the road), and a bushbaby in a tree. The bushbaby is a small prosimian primate that lives in bushes and has a cry like a baby, thus the name. It was getting late and time to get serious about finding the sign to this park. We finally discovered the sign, about four hours after we had intended to, now approaching midnight. The rusted and barely legible sign was buried under a mat of vines. Nevertheless, we kept up our barrage of abuse on Peter (now called Chief Fuckwit), who had been acting as navigator while Gary drove.

We were all tired from the long drive through endless bush while trying to feel our way along through the dark to our unguarded campsite. We would be the only visitors to Lochinvar that were not there to poach or to trade fish. Kurt ignored my announcements about our altitude and location from my GPS readings. He said sarcastically that it was unfortunate that we didn't have a GPS fix for our *campsite*. After the elephant charge, Kurt went on obsessively about what it was all about when it could have nearly been "all over" as he was contemplating the Great Void.

We unpacked as quickly as possible. The tent was pitched, and we had a quick dinner. I crawled into my sleeping bag to sleep soundly in anticipation of the new events the morning would bring. As I drifted off, Kurt was still going on about the meaning of it all. I was on *vacation*. It was time for sleep.

The next morning when Gary asked him casually if he had slept well, he said, "I just had one of the most appalling nights of my life." All night long, he stared into the psychic void and had to confront his own fear of oblivion after witnessing my close call with death. The near miss had terrified him more than me. Maybe the combination of Jack Daniels and mefloquine was not a good one. My close call with the enraged bull elephant remains one of my more lucid impressions among the memories of this trip. It made an even greater impression on Kurt, an individual who was not the target of the rogue bull's charge.

A WALK ON THE WILD SIDE THEN A LONG BIRD DRIVE TO CHUNGA LAGOON TO SEE THE ENDEMIC HERDS OF KAFUE LECHWE

July 27, 1998

The ThinkPad's black traveling case now looks exactly like the dry sand flood plain of the alluvial fan of the Kafue River. I hope the sand and grit has not made it through the protective cover. I plugged the machine into the cigarette lighter of the Toyota Hi-Lux and it works well. I may try to do some typing during daylight tomorrow as we go north to another Zambian "National Park." There is not much distinction between the vast trackless bush and what they call the Lochinvar National Park except that there is a gate where we woke the guard to enter. We returned today to pay the fee for foreign tourists visiting the park— the only ones that we have seen registered or present here. The last people that registered came three years ago to hunt the special Kafue lechwe that is found nowhere else on earth. Lochinvar is not Yellowstone National Park in August.

With so few paying visitors, the park seems to have been designed as a private poaching preserve for the indigenous people, who continue to poach despite the large warning sign on entry and "community development center" with the World Wildlife Fund (WWF) logo on it. Obviously the WWF financed the start up of this park for conservation but has pulled out entirely after putting together a little display on Stone Age artifacts found at Gwisho Hot Springs, a small thermal spring which we will walk to this morning in this very large flood plain. A sign at the park entrance warns that poachers will be fined 50 million kwacha, an absurd amount given the poverty here. There are graphic pictures of what will happen to apprehended poachers and a written warning: "Your Family will Starve to Death!"—if you are caught and jailed for poaching. The poachers understand probability theory. "Do not get caught. If you can regularly poach without getting caught, your family will eat quite well. After you inevitably get caught, however, they will get quite hungry."

I have mixed feelings about saving the Kafue lechwe at the expense of the indigenous inhabitants, both species overpopulated just now, but each subject to attrition. The entrance fees that we paid, the first in several years, provided a welcome addition to the local economy. When we went into the park and paid our fees, which amounted to something around $ 100.00 (if our "change" was not returned, which, of course, it wasn't), the village around the entrance was almost deserted and quite inactive. On the way out, the visible local population had grown by an order of magnitude. The village sparkled with a party atmosphere. There hadn't been that much cash around in a long time. The indigenous people were celebrating.

A WALK ON THE WILD SIDE

This morning we took a walk before breakfast. About half-way through we recalled that another part of that sign told us that we were required to remain in a closed vehicle unless accompanied by an armed escort from the Parks Board. Escorts were unavailable, so we couldn't follow the rules. On the other hand, there is zero possibility of them catching us and prosecuting some foreign naturalists who know more about the flora and fauna than the untrained and unavailable gate attendant could offer. They had no vehicle to come and return us the change from the overpayment of the fees, so, presumably, there were no patrols either. They had little incentive for bothering the only paying, nonpoaching guests the park has seen for years. They let us come in and do what we want to do since we were paying full fare.

We walked a long way over the vast flood plain and saw the dry alluvial fan and a few birds, including an uncommon Collared Palm Thrush (*Cichladusa arquata*). This brown-backed passerine has a striking yellow eye, and a buff throat patch outlined in black on an otherwise gray underside. When Gary spotted this unusual bird in a *Borassus* palm, he told us to keep an eye out for the Red-necked Falcon (*Falco chicquera*), an elegant little falcon that favored the same kind of palm tree. Only much later did we see the first game. These were a couple of antelope in the distance, which were probably oribi (*Ourebia ourebi*) We also saw what were probably Kafue lechwe, an endemic subspecies of the lechwe (*Kobus lechwe*). Far away we saw a few Burchell's zebra and then a large herd of Cape buffalo. All of these were perhaps 1000 meters distant across huge flat spaces with no water. I could not imagine what the Cape buffalo, who each require about 35 liters of water daily, were doing in this near-desert habitat.

We then saw the first green, which was not in any depression, but on a rocky hillock. The kopje had what seemed to be artesian water pressure. Then I could see bubbles, and realized that this was a hot spring with some algae that show by their color that the temperature is 94° C., nearly boiling. These are the Gwisho Hot Springs. Relics of Stone Age culture had been found in the vicinity of these springs.

As I reached the springs, I looked to my right and saw a group of eight greater kudu (*Tragelaphus strepsiceros*) that simply materialized in the dry plain. One was a bull and oddly had no horns. The large antelopes have gray and tan bodies with prominent vertical stripes. Their large horns form a long, elegant spiral. They watched me as I walked away, and then I looked up and saw the herd of about 100 Cape buffalo, now half the distance they were before. With the new and powerful Swarovski binoculars on loan from Gary, I could see the tears in their ears. We retreated slowly, watching birds and hearing the bark of Chacma baboons on the kopjies. I had just said that this would be ideal habitat for baboons, and therefore for leopards, when, as if on cue, we crossed a large set of *chui* tracks. We made it back to camp by the time the temperature rose, so we merely sat around after breakfast and vegged as the warming sun climbed overhead. You are reading these observations of the morning's activities of both man and beast, before the later heat of midday put each species into a lazy haze of enervation. Only the ThinkPad is now replete with energy.

A BIRD DRIVE TO THE CHUNGA LAGOON
WHICH FINALLY RUNS INTO THE HERDS OF GAME
THAT SHOULD HAVE FILLED THE PARK—
NOW CONCENTRATED AT THE WATER

While the others studied bird books and made notes on the morning's sightings, I went on one of my solo bush walks amid a large herd of Kafue lechwe wading into the Chunga Lagoon, part of the Kafue River's flood plain. The rest of the park looked ravaged by the dry season. At the lagoon, the overgrazed terrain now became lush with tall green reeds. I found three desiccated carcasses, two zebra and a Kafue lechwe. There were "scouts" at a hunting camp where the skulls of several large lechwe were stacked up and a lot of throwaway bones and hide samples seemed to be stacked up along the campsite. There were also some large fish skeletons.

I saw a strikingly large heron that I measured by comparing him against the lechwe that were standing around in the area. He flew away after I got a few pictures of him standing. I recognized him through the binoculars as the Goliath

Heron (*Ardea goliath*, at 140 cm, the world's largest heron). When you look at it, you wonder how a bird can be this big and still manage to fly. I also saw the Saddle-billed Stork (*Ephippiorhynchus senegalensis*), Red-knobbed Coots (*Fulica cristata*), and African Spoonbills (*Platalea alba*) that look a lot like those in the Everglades except they are white instead of pink. I heard African Fish Eagles (*Haliaeetus vocifer*) overhead. The other raptors circling above them include a Martial Eagle (*Polemaetus bellicosus*) and a Bateleur (*Terathopius ecaudatus*). This elegant raptor has a very short tail and long, thin wings. When in flight, it tilts its wings up and down to steer itself, resembling the balancing movements of an aerialist tightrope walker with a balancing bar. I have been told that the French word for an aerialist is *bateleur* but my modern Larousse dictionary defines this word as juggler. Maybe in Flemish (and therefore perhaps also Afrikaans), *bateleur* means aerialist. Maybe the bright colors of the Bateleur are reminiscent of a medieval juggler's costume. Whatever, the Bateleur is elegant as it soars and strikingly beautiful close-up (**Figure 35**).

I marked Chunga Lagoon at 15° 50.34′ S and 027° 14.78′ E and noted the high water of this dry season. I trekked along the side of the lagoon, shooting photos of unidentified coucals, pratincoles, and ibises. I also spotted a pair of Pygmy Geese (*Nettapus auriatus*). This most diminutive of African geese has a golden belly, dark green back, and black and white head. The male sports a handsome green and black-fringed patch on the side of his face. These birds were a delight to observe.

I saw a big lechwe ram at a distance. He was a frantically busy fellow, trying to keep a large herd of ewes in control. Paradoxically, they ran with their heads down as though this sneak posture made them invisible in the wide-open, flat, dry pan, like the proverbial ostrich with its head in the sand.

I tried to stalk the big ram, even reloading film on the run using the anthills along the way as cover through the parched and desiccated conditions of the overgrazed area. I shot a photo of the beautiful oribi, a small antelope with barred stripes on the inside of its long ears. I had seen red lechwe in the Okavango Delta in Botswana. Kafue lechwe are similar to the red lechwe there but these are an endemic subspecies that is so numerous as to have overgrazed this small park. It is probably a good idea that there is a hunting season to limit these prolific lechwe, even in this game preserve. Whatever its current status, having once been financed by the WWF, Lochinvar National Park is now a bit of an officially sanctioned extractive reserve for poachers and fish traders. Without the pressure from these hunting camps at Chunga Lagoon, the whole park would most likely look like the devastated near wasteland we had seen everywhere but at the waterside.

We returned in what would be a spectacular sunset to see the birds retreat to wherever they can find cover in this dry season desert at night. We felt the temperatures drop from the dry heat of the afternoon to the desert chill after sunset. It was a good day around Chunga Lagoon. We would have written off Lochinvar as nearly lifeless early on and completely overgrazed and devastated as we drove and walked farther. The explosion of life that the Chunga Lagoon produced rewarded our persistent exploration.

Africa is really the continent of contrasts.

FROM LOCHINVAR NATIONAL PARK
TO KASANKA NATIONAL PARK

July 28, 1998

This is beautiful! We started out in the cold and dark, breaking camp before an extraordinarily beautiful sunrise. We drove as far and as fast as we could over roads being paved and improved by a Danish development group. We noted one extraordinarily sun-burnt, over-heated Danish man supervising road construction and imagined what his wife thought about their posting here in the middle of nowhere. Shopping probably wasn't that great around here. We were stopped frequently by police roadblocks, to show our customs declaration for our vehicles and camp kit, and the Zambian insurance purchased at the Kariba entry. We were headed northeast to Kasanka National Park, a 420-km^2 park with rivers, riverine woodlands, and a large papyrus swamp. It represents a different ecosystem where we would presumably find some new birds. Gary and Peter were excited by the prospect of enjoying the birding in a new habitat. They are both keen birders with a lot of experience in Zimbabwe. Last year, we beat the bush in the Eastern Highlands on Zimbabwe. During the week, Gary listed only one new life bird, the obscure Marsh Tchagra (*Tchagra minuta*). This little black-capped winner is a tough bird to find. It is endemic to the Eastern Highlands of Zimbabwe and adjacent areas in Mozambique. Peter had picked up perhaps six new birds for his life list on that trip. Both men were full of high energy and clever good humor about the frequent ironies, a part of adaptation in Africa. They delighted in showing us what were for them familiar birds. They took vicarious pleasure from our delight.

Zambia was a whole new birdgame for all of us. For starters, there isn't a proper field guide for Zambia. Gary found a published but out-of-print book of detailed field notes on Zambian ornithology. Unfortunately, it had no illustrations. We had along copies of Newman's *Birds of Southern Africa* and Zimmerman's *Birds of Kenya and Northern Tanzania*. Kurt had also brought along notes gleaned from the scanty descriptions of Zambian sites in Wheatley's *Where to Watch Birds in Africa*. Using these sources, Gary and Peter were able to sort out nearly all birds observed. The bird listers were in hog heaven

We traveled over 800 km today. The map would show 341 miles between Lochinvar and Kasanka (at 12° 33.37′ S and 030° 17.68′ E from the GPS as the Ross's Turaco would fly. In Kasanka, we realized we were only about 20 km from the furthest southeast extension of Congo's Shaba Province. The roads were indirect and often in disrepair.

We would have made nearly as good a time as we might have if traveling on the US interstate highway system, if we hadn't spent so much time showing our credentials and getting our possessions eyed by the uniformed guards at roadblocks. Kurt is still perseverating about the last one who took his Zeiss binoculars, carefully examined and admired them and did not give them back any time soon. Besides costing the guard's lifetime salary and that of his village, Kurt would rather give up both testicles than part with his binoculars. Without this important tool, the bird watching for him would be seriously undermined. We managed to escape the roadblocks by giving up ballpoint pens or a few dollars to the "inspectors" checking papers. How many times have you been stopped in long-distance travel across the USA? There is no particular war threat here. This is just African SOP, so that the local "authorities" can examine and see what plunder is slipping through their temporary jurisdictions that could be viewed as manna from heaven.

So, if the people we were driving by and the petty shakedowns were not an adequate indicator that we are in the third world, one checkpoint we encountered was. Just before the entrance to the Kasanka Park dirt road, we saw three guards in the green fatigues with orange pinstripes that I recognized as Eastern Europe castoffs from, I believe, the Czech Army, along with Chinese machine pistols fitted to wire shoulder mounts. Ralph Lauren could have added to his fortune by using this fabric for shirting. Kurt began worrying about the possibility of losing the Ray-Ban sunglasses he loaned to me (his backup set) since mine had become Sasa's new status symbol in Assa. I assured him that if they were shaken down at the checkpoint, I would replace his sunglasses on return to the land of shopping malls. Then the guard put all of Kurt's sphincters into spasm, by spitting a shell from the clip into the action. I remarked later that the performance was not all that impressive, since he had to look at the weapon to work it. A very experienced fellow could have done that without looking. Since this was Kurt's first encounter with automatic weapons he was impressed enough to forget his worry about his Ray-Ban sunglasses!

LUNCH UNDER THE BLUE SKY HABITAT OF A GYMNOGENE

We had broken camp in the dark and had pulled out, leaving the Kafue lechwe ram skull I found at Chunga Lagoon (**Figure 38**) as our Lochinvar souvenir at the campsite, just as we saw the sun rising. In the early light, we had found our way down the dirt roads that we could not see as we came around midnight. We slid down the road in daylight until we reached the main paved road. We went north and arrived at Lusaka, the capital, before noon, and saw the crowds in urban Africa, looking a bit like the sprawl of Nairobi. On the northern outskirts of Lusaka, we passed through a depressing shantytown. Huts were constructed out of reeds, sheet metal, and discarded plastic.

There were a lot of people living on the edge here. The main industry appeared to be "entropy" factories. In these, people were taking large boulders, cinder building blocks extracted from decaying buildings, bricks, and the hulks of burned out trucks and reducing them to piles of trap rock, brick sand, and small scraps of steel. The product of these manual reductions was then loaded into burlap bags. The purpose of all this was unclear to us. Can you reduce bricks to clay and then remanufacture the bricks? If so, why not just use the bricks again? Presumably, the wrecked trucks represented high-grade ore and they were being reduced to make then portable enough to be loaded on porter's heads. Pakistan, which has no iron ore, is a principal steel producer from the manual labor of "ship breaking." The most memorable sight was an old woman (50-80) sitting beside a gray boulder perhaps three meters high, slowly reducing it to pebbles with a hammer. The amazing part was that all this was being done in Zambia with simple hand tools.

We crossed out of town and headed up to Kabwe, the third largest town behind Ndola, the second city of the North. These are the urban centers of Zambia. The copper belt around Ndola produces most of the extractable wealth of the Zambian economy. Unfortunately, copper prices continue on a decades-long slide. At present, the vast copper reserves can't even pay the cost of extraction, even with the pitifully low wages paid to Zambian miners. This copper belt extends to the Shaba and Kasai provinces of Congo.

When we got past Lusaka, we headed toward Kabwe. About 20 km beyond the urban squalor of Lusaka, we pulled off very briefly on a dirt road at a place called Blue Gum Farm for "brekkie." We had hardly pulled into the dirt road when a big gray hawk floated overhead. We parked in the shade of the only nearby tree and ate our late breakfast of Pro-Nutra, an instant cereal product most like US baby cereal. When you are hungry and it is supplemented with fresh apple slices and a dash of yogurt, it tastes remarkably good. We kidded Gary (the cook) incessantly about the food, bitterly complaining that "Comandante Bird" would make us wait for food until we were nearly ready to gnaw at our own extremities and then feed us with curried road kill to make us think it was suitable sustenance. In truth, the food was delicious and probably even good for us, but we never let on to Gary.

What is that? The large, gray, broad-winged raptor with long yellow legs and a yellow bare face and bill is a Gymnogene (*Polyboroides typus*), a prime raptor near the top of Kurt's wish list, so we had perfectly timed our good late brunch stop. We stopped for fuel when we reached Kabwe. I ran around the corner down the middle of this town's streets and found the post office. Kabwe was once called "Broken Hill." There are lead mines here with plenty of galena, the lead sulfide ore. Aerogramme postage was 700 kwachas, to the best of their information, since they did not know of anyone who had sent one before. There should be 600 kwacha stamps for the postcards. Now the bad news is they had neither 600 nor 700 kwacha stamps. "But if I would come back later...." This was the same statement we had heard at the Lochinvar National Park, where they did not have the correct change. They would return at 6:00 AM to bring the $15.00 US change, from the $100.00 fees. Of course, there was no man at 6:00 AM, nor could they find where "he stays." There are 2200 kwacha to the dollar, so we drove off leaving a relative treasure for the impoverished guards. I ran back to the refueling truck, borrowed some kwachas from Kurt, bought my stamps, and mailed my letter and postcards.

ARRIVAL IN THE PLUSH COMPARATIVE LUXURY OF THE "CHALETS" OF WASA CAMP IN KASANKA NATIONAL PARK

I am now parked at our encampment in Wasa Camp in Kasanka National Park. The ThinkPad is now charged up as I sit by the side of the watercourse in which I have just spotted a number of species before the sunset. This is Wasa. The Luwombwa River is where we might be tomorrow night and the Kasanka River will be crossed. These rivers do not connect with each other. This is a watershed divider, from which some of the flow goes north into the Rift and out the Nile; the remainder contributes to the westward flow of the mighty Congo.

Just before reaching Wasa Camp, we crossed a small bridge constructed of interlaced branches over a small stream. We carefully lumbered over the narrow bridge. We stopped to look and immediately saw a marvelous bird, Ross's Turaco (*Musophaga rossae*). There she was, in all her gorgeous splendor, the last of my turacos of Southern Africa.

From the common Grey Go-away Bird (*Corythaixoides concolor*), that I first got to know, I have moved up to the top of the line. At Sodwana, in KwaZulu/Natal, I had spotted the Knysna Lourie (*Tauraco persa*), with its spectacular red flashes of underwing. Last year, in Zimbabwe's Eastern Highlands, I saw the Livingstone's Turaco (a different subspecies of *T. persa*) and the Purple-crested Turaco (*Musophaga porhyreolopha*). Next year would be the right time, we had figured, when we would try for the last of my Southern African turacos, namely Ross's Turaco. In Southern Africa, this is the most spectacular but rarely seen turaco. Ross's Turaco is found only in the Okavango Delta in the countries covered by Newman's *Birds of Southern Africa*. It is more widespread in Zambia and the Congo, but never easy to find. We assumed that it would be very unlikely that we could ever see the Ross's Turaco.

The turacos are large, usually dramatically colored birds. They have brilliant red panels at the tips of their wings that become conspicuous when they fly. Their bodies are often rich greens or blues. These are not structural colors, formed by diffraction gratings of melanin granules in the feathers. Rather, these colors are pigments formed from copper-containing porphyrins excreted through their skin. The red of vertebrate blood, the blue of horseshoe crab blood, and the green of plant chlorophyll are each due to iron-, copper-, and magnesium-containing porphyrins respectively. Similarly, the red of the wings is due to a compound called turacin or uroporphyrin III, an unusual copper-containing porphyrin. The green of these birds is caused by turacoverdin, another porphyrin with uncertain chemical relationship to turacin. The books said that Ross's Turaco is rare and could not be predictably seen and that, of course, made it all the more desirable for the birders.

Can you believe, I have now seen all the turacos in Newman's book? There in the tree over us was a pair of Ross's Turacos! These birds were large and predominantly blue with a prominent red crest and a bright yellow bill. When they flew, their wings have a panel of brilliant red with an iridescent blue border. The bird is unmistakable in the field. As Peter stared through his binoculars, he whispered, "Lady Ross's Lourie, you fucking beauty," in rapt awe. We were all thrilled. It was even a "lifer" for Gary. We exchanged jubilant high fives. I took the binoculars down and raised the camera—just too late. But a Lizard Buzzard (*Kaupifalco monogrammicus*) came in and a little later a new large hornbill, the Pale-billed Hornbill (*Tockus pallidirostris*) came along with a half-dozen other birds to round out the day. So the bird listers were in nerd paradise.

We drove about 10 km farther along a rough dirt road and finally arrived at the Wasa Camp. An Englishman named Edmond Farmer here from Volunteers in Service Overseas met us. Ed and a group of indigenous people were guarding and maintaining the park as a private concession for a trust. Some of these volunteers are passionate about stopping poachers. Tough animal conservation measures are not popular here. Native people have been living off the game here forever and are not moved by the designation of their food supply as a game preserve. Hunters, paradoxically, are among the best conservationists. Newcomers, funded from some preservation trust a world away who arrive with inspired mandates about "saving" anything are not well-oriented in the ways of African bush life. There must be some kind of compromise to make game management and survival of indigenous people work.

ARRIVAL AND GAME VIEWING AT WASA CHALETS OF KASANKA NATIONAL PARK

Soon after arrival, I found my way to an observation platform perched in the crown of the tallest tree in sight. I climbed the tricky ladder of boards and sticks nailed to the trunk until I got up to the canopy and looked over the Wasa marsh and river, and saw—nothing, at first. Then scanning it with the Swarovski binoculars, I started seeing things: an African Fish Eagle, many Yellow-billed and Marabou Storks, and a lot of Spur-winged Geese, Africa's largest goose. Then I saw the other animals. One was a big hippo in mid-river. I had localized him with the help of his grunting bellow. Then I saw several antelope, which look like the lechwe we had seen yesterday, but here the niche is filled by pukus (*Kobus vardoni*). Then I saw an animal I was really eager to see. The sitatunga (*Tragelaphus spekei*) is a beautiful dark brown antelope. Ed told me that Ross's Turacos were as common as sparrows and he added that this is one place I could be guaranteed to see sitatunga. He also mentioned that Black Mambas are common and a real problem around here. This is a highly venomous and extremely aggressive snake. When threatened, it attacks and bites repeatedly. I once heard of seven people dying in an incident in South Africa involving a cornered Black Mamba.

I am chilled out now as the sun had set and I learned more about this privatized park from the locals. They are very keen to compare notes with our Zimbabwean guides who are here with us to find out more about this totally different ecosystem. So, we have a busman's holiday for them, and a focused natural history tutorial for me, while Kurt obsesses over his life list, and how many years it will take to list the one half of the species of birds on earth that is his goal. He has observed and identified about 1,300 species of the required 5,000, and unless he picks up the pace, he will be 98 and unable to put up with these hardships and he will still not have crossed the halfway point in his list. I have been without power and plumbing most of this month and I am now in a thatched chalet with a bed, mosquito netting, and hot water. I am sitting in a spot like the San-Ti-Wana Lodge I had visited in the Okavango Delta in Botswana. This is comparative luxury for me. I'm on *vacation* in the African bush and couldn't be much happier.

So, we have arrived at "destination travel." Edmond Farmer advises against a one-day expedition into the swamps of Lake Bangweulu. In that short time, we have no possibility of seeing the central swampland of Lake Bangweulu and the Shoebill (*Balaeniceps rex*) that was our next target. The Shoebill is a one-meter-tall gray stork. It has a huge bill, literally the size and shape of a shoe. Lake Bangweulu is 140 km but over eight hours away. Then we would need to round up guides and a boat, and then actually find the bird. All this simply won't fit into one day. I am keen to see the place where Doctor David Livingstone died near here. So, I have arrived where I would like to be. I am in the swampy headwaters of the vast Congo River basin. These streams here join the Congo River and eventually flow over Stanley Falls, named after the New York Herald reporter Henry Morton Stanley. In 1851, Stanley finally came upon Livingstone and said "Doctor Livingstone I presume." —nearly the same line that has been applied to me several times recently in various paths of the good Doctor Livingstone that I already crossed.

41 WASA WALKABOUTS

A DAY OF WASA WALKABOUT EXPLORING THE BIRDS AND BEASTS OF KASANKA NATIONAL PARK

July 29, 1998

At dawn this morning I clambered up to a platform overlooking the Wasa marsh in front of camp to see the orange sunrise before it disappeared into the clouds that cover this part of the swampy interior of Zambia. Here the headwaters of the Congo start trickling through the bush to the mighty river that gives its name to the nation in which I spent most of this month. We are only 20 km from the southeastern border of the DRC as dusk falls on another eventful day.

WALKABOUT NUMBER ONE

The birders went for a short walk through the miombo woodland hoping to sight new species for their lists. I took off six km down the road to see a large flood plain studded with "termite tombstones," the hills that extend to the horizon from the lateritic base. The burned-over swampy grasslands are now powder dry and marked with cemented-in footprints of everything from elephants to African civets and genets, and the most frequent species of antelope here, the puku, (*Kobus vordoni*). This middle-sized antelope is tan above and white below and has black spiraling horns that curve like half of a recurved hunting bow

I then walked toward several herds of these antelope. The puku is almost as characteristic of this park as the Kafue lechwe was of the Lochinvar Park. They are each about the same size and inhabit flood plain systems. Lochinvar's Kafue River drains to the Zambezi River and eventually flows out through Mozambique into the Indian Ocean. The rivers from the Wasa area of

Kasanka are part of the Congo watershed. They arise from a much higher altitude than those of the lower Zambezi watershed.

I stalked a herd of puku ewes, and could actually get reasonably close to them, within easy rifle range. I saw another herd in the burned over dry season swamp, and stopped under a tree, with the local name "*Wasa wachi Congolo.*" In it were the first Green Pigeons (*Treron calva*) I had ever seen —but then I saw 40. I took a picture of a lourie (another name for the turaco group) but after taking a picture of it I realized that it was the ordinary Grey Go-away Bird not the spectacular Ross's Turaco.

I turned to see a group of pukus. Behind them perched a pair of Ross's Turacos. This bird certainly isn't scarce in Kasanka National Park. I took a few photos and then advanced on the pukus as they were looking in the opposite direction. As I got closer, they still looked away, and then ran toward me. I wondered what had startled them. As I walked back across the flood plain, I saw a lone puku ram sitting in the middle of a large burned area looking away from me. He did so consistently, and I used the trees and termite mounds to cover my upwind approach to within bow range. I took several good photos that I hoped included the termite mounds, reminding me of tombstones in a cemetery. These would provide a special backdrop. I then saw the puku ram stand up and still looking away from me, he ran as he pronked with the startled four-footed springs that are characteristic of this antelope and the mule deer in the Western US. He ran over the termite tombstones of the "cemetery in the flood plain" as the tangential light of dawn arrived. I was dive-bombed by Wattled Plovers (*Vanellus senegallus*) who were trying to distract me from their nesting site nearby.

I walked back in a "happy camper" mode from my solitary walk in the African bush, the kind of thing I had done so often and missed so much on this trip to Assa. On my previous visits, I often did it with a rifle in hand, checking the natural history around me for good reason, dinner. I returned to camp and ate Gary's healthy brunch prepared as we packed up for what would be the second birding foray for the group. We took a little while to get organized. We first set out on foot around camp, but Kurt had a suggestion, that they get together a better accommodation—two lounge chairs in the back of the pick-up truck bed, and a "cooler box" filled with cold beer and lunch. He would sit with the Zeiss binoculars that nearly left his hand for good at the roadblock checkpoint. The slow start began with a roll forward while Gary listened for birdcalls. By using incredibly accurate imitations of these calls, he attracted a few of the calling species in for closer observation in the canopy of the miombo woodlands. He may have initiated bird parties of his own through excellent mimicry.

HIKING THROUGH THE BUSH TO A PLATFORM HIDE
OVERLOOKING KAPABI SWAMP

As the rest of the group pursued little brown birdies to differentiate, I wandered forward on foot. There were no mosquitoes—good news; there were lots of tsetse flies—bad news. I walked along while the blazing sun baked the exposed cement-like terrain with its dry, lateritic base with sparse, hard-scrabble, burned scrub. The sun is ferociously intense in such places, where the air is very clear and dry. I saw large termite hills, tall enough to climb and use as observation posts. I saw a breeding herd of the puku and crept relatively close. I was also on the lookout for the Black Mamba, the most frequently seen snake here. The Gabon Viper is also common here. It is a large, thick, sluggish pit viper with a brown and gray pattern on its back that is nearly perfect camouflage for the dry leaves that litter the forest floor here. When stepped on by mistake, it swiftly delivers a massive dose of potentially lethal venom. Neither reptile should be stumbled over unannounced.

I passed a few forks in the road on my way toward the Fibwe Hide, since I wanted to look over the large Kapabi Swamp where there was an assurance of seeing the rare sitatunga (*Tragelaphus spekei*), the last of my "twist horns." After about 45 minutes I happened upon an endless expanse of mature papyrus fringed by tall *Phragmites* (grass) that had no visible limit. I scanned the hummocks and the edges where vegetation met water and saw the splay-hoofed tracks of the sitatunga. This low-slung antelope has shorter legs than its open-country counterparts and long, broad, splayed hooves that hold it up on the floating mass of reeds.

At the edge of the stream that drains this large swamp toward a river we will see tomorrow, I saw a huge *Khaya anthotheca* tree, and in it I saw a platform. I turned to climb up into the enormous tree overlooking this swamp and found myself on the Machan Sitatunga Hide. And, I saw them.

At first, I saw them a long way away. They are so well-protected in their swamp world—in which I had first indistinctly spotted them in the Okavango—that they are nearly impervious to invaders. I saw a male, and a few females, one followed by a lamb. I spent a long time watching them, spoiled by the powerful Swarovskis that make them so clear and close.

I spent two hours in the canopy, making observations and enjoying the cool and relatively bugless altitude with a huge panorama of swamp over which I was watching, very much like a number of deer stands I have been in 'at quite different temperatures and latitudes. I was wondering about the following bird watchers when they drove up in their diesel vehicle. They went nuts about the size of the tree and the number of species flitting around in the canopy. A number of times I had heard a loud startling "pop," as the large woody seed pod of the *Khaya anthotheca* opened explosively to spread its seeds, leaving behind a hard, "star flower" as a husk. Last year, in the Chirinda Forest in the Eastern Highlands of Zimbabwe, we had all hiked to "The Big Tree," a 65-m specimen of *K. anthotheca*. This is said to be the tallest tree in Zimbabwe. Along the way, we spotted Swynnerton's Robin (*Swynnertonia swynnertoni*), a difficult species to find, which is restricted to secluded montane forests in East Africa with an isolated remnant pocket population much further south in Eastern Zimbabwe.

I explained to the newcomers the wonders I had seen, and they decided to come up to the platform for a while. The platform was perhaps 30 m up a twisty ladder of boards and branches nailed to the trunk. It was a bit daunting, especially if you thought about breaking a leg out here. Also, encumbered with lunch, books, binoculars, and a spotting scope, it took everyone about 10 minutes to clamber up to the platform. We saw lots of good birds up there, including a barbet that we couldn't identify. We gathered a complete field description as a team, calling out observations as Kurt recorded them. Later, he was able to sort it out as the Black-backed Barbet (*Lybius minor*), a lifer for everyone. The prettiest feature of this black and white bird was a delicate wash of peach color in the middle of its lower belly.

We took a break for lunch. The salami had "gone off in the fridge." The extremely bumpy bush roads bounced the gas-fired refrigerator around enough that it barely worked. After an extended consultation, we decided that the salami just barely passed the "whiff test." We were all hungry so we ate it anyway. Soon after lunch, Gary heard a commotion in nearby trees and said, "We better leave because that might be a Black Mamba." Our exit from the platform was considerably more rapid than our ascent.

WALKABOUT NUMBER THREE

The next order of business was to trek through a climax forest at the margin of the swamp. We heard the cries of the African Fish Eagle (the national bird of Zambia) and saw other raptors as well as Woolly-necked Storks (*Ciconia episcopus*). I walked ahead, while Kurt worried about Black Mambas. Gary walked with his sandaled feet through the trail—and abruptly began stamping his feet and howling. Somehow I walked through a huge army of driver ants, who were ready to latch on to Gary when he came by. They are called "driver ants" since they push everything before them. Earthworms and other creatures will get right out of the ground ahead of an advancing colony which can number over 20 million individuals.

As I was watching Gary do his dance, I thought of my similar dance when I had changed film in the Ngong Hills only to find out that I was doing so in the middle of a colony of very aggressive ants. Suddenly, I looked up and saw a flash of red and blue as a Ross's Turaco came through the treetops and I tried to photograph it. But I noticed also that there were splash marks of an even larger bird. I was standing near his perch beneath the area from where the turaco had flown and then called out as it flushed. A sudden swoosh revealed a large Crowned Eagle (*Stephanoaetus coronatus*), who flew out ahead of us. We heard several mewing calls from the eagle. It sounded a lot like the Osprey's call. Then I looked down. It was like finding the best of emeralds: I found a complete wing flight feather of the Ross's Turaco! It is stained with the bright red turacin that these birds excrete in their wing feathers that gives them the surprising flash of crimson as they fly. The feather also sported an iridescent blue-green patch near the base of the shaft. It was remarkably beautiful, a collector's keepsake (**Figure 42**).

Kurt was running out of energy and wanted to call off the rest of the day. Gary was still keen on going off to another site and seeing what could be found there in the prime birding time when the "bird parties" occur. These consist of mixed flocks of vocal birds, often following the White Helmetshrikes (*Prionops plumatus*), Fork-tailed Drongos (*Dicrurus adsimilis*), Rufous-bellied Tits (*Parus rufiventris*) and others depending on the waves of the termites beneath them, some as flushers and others as gleaners. Kurt called all this the "Comandante Bird's bloody Zambian death march." He voted that we collapse with a cold beer or two and beg out until a catered dinner. Although I was eager to use the last of the light—a habit of recent desperation in the Congo— we turned back toward camp.

As unexpected as it was prehistoric, out of the tall dry brown grass, a large, lone, tusker bull elephant came marching into the tangential twilight of the African flood plain. He had once been shot at or speared and had a wound behind his left eye in front of his ear. He had a broken off tusk on the left, with about twelve kg of ivory on that side still left—enough to make him a target for poachers still. And he was huge. He weighed about the same as the five tons of the enraged bull elephant that decided to squash me flat at the Kariba airstrip, but this bull was much more skittish and spooky. He knew we were there, so he snorkeled the air repeatedly with his trunk upraised high and his ears fanning. We had shut off the engine and rolled slightly as I was snapping photos of him. He came up and turned with his ears flapping and stared in my direction.

As we watched him in his threat displays and his warning motions of ears and trunk, we started the engine. And here he came! With a shuffle of dust and a wide, spread-eared, head-on view which made him look twice as wide as a freight train and at least four times more menacing, he charged the vehicle (**Figure 41**)! Gary had it rolling as I was shooting—this time from a vehicle and this time with a telephoto lens at a range of 100 meters—instead of at a range of two meters and with wide-angle lens. We drove away before he could reach our vehicle. I preferred this elephant encounter to the one in Kariba but the event and the photos of the latter were more exciting at a close-range near miss.

42 ROAD TRIP TO LAKE BANGWEULU

THE BIGGEST BRIDGE IN ALL AFRICA
THE MIDPOINT IN A LONG ROAD TRIP FROM WASA CAMP TO
LAKE BANGWEULU, TWINGI, AND LAKE KAMPOLOMBO

July 30, 1998

SAMFYA, ZAMBIA

It is hard to believe that we have pulled off another winner of a day in northeastern Zambia, starting off early at dawn from Wasa, covering over 360 km *one way*! We had been warned that our target destination, Lake Bangweulu, is way out of range for a day trip. Given this challenge, it only seemed reasonable to overshoot this large lake to have our lunch in a grove on still further Lake Kampolombo in a mission station named Twingi. Along the way, we spotted birds, including a large flock of Hammerkopf and Marabou Storks even before getting out of Kasanka. I loaded cameras to record what I hoped would be a stop at Chitambo Station, David Livingstone's Memorial. I wrote the first postcards of the trip into upper Zambia while bouncing around in the back of the truck. I later gave the postcards to a hitchhiking Peace Corps volunteer (PCV) and his girlfriend, trying to make it to Lusaka to catch a plane on the weekend.

What also transpired turned out to be brunch on and then under the four-km Luapula River Bridge on the long, straight, paved, Chinese-built highway on which much of today's 750-km, high-speed road tripping was done. What further happened was the "puncture" and changing of a tire among an appreciative audience of a bush crowd, picking up a Peace Corps Volunteer and his girlfriend, the running out of fuel, the running across a large herd of rare black lechwe at the last moments of light, and catching the sun setting over the Luapula Bridge. And, now for the details.

THE LUAPULA RIVER BRIDGE AND ENDLESS FLOODED GRASS-LANDS OF THE BANGWEULU SWAMP

This is a wonder! A long straight road up through the middle of what Peter called, "miles and miles of bloody fuck-all." The Chinese constructed this road in the 1980's with the then left-leaning socialist government of Dr. Kenneth A. Kaunda, a proud graduate of UNISA (the University of South Africa), the largest correspondence school in the world. On August 19, 1983, Dr. Kaunda dedicated the Luapula River Bridge, according to the sign posted at the guardhouse at the end, a product of the Chinese-Zambian Economic Cooperation Council. This four-km bridge, longest in Africa, crosses a wetland that stretches to the horizon in all directions. This is another *River of Grass*, the title of Marjorie Stoneman Douglas's book on the Florida Everglades. There are long stretches of reeds and a lot of birds, a few large fish, and one crocodile head poking up for air.

We chatted up Emmanuel, the crossing guard, as he checked each crossing vehicle—(two in the course of our being there, the other being an overloaded, top-heavy combi, with dead bream hanging from the wing mirrors). He had a uniform and a Chinese G-3, a cheaper version of the 7.62 caliber SKS with a 20-shot clip and full automatic capability. Emmanuel allowed us to pack out our cooler boxes and even the spotting scopes and carry this arsenal of optics down to the water and around the bridge pilings. He let us know that this was all a special favor for which we should do something nice for him, and to come back quickly if the "big boss" comes. So, we had our usual on-the-road Pro-Nutra brunch with fresh fruit topping, this time as we sat under the bridge and watched men poling their dugout canoes to haul up fish or firewood, as we bagged six new species (**Figure 46**). We added the Blue-breasted Bee-eater (*Merops variegatus*) who posed for me in photo range, and a lot more that were in range of our binoculars. This immense wetland is similar to the Everglades in its species and niches, e.g., the Fan-tailed Widowbird (*Euplectes axillaris*), is almost identical in appearance, behavior, and niche to our common Red-winged Blackbird in the US.

Emmanuel was quite friendly and had done us a favor, so we gave him a few dollars. He worried as we set up the military-looking Swarovski spotting scope. He let us eat breakfast and look for birds as long as he dared but then wanted us out of there. To return Emmanuel's kindness, we gave a lift to some of his relatives, a man and his daughter with the man's nursing grandson clutching her torso. They threw a sack into the back of our truck and piled in as we moved on—and on.

We headed toward Lake Bangweulu, which we had been assured, was out of our range, but was at the end of an excellent tarred road. Most of the traffic was pedestrian as we raced down between walls of elephant grass, which had been burned over or harvested for thatching everywhere except immediately adjacent to the road, where it obscured our view of the surrounding wetlands.

We drove on to the odd town of Samfya, where a sign advertised it as the "tourist capital" of the Luapula Province. From there, we saw Lake Bangweulu. It was fringed by immense sand dunes, and even had a little harbor marina with four large pleasure boats now rotting in ruins on the bottom of the harbor. There was not a lot of luxury around Samfya. It looks like any other down-market Central African town. We saw little roadside piles of cassava for sale.

One fellow attached himself to us, saying he would be our escort since he was suffering severely from hunger and needed our help. For the cost of several pieces of hard candy, we got the door closed on him and went on our way. We left behind what looked like the great lakes of the Rift Valley, southernmost being Lake Malawi. Lake Malawi was formerly Lake Nyasa. David Livingstone asked the Jao-speaking Nyasaland people (in what is now the Niasa Province of Mozambique) what it was called. They told him it was called *nyasa* = "lake." Livingstone dutifully named this body of water "Lake Lake."

We went forward to get a GPS fix on the outlet of Lake Bangweulu at the origin of the Luapula River in a town named Mpanta. We kept on going over a hand-dug canal connecting Lake Bangweulu with Lake Kampolombo, lying to the south. We drove along a long road improved by the Chinese, presumably for the harvesting of fish from the lakes. We passed several large groups of seated people, possibly funerals. All the people were doing daily chores—grinding cassava on stones, mending nets, weaving fish traps, doing hairdos, chasing kids, and waving at the unusual passing vehicle.

TWINGI LUNCH STOP UNDER THE ARBOR ON THE LAKE PICK-UP OF HITCHHIKERS, SPOTTING THE BLACK LECHWE, AND THE LONG HAUL BACK TO WASA CAMP

We drove farther on a dirt road along Lake Kampolombo. We finally came to a mission station where we met a school teacher to ask if we could make a circuit forward to Mpanta, a river port that is seen on the map. The ferry was not working so we would need to backtrack. Bummer! We were all hungry now so we asked him about where we could stop for our late lunch. We got directed to an arbor along the marshes of the lake. We gave him a small donation for the church and tried to get him to keep the rest of the village from closing in on us.

He was halfway to being successful, since we only had a few hundred observers, all intrigued by our appearance, our vehicle, and the idea that we were talking about and looking in the sky and trees—for they knew not what. "Don't the birds come to you? Why should anyone have to go to them?"

We had a lunch of canned ham and crumbly bread, the scraps of which we turned over to the gathered crowd, which, as we knew it would, induced a feeding frenzy. The remains of lunch were spilled on the swampy ground but eaten in any event. While standing there, we were treated to a dissertation by Kurt about a certain visceral urgency he had and about the sundry inhibitions he had about resolving that problem. We gave him suggestions about what he might do for relief. In spite of Gary's helpful warnings about Black Mambas, Kurt took some TP and left his spoor in the elephant grass. While this drama was going on, five raptors appeared nearby, several of them new to the group, including a pair of Red-necked Falcons (*Falco chicquera*). These look quite a lot like Peregrine Falcons, but have a handsome rust-colored collar. We pulled our kit together and packed for the long road trip, and had pulled out on our way when we heard a soft flapping noise on the dirt road.

We had "got a puncture." Not the "slow puncture," which is the Zimbabwean euphemism for AIDS, a rather good description of the slow deflation that happens in "slim," in which the "air is let out" as the person vanishes by inches. We lowered the spare after checking to see that it had not been stolen. It was fastened with a chain to prevent that inevitability, at least temporarily. Our kibitzing audience grew, and all stood around in fascination as we turned the lug nuts and fiddled with the new screw jack. When we completed the operation I turned to the audience, took a bow, and received their applause as I shot a picture. This was the biggest entertainment that they had seen in this community from Twingi to the great Lake Bangweulu in all of the province to Samfya for the first vehicle that had come down the road for a long time.

We drove on to Samfya, the corner we had tried to pass through quickly when Kurt was hiding his Zeiss binoculars and Ray-Bans under the seat. Ever since the earlier encounter with an interested checkpoint guard who admired his most prized possession too much, he had taken to sporting his small, chintzy, backup Bushnell pocket binoculars as a decoy when in sight of any indigenous peoples, especially any with a gun or uniform.

On the corner of a forsaken intersection in Samfya, we spotted a hitchhiking, young, white, handsome fellow carrying shades in his dirty white shirt pocket. He came over and spoke with us in an American accent. His girlfriend quickly joined us. They had somehow got here to do his thing—carrying fish as a PCV in a pisciculture project. Besides getting a rapid exhortation from Kurt as to his sanity for importing an exotic species for pisciculture (*Tilapia niloticus*), which had been here for ten years and had got into the lake already from the holding farm pits, he was treated to a dissertation on taking a girlfriend on a holiday through hell. In Kurt's defense, he has a daughter about her age. Therefore, he was acting parental.

Her name is Karen and they are both from Massachusetts, where she graduated from UMass and will be going next to SUNY in paleontology. I took pictures and exchanged names and addresses, and said we were in a hurry, but they could make themselves comfortable in the back of our truck. Despite the wind-whipping they got back there atop our bulky safari kit, she said it was the most comfortable ride they had had in Africa, since they were at least alone without a suspicious group of Africans hovering over them. I said we wanted to see the black lechwe, which we had been told might be seen from the big bridge. I had just said something about lechwe to Peter as the tangential light of twilight was making the likelihood dim of taking photos of the last of my lechwe collection. The black lechwe is a subspecies of the lechwe (*Kobus leche smithemani*) found in the Bangweulu basin. Then, I looked over the vast burned-over flats of the flood plain before the bridge approach and saw a herd of hundreds of antelope. Black lechwe!

BLACK LECHWE IN THE SUNSET OVER THE BRIDGE AND A TYPICAL SET OF AFRICAN STORIES IN FOLLOW-UP

There was a smaller herd of black lechwe on the opposite side of the road. Only a half-dozen rams were visible in the large herd. They were dark and handsome with their long, black, spiraling, swept-back lechwe horns. We next approached the bridge and were waved through by Emmanuel. We stopped to photograph the Coppery-tailed Coucal (*Centropus cupreicaudus*) on the mid-part of the span. When we got to end of the bridge, another guard was checking the sparse traffic. There was only one other truck from the oncoming side as long as we were there, despite hundreds of pedestrians walking along on this high-speed tarred road. The sun was setting over the vast river of grass and this unusual artifact—a four-km, Chinese-built bridge in the middle of what seemed like empty Africa.

We dropped off the PCV and his girlfriend as we came to the Kasanka turn-off, just past the turn-off to the Livingstone Memorial that was my primary objective of the day. My pilgrimage was put off until the next day. We flagged down a huge but empty tandem hauler with an open back, headed to Lusaka. The PCV and his girlfriend decided to take this ride rather than wait on the side of the road or come into Wasa Camp with us. The truck was going to Lusaka so they piled in to the empty trailer with their baggage. Kurt remarked wistfully that this woman must really be in love with the guy to follow him out here. The truck driver was excited about having a pair of *Wazungu* bouncing in the bed of the empty bulk carrier. So, we parted as I handed them my letter and cards to mail on the pass through the Lusaka Airport. She is going to Madagascar and he will return to his duties in Samfya.

Here are two more stories as addenda to this day trip to Northern Zambia. I had asked the PCV, "How was it that you got up to Lake Bangweulu in the first instance and what for?"

He said, "I was transporting live fish to start a fish-farming operation."

"Well, how did that go?" I asked.

He replied, "This is Africa. They were in a tank with an aerator, and the fuel for the pumps ran out. The fish all arrived dead."

Story number two follows. We picked up one of Emmanuel's relatives who had been taking a trip by bus, but was robbed of his money and could go no farther. So, we gave him a lift to Samfya which was a big favor, considering he then waved to have a woman with a small baby and a large sack of some unknown cargo join us. We drove them several hours, farther than they ever thought they could go especially since it would have taken forever on foot with a baby. When we returned to Wasa Camp, we looked into fixing the punctured spare tire. The camp workers did this by *sewing* the inner tube with thread—like the bicycle tire repairs in Assa. We had to check to see if it could hold up under the inflation pressure that would be needed for a trip with a functioning spare. We went into the bed of the pick-up to get the foot pump for the tire—an essential bit of equipment Peter had packed back there. The pump was gone, probably stolen by the fellow we had carried to Samfya. This all too typical story might be the prototypical African return of a favor!

43 LIVINGSTONE'S MEMORIAL

EARLY IN EDEN

July 31, 1998

I did not expect too much out of what was coming up today. I knew that one thing I was going to do for sure was to visit the site of Livingstone's Memorial. The guides and Kurt did not place it high on their list of priorities. They had every intention of blowing off that "must-see" event to go in pursuit of still one or more other new bird species to get another "lifer" for themselves—typically, some little cisticola or bulbul which is indistinct from the others to all but an amorous cisticola—but a new "listable" species. As Kurt would say often, some obscure little brown job "Counts just as much as a Harpy Eagle!" He was trying to make himself feel better about bouncing around in the back seat of the truck, covered with dust, and bitten by tsetse flies, all for some obscure little brown bird. Peter spoke derisively of the cisticolas as "The Seven Dwarfs." Their common names are e.g., Bleating Cisticola, Wailing Cisticola, and Lazy Cisticola. Peter called them the Dopey Cisticola, Sneezy Cisticola, and Grumpy Cisticola. They all look alike and can only be distinguished in the field by fanatical experts based on call, habitat, and behavior. Gary was such an expert who was keen to sort out more of them. Everyone else was rolling their eyes at this point. We took off after a somewhat more leisurely morning, with the plan for stopping long enough for tea and packing along the "road brekkie" which would include pancakes and fruit when we eventually stopped to have it in the bush.

We stopped to see a "bird party" in which a group of insectivores are feeding at various levels, following the hordes of termites. Termites not only account for the highest animal biomass of the African bush, but also contribute to the desertification of sub-Saharan Africa. These highly organized social insects dig subterranean tunnels and bring up dry sand that shapes termite mounds as far as the eye can see. One group here is named generically

Macrotermes, reflecting the size of the insect. It could just as well apply to the size of the termite's mound, which is bigger than most of the huts around here. I stood upon a couple of these mounds to observe and to cover my approach to a group of puku I saw in a cleared and marshy pan. As the birders followed the bird party through the bush trees, I went the other way into the pan, looking at two birds of my own interest in a mixed community grouping.

CHISAMBA PAN:
MY "GARDEN OF EDEN" EXPERIENCE

I walked forward toward a different-looking antelope along the edge of the reeds. The puku were at first nervous and chirped their whistling calls to alert the others that there was a stranger wandering around their breakfast club. I eased in slowly toward a couple of termite mounds that were higher ground off the center. I was trying to get closer to the two birds that had been spotted earlier by Peter and identified as Wattled Cranes (*Grus carunculata*). They were tall, elegant black, gray and white birds with a bright red and white wattle (**Figure 36**). Peter aptly compared them to tuxedoed waiters in a formal restaurant. They were dancing and preening as the wind ruffled their feathers. I advanced on them by using the termite mounds as cover, then walked around to the far side of the mound to stand on it to look over the group with binoculars.

I advanced into the marshy area, getting my feet wet in the soft reeds that often sink a little as you step on them. I also identified the one antelope at the edge of the reeds as a sitatunga, and wanted to get closer. The sitatunga was aware that I was advancing but did not feel too threatened since he could see that he was better at moving over the reeds than I. So, I continued to ease forward among the antelope that formed a large ring around me. Perhaps 60 puku in small scattered herds looked in my direction, having been alerted by the chirping of those on the downwind side. I slowly moved toward the center of the pan as far as the marshy ground would allow, heading toward one termite mound I hoped to use as a platform from which to make the viewing of this collection of game all around me.

I made it to the mound, and found I was not the first. There was some carnivore scat at the top, possibly leopard. I stood there and glassed the area. The more I looked, the more I saw. I was alerted by the "mewing call" of something in the trees behind the Wattled Cranes, and looked to see an African Fish Eagle. It looks like an American Bald Eagle that got too careless with a spilled peroxide bottle. The cranes continued to prance and preen in front of me, actually moving closer. I saw another sitatunga, which I watched moving slowly around the reed beds, never completely exposed for a really good photograph, but as close as I would need if it walked into the clear. The puku around me started getting used to me and did not pay much attention other than to keep their distance. I then noted that they were alerted to the birders approaching the far side of the pan from the bush land. They had already become accommodated to my presence.

Two puku rams ran away from the birders, directly at me, bounding over the marsh and the smaller termite mounds. I caught them on film in full run, and then turned to see that the Wattled Cranes were airborne. They too were flying at me, so I used up a lot of film quickly as they soared into view over the antelope, with the eagle still perched behind them. It was one of those kinds of Sir Thomas Browne's "O Altitudo!" experiences. Chisamba Pan is a pristine part of Africa, which has not been sanitized or packaged, and that I was able to wander into on my own. This kind of experience furnishes no excuses and needs no explanation. It simply *is*, and is beautiful, unapologetic, and in a not very obvious harmony with a harsh and unforgiving environment.

At that moment, another sitatunga female came out of the reeds, not very far from me, and exposed enough of herself to have me photograph her. Behind her was a dark small bundle that looked like a stump. I recognized that the dark blob shadowing her was a sitatunga lamb, as I had seen in the Kapobi Swamp, which followed the sitatunga ewe there. I then saw that the "stump" had not moved and I looked again to see that it was another sitatunga lamb, this one struggling to catch up—*twins!*

I was told later that it is highly unlikely for a sitatunga to have twins but rather common for the deer-like puku to have twins. This is why they have come back so quickly in naturally repopulating themselves after an armed guard was put on Kasanka (**Figure 40**). The only way that could happen is to take a very depleted small park and privatize the protection of it. I remember the statements of two of the roadblock police guards along the way: "Oh, you are going to Kasanka? Bring me back the leg of some nice animal!" They had obviously been paid quite often in that currency. There is a nearby park east of the "Chinese Highway" that is several times the size of Kasanka. It could be mine for the asking if only I would guard it and protect it. It receives no visitors except for poachers. The sound of their home-made guns is encouragement enough to think that there is still something left there to poach. The name of this plundered area is Lavushi Manda National Park, which is as much a national park as would be Yellowstone if it were an open pit mine.

My "Garden of Eden" moment was awe inspiring as I stood where the animals and I were wary of one another, yet alive together with our different purposes for the moment, each without threatening the other. I enjoyed their company and they at least tolerated my presence. I returned to the vehicle some distance away only when I had run out of film. The birders had missed all of my exaltation, since they were set on getting to the Bifumo Forest to see an unusual ecosystem in which we might find something new, one of the desiderata being the uncommon Boehm's Bee-eater (*Merops boehmi*). To get there we had to go across the Kasanka River on the pontoon ferry that would just hold the Toyota. The ferry is pulled across with a rope by the fellow you wake up to do that at a hut on our side. He requires "hooting" in order to rouse him on our return over the same ferry.

KASANKA RIVER PONTOON FERRY
AND THE BOEHM'S BEE-EATER

Waterberry plants lined the sides of the river. If the ferry had a few more 55-gallon oil drums, it would have been a pontoon bridge (**Figure 43**). As we were loading the Toyota on the ferry, we looked up and saw a little green bird, a bee-eater with an unusually long pair of tail feathers. It was unmistakably Boehm's Bee-Eater *(Merops boehmi)*, so each of the "listers" had their moment in the sun following mine. Once again, Peter whispered, "Boehm's bloody Bee-eater! You bloody fucking little beauty!" to show his appreciation. Again, we exchanged elated high fives. If we had had an elevated air intake for the vehicle and rubber door seals, Gary was thinking of trying the "ford" near the ferry but it looked steep and muddy enough to sink the vehicle without a winch to help get it through. If we had not loitered while loading the vehicle on the pontoon ferry we might have missed this prized bird.

I marked this site on the GPS, when we pulled just a little further ahead and stopped for our "brekkie break." We pulled out the table and our cereal with fruit, and rejoiced at our sightings so far, now moving into the new ecosystem of the Bifumo Forest, a wood of stunted trees, and one other very notable form of wildlife. This particular wildlife is a flying pest that had made this area nearly unpopulated by humans for a long time. No cattle are seen in our trek and we soon found out why. The vehicle filled up with the biting and nasty tsetse flies (*Glossina sp.*).

I had just seen a rather large, dark male bushbuck, and told the others that because of their close proximity to man, these secretive antelope often serve as the reservoir for a pathogenic microorganism causing the Rhodesian variant of African sleeping sickness. Here we were right next to the bushbuck with a swarm of the pesty and hard-to-kill tsetse flies biting us, in what was once known as Northern Rhodesia. Suddenly, we got much better at killing the tsetse flies and forgot about the heat of the day, opting for travel with the windows rolled up.

We swatted our way along for several miles and tried to defend ourselves from tsetse flies. Their bite is bad enough but they also carry an awful disease whose treatment is just as gruesome as the disease itself. Flycatchers are an aerial part of bird parties, and their generic name *Muscicapa* says that they catch flies. I would invite quite a few of them to be my guest in feasting on the tsetse flies, which had been feasting on us. They are persistent little devils and their bite hurts. What we really needed at this point was some aggressive bird named *Glossinaphaga gluttinosus*.

We got out at one point and walked along to see a new primate species for me, the yellow baboon (*Papio cyanocephalus*) or "dog-faced baboon." The local name for the baboon is "Babba John." They ran away barking at us. The females carried underslung babies. I taped their barking and also the chatter of the Sharp-tailed Glossy Starling (*Lamprotornis acuticaudus*), all iridescent blue and green with a russet shoulder patch. Newman's *Birds of Southern Africa* says the call of this species is "unknown." If some professional ornithologist would like a lot of noise from the chattering birds to make it known. I have lots of it on tape.

A SECOND DRAMATIC MOMENT OF MY AFRICAN EXCURSION INVOLVING A KILL BY AN AFRICAN CROWNED EAGLE

Recall that as I left the Assa airstrip, after waiting most of the day for the Cessna flight that never showed up. I saw a big African eagle. It was probably the Crowned Eagle. It struck and killed a Green Mamba in the trees as I walked the path under the equatorial canopy. An amazing sight!

Ex Africa semper aliquid novi, remember? I am not through relating unusual stories associated with this big raptor. We had been walking and talking and probably had alerted every one of the baboons and other animals to our presence. For at least one of the observers, this distraction was lethal. Gary mentioned that the baboons seemed unusually agitated but chalked it up to his unfamiliarity with the species. We soon found the reason for their agitation.

We flushed a Crowned Eagle as we rounded the bend in a road, and he flew off sluggishly from ground level to a tree not far away. We got an unusually close view of this magnificent raptor and vice versa. We jumped out of the Toyota to look around on the ground where he had been. I spotted a streak of droppings from a perch he had occupied, but it was Peter who advanced and said, "There he is!" I rushed forward, and there was an immature, but large, yellow baboon, which was still warm and supple. The gaping hole in his chest where his heart and lungs had been ripped out showed his still-twitching diaphragm. He died clenching what Gary called a mbola plum (*Parinari curatellifolia*) in his

311

teeth (**Figure 44**). The local Bemba people call the tree that bears this fruit the mpundu tree. The young baboon was probably distracted by our noisy approach. The Crowned Eagle hit him, killing him on impact, and then rode the victim to the ground from the canopy. The baboon had died with his mouth full!

Remember two things about this incident. One was the name of the mpundu tree and how it figures prominently in the names and significant events of this area. Second, a Crowned Eagle had just killed a primate larger than a human infant. Last year in Zimbabwe, there was a confirmed report of an attack on a nursing mother. A Crowned Eagle snatched her baby from her breast. The nursing mother sustained a serious chest and lung puncture, but the baby was carried off and devoured. Skulls of up to 12-year-old children have been found in Crowned Eagle nests. Some say that this is a second order phenomenon, i.e., scavenged carrion. But the dead baboon is proof that the eagle is an effective predator and raptor for human-sized primates. His large crest and immense size resembles that of another immense, primate-eating raptor, the slightly larger Neotropical Harpy Eagle (*Harpia harpyja*).

This bird had eaten the heart and lungs of the baboon, and only reluctantly left his kill when we came by. His quick departure allowed us to obtain photographic proof of his predatory skill. He would no doubt return to do his own thing.

The Lammergeier is said to have carried off children (the name alleges that it does it to lambs), but that is probably folklore. This kill was for real. In the two halves of my African excursion I saw an eagle kill a very poisonous Green Mamba that could (and does) easily kill a man. Then the same raptor killed and partially devoured a young, human-sized primate.

LUWOMBWA RIVER AND THE
MUSANDE CAMP

We spotted a group of Kasanka guards at the Luwombwa River station who were trying to start a tractor by pushing it to start—like the garden tractor at Assa in its episodes of starting up and interrupting the sentiments at the time of departure. I went down to the river, at a site from which I could take a canoe ride and would be assured of seeing crocodiles. The birders had already gathered the bird species they needed from along the rivers, so we passed on that potential mini-adventure. We stopped here for lunch and Kurt bought two realistic carved puku heads. They were made from a single piece of dense maroon and white wood that was artfully carved to mimic the facial color patterns of the puku. The horns were stained black with some unidentified pigment. Kurt paid $ 20.00 US for both heads. I don't think the sellers had much concept of the value of what they received, but they knew it was a good deal for them.

We then went over to the Musande Camp to which we were headed on the day of our arrival at Kasanka. It is a good thing that Edmond allowed us to establish our base at the Wasa Camp because the entire campsite consisted of several partially finished grass huts and a partially dug latrine. There was no running water except for a stream. The trees had birds in them that were no longer needed—including the Boehm's Bee-Eater that had occasioned such ecstasy earlier. Now, on its second sighting, it was nothing but a "trash bird."

I examined the bright red stain that occurs in the new leaves of the waterberry (*Syzygium*), a brushy riverine shrub. The anthocyanin pigment protects the tender leaves from sunburn and browsing. The fruit of this plant is probably food for Ross's Turaco. This is why we first spotted this bird along a rivulet.

I marked the rivers and the other features around our camp with the reference point of Chitambo (**Figure 37**), only 17.1 miles by GPS from my goal, Livingstone's Memorial. I was startled when we pulled into camp early to hear that the birders had had enough for the day. They were too tired to see the Livingstone Memorial. Kurt had made a deal for some local Mosi Lager, and planned to sit in camp, scope the marsh in front of camp to confirm a possible sighting of a Lesser Jacana (*Microparra capensis*) and suck beer, blowing off the Livingstone goal I had, with a "Fuck that!"

I was not about to get within striking distance of the last bit of Livingstoniana and pass it by because the unenlightened preferred to suck beer and quit. I convinced Peter that this was an important mission. We took off in order to get there while there was still light.

THE LIVINGSTONE MEMORIAL
CHITAMBO, ZAMBIA

It was relatively easy to get to the Memorial. We had driven right by it on a 750-km excursion for a lesser yield the day before. The sandy road was easy to navigate. We picked up some suppliers of mealie meal (ground corn) and carried them to their destination at the Chitambo School. The heavy bags of mealie meal in the back of the pick-up bed added to our traction. We passed the palace of the Chief of Chitambo, the great grandson of the chief that had welcomed David Livingstone on his trek to get to Lake Bangweulu, which we had seen yesterday.

Livingstone arrived at Chitambo while searching for the origin of the Nile, a great challenge to explorers of his day. He heard stories of great lakes farther up the rift. He almost made it. He arrived in Chitambo weak and sick and went to the shores of the marsh to pray. While kneeling, he fell over dead. His followers buried Livingstone's heart under a mpundu tree, with an inscription on it that he had chosen. His faithful retinue salted and dried his body to a mummified corpse, protecting it day and night from the vultures as they suspended it in the bushes. Later, they carried it all the way to the Tanzanian Coast where it was put on a steamship for England. His corpse was positively identified by the poorly reduced fracture of the humerus caused by an earlier lion attack.

On the centenary of his death, the city of Barcelona erected a monument over this site, indicating that he was a worldwide hero, and not just to his native Scotland or the United Kingdom. His inscription in Westminster Abbey, where he received the full honors of the nation, attributes to him the eradication of slavery as a curse lifted from the world. The US Civil War and Livingstone's efforts to end slavery in East Africa overlapped. I took pictures of the marker at the place where Livingstone died (**Figure 45**) to add to the one that I had taken years ago (against all rules regarding photography in that shrine) of his final resting-place in Westminster Abbey.

Now, let me tell you a less sentimental and more typical true African story than the lore of his death conjures up. The tree under which his heart was buried died. It once bore an inscription to Livingstone. The tree is gone but the inscription was removed and sent to the Royal Geographical Society Museum in London. I imagine that the rest of the tree was chopped down and burned. This is the fate of most trees in this land. Nonetheless, a cutting from the tree now survives over the site of his last moments and his heart. This is Africa, after all, and old habits do not die. In fact looking around, I could tell that there were few changes from the time when Livingstone preceded me to this spot. The same people are still chopping down lots of trees, one of which sheltered Livingstone's buried heart and that bears the fruit the baboon had eaten as his last interrupted meal. The Livingstone Memorial is 80.6 miles from Lake Bangweulu, his intended destination.

I went to the Chitambo Clinic to sign the guest book, and to write some comments. I was the third visitor of 1998 to sign in. On the preceding page for 1997, the prior visitor was Wilbur Smith, the author who lists his nationality as "UK" although he is probably South Africa's best-selling author. I talked with a number of people at the clinic, including Frederick Mutoba, a medical assistant, who has made an earnest effort to work in public health with the community. He displays and promotes family planning devices and other supplies for birth control and AIDS prevention, but has pitifully few medicines. I arranged to send him all the antibiotics and antimalarials we had brought with us but not used. I relayed them through a woman named Cornellia at the Wasa camp. She is Edmond Farmer's right-hand woman. She is also the one who will carry the mail I had written on the Zambian experience. If it gets out at all, it will be because she hand-carried it while hitching a ride on a truck to find her way to some town.

I promised Frederick I would be back in touch with him, gave him my card and will send him his photo. He continues the struggle on the front line of rural tropical medicine that had been pioneered by a prior selfless explorer.

These thoughts were on my mind when I returned to camp to find Kurt either in his Mosi cups or suffering from mefloquine-induced psychosis, because he lit into me for saying any good thing about Livingstone. He believes that most colonists come for riches to exploit, proselytizing the Africans with a false religion. Since I happen to disagree with him, I was obviously a religious zealot, and there was no hope for me either. I was looking for martyrdom like Livingstone, which, according to Kurt was just idiocy. When I asked him what he would do about conditions in Africa, he said, "Leave them the fuck alone. Throw them all condoms and run for your lives." In a cooler moment, he explained that he thought that missionary colonial interference in Africa had created as many problems as it had solved. We, of course, are not exploiting Africans, but helping them, merely since we have spent money here coming to look.

A man who has spent money to holiday on three trips to Africa to watch birds should not be telling the real story of what Africa is all about to me, a man who has been coming to and working in Africa for thirty years this trip. I have donated over two years of my professional life in this continent. During the first restless night he had in the tent at Lochinvar, Kurt was searching for the reason I have come back consistently to this misery, and what is the meaning of it all. Why should you risk the Great Void, when all that you have to look forward to is rotting in some forgotten place? For me, the reason to be in Assa is because I have carried desperately needed skills that can improve people's lives. I couldn't cure all the ills of Africa, but I could do *something* that would help *someone*. I also hoped to create the means for self-help initiatives.

I have found that there is a lot more to Africa than its birds, however interesting and exotic they may be. I certainly have put a lot of my professional life into Africa. I have carried out very little in the way of the material riches I keep getting stripped of when traveling this continent. But, I have carried away a lot of inspiration and it has come from giants—like Livingstone, and like the Congolese colleagues I have as close friends—who can teach more about life than the Audubon Society can. There is a big difference between Livingstone and the exploiters who have come to the continent from time to time to be defeated by it. Bird watching has turned out for them to be "mind-blowing" when they could not ignore the human backdrop behind their feathered friends.

Livingstone had a great soul, and could encourage those he freed here to develop their own souls. Livingstone's exploits have stimulated others who have followed, perhaps at some distance, but at least every bit as far as the monument, once a mpundu tree, over his heart at Chitambo, 17.1 miles from Wasa Camp, even if it is stocked with the wretched Mosi Lager.

44 RETURN TO HARARE

LEAVING ZAMBIA

August 1, 1998

The setting of this tale is odd and unusual, so I will describe it. We are barreling down the Danish highway, having turned from the Chinese highway, listening to Tina Turner belting out her soulful songs. Kurt is grooving on Gary's tape of Motown songs with his decoy Bushnells around his neck and his goofy hat on his head, with a Rapala fillet knife dangling from his belt. He is explaining to "Golfie" Gary Douglas, and "Chief Fuckwit" Peter Tetlow who the Supremes were, as "miles and miles of endless bloody Africa" are rolling away in our 1000-km dieseling day out of Zambia through Zimbabwe and closing out the birding safari. Try to figure, I am typing up this narrative plugged into the cigarette lighter through my D/C charger in the cramped backseat of the Hi-Lux pick-up. We are hauling the camp kit and several jerrycans of diesel fuel that we stop to use to top up our fuel supply every once in a while. Rod Stewart is crooning to Kurt who is doing his dead American imitation at each roadblock stripped of his Ray-Bans and looking like a very good resemblance of road kill.

Periodically, the party closes down as the roadblocks check out this bizarre entourage, to see what kind of pickings could be gleaned from the Toyota carcass. When we have stopped to set up our formal table for "brekkie," complete with a newly washed table cloth (courtesy of Gary) in the highveld predawn chill and even the first drizzle of the dry season, people have materialized out of the trackless bush around us. One of our battle cries of the trip so far has been "Bring out your dead!"

The dead have more frequently been on the inside of this, the "Fuckwit Safaris, Inc." vehicle. In preparation for this trip, Kurt had waded through both volumes of the Dover reprint of Stanley's *Through the Dark Continent*. During his explorations along the Congo, Stanley would impress a local interpreter who was brought along in the canoe. They had heard a call from each bank of the river announcing their presence with a particular word, that Stanley had the curiosity to ask "What does that word mean, which I hear so frequently applied to us?" The interpreter said the word meant "meat," giving more credibility to rumors of cannibalism. This answer became the second watchword of this excursion of the Fuckwit Safaris, Inc.

The third watchword might be one of the most frequently heard short utterances of Central Africa. It had to be one of André's more frequent comments. It is the response to most all the mendicants coming to ask for lifts, cash favors or most of the functional implements that we have packed along. My useful computer could have been one of the highest targets, had it not been obscured under road maps at most slow-down points and roadblocks. The response to most all questions is "Sorry!"

"Sorry" is said with a quick acknowledgment of the common hardships life dishes up all around—"Sahrdie!" This is not necessarily an acknowledgment of liability for another's predicament or having caused it. It is the generalized fatalistic response to Africa, whether as transient or resident. For example, at one terrifying instant, we rounded a blind curve and had to swerve to avoid collision with a semi-trailer. The narrow road had a steep drop off on one side. Peter was driving and he said "Sorry" as we looked down into the ravine containing burned-out hulks of several trucks. Or, as we rolled into Samfya, a miserable little town, Peter had called out, "Bring out your dead." It was black humor that served to release tension. I should take you back to the beginning of this long day.

THE LONG TRIP FROM WASA CAMP
TO THE ZAMBEZI ESCARPMENT,
ACROSS THE SIR OTTO BEIT BRIDGE
OVER THE ZAMBEZI RIVER INTO ZIM FROM ZAM

The kerosene lamp was still glowing and had not yet used up its fuel as it had by dawn on the other mornings when we got up around 6:00 AM. The lamp hadn't been burning as long as usual, since we were up at 3:30 AM for coffee. By 4:30 AM, we rolled along passing the Chisamba Pan where I had so much appreciated the early morning seance yesterday. I was cramped up in back, with all of our gear packed away last night into the Venter trailer and the Hi-Lux as we were ready to roll, anticipating a 14-hour-long rolling return to Harare, if there were no delays, and only brief "pit stops"—always at deserted places where there would be more birds and fewer people and the dry bush looked like it needed watering.

ALL AFRICA AND ITS WONDERS:
WITH NOTHING BUT A LONG AND WINDING ROAD
BETWEEN US AND THE END OF OUR
EXCURSION

I had packed the ThinkPad in the back where I was knotted up a bit, but it came in handy after midmorning, as you can tell from reading this. I had developed the habit of maximizing the use of the minimal daylight in the antipodal winter. We are in a world without the artificial illumination that we so thoughtlessly substitute for the sun that had been so precious in the Congo. Sunlight had been, at best, an equatorial equinox in powerless and plumbingless Congo, where even the solar panel was stolen. We are now about 15° south of the equator, experiencing the shorter days of winter. To be precise, it is 16° 02.32′ S and 028° 50.41′ E at the Zambezi River Zam/Zim crossing of the 1939-built Sir Otto Beit Suspension Bridge. That 16° multiplied by 60′ = 960 nautical miles or 1,000 miles south of the equator, still 11.5° north of the Tropic of Capricorn. Multiply that into the 1.66 kilometers in a statute mile, and you can tell that even under ideal conditions, as the crow could never fly so far, we have undertaken an ambitious trip for a single day's journey. These calculations don't factor in road conditions, border crossings, customs agents, and roadblocks by various police who have less than the worldly goods in this vehicle in their village. And there are more mountains, rivers, accidents, roadside mendicants, a *big* and wondrous environment—called by Sir Thomas Browne, "All Africa."

ALL AFRICA: IT HAS COME UP THE SCARP
IN ALL ITS EXPANSIVENESS TO WAVE
GOODBYE TO IT'S ADOPTED SON

It is magic! Even our simple luncheon stop on the Zambezi Rift Escarpment on the Zim/Zam border has "my Africa" showing off in all its expansive grandeur in front of me! We could see panoramically to the horizon. All four of us stood in absolute silence over this endless expanse of wild Africa. I think the immensity of the vista was a revelation bordering on a metaphysical experience, even for those who typically reject such sensations.

We pulled up the incline of the scarp of the Zimbabwean side of the Zambezi Rift, a branch split off the Great Rift over which I had been watching in East Africa, walking over at the Ngong Hills in Kenya, and flying over en route to and from the Congo. The sedimentary rocks in the steep incline behind us hold the fossils of *Allosaurus*. The whole area ahead of us is the trackless bush of he Nyankasaka Hunting Area. I took in a vast sweep in a single wide-angle shot overlooking the Mana Pools National Park along the Zambezi River (**Figure 47**). It is Africa in all its grand sweep—huge vistas, insurmountable problems, helplessness and what looks like all the signs of hopeless entropic collapse but for one thing—the magic and beauty of life, in all its variety and persistence against all odds, and not simply surviving but somehow flourishing! *Oh, Africa!*

I reached for the peanut butter and jelly and looked up with the jars in hand and saw him—a huge elephant. He was a long way off, but somehow I knew he would be there. The elephants would not let me leave or enter Zimbabwe without saluting so we could enjoy each other's contemporaneity. A lone bull elephant, a thousand meters away, was looking up the scarp and waving farewell with his ears as he sidled away into the bush. They know me, and I know them. We will be back together again soon, bush-bashing this haunting African environment.

"OH, SORRY!"

As we drove up the switchbacks from the "lay-by," I would hear Gary say, "Oh, Sorry!" at each turn. Some of these are serious "Sorries." At each turn there are vehicles that have rolled off the unprotected road and fallen down the scarp. They were serious accidents, so that there is not much to salvage. Golfie said, "We have to be careful on these switchbacks, since if you run off the road, you would be likely to hit another vehicle falling down the scarp."

Gary worked as a park ranger around here in 1983. His earliest interest was in fishing, but now he is probably second to none in his knowledge of Zimbabwe's birds. Last year's excursion to the Zimbabwean Eastern Highlands had "listed" 289 species, this year's total stood at 226 species. Many of these were lifers for the birders. I have already described the major species of mammals although, most not my first, were some of my best, or my most numerous individuals of only a couple species. They are endemic to these small and isolated "parks"(in name only). These parks are a little short on visitors' centers, maps or postcards. They were very long on poachers, tsetse flies, and obstreperous personnel and conditions.

In Lochinvar, the Kafue lechwe, is endemic, and numerous. It is a dominant species of over 30,000 individuals. They are even hunted in this preserve, which I could have done myself if I had gone through the permits and the firearms—I even picked the herd ram that I would have pursued, and got him on film. They looked like the red lechwe I had seen in Botswana.

In Kasanka, the dominant mammal is the puku, which is a relative of the Uganda kob (*Kobus kob*), which I had even hunted in Assa. We sighted many sitatungas, including a ewe with twin lambs, but I had not seen a good ram. There were two new primates on this trip: the yellow baboon and the blue monkey, and over the Luapula River I had seen a large herd of the black lechwe. So, I have a lot of film on these animals, and even tried for few pictures of a few of the pretty birds.

So, I had "listed" the summary of the Congo excursion in three parts: 1) Author in Africa function and the production of the manuscript for this book with my jury-rigged charger on a storage battery, 2) the linguistic study in anthropology of color discrimination, and 3) the medical work and 21 surgical operations. This book also describes some of the birds and the mammals and the visits to the two isolated and very unusual Zambian Parks. A few serial letters have been added as well as a number of tapes. I have used up the blank tapes I carried, all of the slide film (I still have some print film because of the earlier death of my flash camera), all my stamps and most of my postcards. I have enjoyed the company of good-natured, competent and knowledgeable guides with a good camp kit. Kurt and I will recover from our little spat.

I am signing off because of a meltdown. The D/C charger had been installed in the cigarette lighter. Something just happened at the lay-by where we had lunch. The adapter was knocked about and shorted, melting down the plug I had bought just for this trip at about the right time for it to be no longer useful. So, I will now try to use the other charger that will be useful as soon as I get to the land of electric outlets.

Here we are in Harare at the Bronte Hotel, site of our check in and group dinner with the Fuckwit Safari, Inc. and regrouping with the left luggage, calls home, and a real shower. It is 17° 45.67′ S and 030° 52.87′ E or only 362 miles from the Wasa Camp we left at 4:30 A.M., even though we had traveled all day to reach about 1200-km total. We are now in Harare, 185 miles from the crossing of the Zambezi over the Otto Beit Bridge into Zimbabwe. I am 1,584 miles due south of Assa and 7,939 miles from home at 315°. Tomorrow I will fly to Jo'burg and then on to Umtata, Transkei.

PART IV

OUT OF AFRICA

45 WORK IN TRANSKEI

August 2, 1998

I am sitting in the comparative luxury of the Guest House for the volunteers who come to the Umtata area where Chris MacConnachie and his wife have just hosted me and a number of other volunteers at their traditional open house and dinner on Sunday night. This is a very good place already set up for volunteers, with a particular interest in and experience with orthopedic and physical therapy volunteers.

BACK TO THE BRONTE FOR THE FINAL LEG OF MY EXCURSION TO THE TRANSKEI

I rose early at the Bronte, probably too early, since I felt weary all the rest of the day. I dressed in my well-worn and grubby bush safari outfit. I had felt considerably overdressed for the last month in places where such luxury being flaunted would cause a large cluster of hangers-on to badger me. Today, I entered a different world in which I was sure that people from the smart set would be tossing me a crust of bread because of my obviously distressed financial status, being the proud owner of a single (dirty) outfit.

I took a taxi from the Bronte to the Harare Airport and made it through the melee with relative ease to board the Air Zimbabwe 737 for the 90 minute flight to Jo'burg. Use of personal electronic devices was not allowed on the flight so I didn't use the ThinkPad. Instead, I listed the 15 GPS fixes I had made throughout Zambia and their relationships and busied myself with other details.

I arrived in Jo'burg feeling tired and a little ill. I checked in for my next flight on South African Airways (SAA) to Umtata and phoned Maeve and Gordon Hersman and arranged to meet them in downtown Jo'burg. I then took the "Magic" Microbus downtown to the Sandton Sun Mall, where the beautiful people come to do brunch, and stroll and flaunt the fact that they obviously have three times more disposable income than I do. I arranged to meet Maeve and

Gordon at the base of the waterfall in the Sandton Sun Hotel. I worried that the guards would throw me out. I looked very like a highveld bush rat coming in to sit in their luxurious lobby. I pulled out the ThinkPad to make a copy of the manuscript disc to give Gordon. I hoped this subterfuge would make the security guards think that I was not a degenerate street person.

When Gordon and Maeve arrived, they filled me in on the South African news and American gossip—including the fact that Monica Lewinsky seems to hold it in her power to shake up the stock markets and the value of the dollar on international currency markets. Nelson Mandela attended the convention of the South Africa Communist Party, still paying political debts. We talked about Dr. Zuma, the South African Health Minister and the carnage she has wrought in the health care system with her denial of all ex-patriot physician qualifications except for the Cubans. She has done one thing in my opinion that may even rescue her from all the other harm she has wrought—only someone as doctrinaire a totalitarian as she could ban all advertising of any cigarettes—period.

We strolled the Sandton Mall among the Sunday brunch set, and then went to Facts and Fiction, an upscale bookstore where we can have coffee and fancy pastries. There sitting across from us is someone that Gordon recognized as "Sandy"—the former Miss South Africa, whose legs are still used in advertisements as the world's most perfect lower extremities. She was there with her father, and has been divorced from her second husband. The first was found dead in an apartment after selling "red mercury" to the Arabs in a scam that someone had apparently settled by killing him.

It turns out that Gordon also knew the author Wilbur Smith, who lived in his same building at University. Gordon has autographed copies of all of Smith's books. One book dealt with the diamond trade. The companies that mine and cut diamonds treated him to a deluxe tour. He made notes on a tape recorder to keep his facts straight. He had used the same techniques for a book on international merchant ships. Gordon insists that he does what I do, and makes novels out of the extensive facts of his travels. Gordon asks why I do not publish these adventures and collect the 10 million dollars annually that Wilbur Smith does, with his books translated in 38 languages? Be patient, my friend. Smith apparently had several earlier marriages and lots of kids by these marriages, with attendant domestic problems. I do not need to be in that line, but sign me up for the successful author gig. As before, I gave Gordon some of my writings. Gordon wanted this material to resubmit a Nobel Peace Prize nomination for me. I promised him a copy of *Out of Assa* when it is published.

OFF I GO TO THE LAST STOP ON MY AFRICAN TREK

I flew Air Link of SAA to Umtata, the only major town in the Transkei, one of the poorest provinces in the relatively rich South Africa. The captain of the plane came back to talk to me about the interesting things to be seen there, and compared notes with my GPS.

After an uneventful flight from Jo'burg, Dr. Chris MacConnachie met me and drove me to a convenient cottage they have for the visiting volunteers of the African Medical Mission (AMM). They are missionaries supported by the Episcopal American Church. They have an open house every Sunday evening, so I was invited down to dinner. I met a number of folk who were coming through including a grandfather orthopedic surgeon and his "medical student" grandson. When I asked where he was in medical school, it became obvious that this was a nice idea yet to come to the application stage. The grandfather was trying to get his grandson interested in medicine, and was encouraging him to apply to medical school while getting the kind of exposure and first hand introduction he would not be allowed in the US. Fair enough, but it is safer to tell the story straight among folks who do this for a living.

I am wearing down. I am now febrile and weary on this my last stop in my African Odyssey, and I feel a little out of place and apologetic standing about in dirty bush clothes, in up-market, winter, socializing conditions. I will have to do what I can to judge the suitability and requirements for Health Volunteers Overseas (HVO) in surgery in this environment. The mission already hosts an orthopedics rotation. Many more pediatricians are volunteering. Unfortunately, the authorities here say that such volunteers are not needed and will be unwelcome. My role, as it often is in such settings, will be three quarters diplomatic and one quarter medical, with a bit of administrative shovel work to be done later right in the middle of my re-entry crunch of catch-up work before packing off on my next long adventure excursion. I will have to get better fast and regenerate the energy to launch not only the start-up of the next trip but also the wind-up of this one.

August 3, 1998

Umtata General Hospital (UGH) would make an ideal site for a General Surgery Overseas (GSO) rotation. It has an established presence in a community already attuned to volunteers coming in programs in most notably orthopedics, but also pediatrics and physical therapy. Its facilities, although not abundant, are funded by the government. It has a relatively well-trained medical faculty in the large provincial University of the Transkei (UNITRA). The physicians here are keen on having volunteer faculty visits, and prefer that they might be at least ten weeks, the term of the medical students who train here. There are undergraduate medical student programs supervised by a staff of 10 staff consultants, four in general surgery. I think that the general surgeons are all expatriate "medical officers," a paid civil service post. They have been begged, from the civil service for rural posting to handle the high load of clinical cases here, regardless of their specific training, for the management of the endless stream of patients at UGH.

As an example of this inadequate training, I heard a medical student, all dandied up in suit and tie, present a case of an eight-month-old child who had suffered trauma with a head injury and shock. My favorite aphorism in such management is that anyone with shock and a head injury has the shock for some reason other than the head injury. This was something this student had not heard, and he called in to the medical officers who were in the OR managing some other trauma cases. They were likewise at a loss to understand, so the student transfused blood to the child too late and without knowing the volume of blood he was transfusing, another error. He added, "When I returned to the ward, the sisters informed me that the child had passed away." The medical student clearly needed closer supervision.

The two medical officers who had been on call in the successive days of the weekend were trying valiantly to manage the surgical load that includes stab wounds and traffic accidents. The cases sounded quite intimidating for me, and I am an experienced trauma surgeon. Another case was that of an intestinal obstruction. The diagnosis of "intestinal tuberculosis" was made after several hours of searching for the bowel amid a lot of adhesions. Any visiting surgical consultant from the more developed world would have been happy to accept their diagnosis. The outside expert consulting surgeons would be clueless to recognize this disorder because they never see it at home but it is common in South Africa. Many physicians in South Africa are expatriates from some other African nation in turmoil, or from Russia or other Eastern Bloc countries. Regardless of their training and background, they often find themselves the only answer to the huge problems presented to them. For example, I had once encountered a doctor trying to do a difficult traumatic Whipple (pancreatic) resection on a patient with a bad abdominal gunshot wound, never having "seen surgery" in his native Latvia.

EVALUATION OF UMTATA GENERAL HOSPITAL

The theatre block at UGH is capacious and well-equipped, thanks to the maternal/child health funding from the government. We general surgeons were "borrowing" the theatre block, and could do so as long as there was no need for it to be used for a cesarean section. Mr. Pandi, a Nepalese surgeon, presented the first case. I greeted him with *"Namaste."* He was surprised to learn I would be leading a medical mission to Nepal next year, before climbing the Kumbu Ice Fall on Mount Everest. The patient was a lucky individual who suffered from a large tumor of the stomach (leiomyosarcoma) without the usual metastases to the liver. It was an advanced cancer that could be removed surgically with a good potential for cure. The next case involved surgical treatment of a complicated pneumonia, an operation called a "decortication", i.e., removing a thick peel over the lung. The surgeon for this case was David Mugwanga from Uganda and within a few minutes we were reminiscing about Denis Burkitt and another colleague, John Ziegler from the National Cancer Institute. John had set up a Cancer Center at Kampala in Makere University

My host is the Acting Chairman of Surgery, a Nigerian named Dr. Adekulene. He is taking over more and more administrative responsibility since the Chairman of Surgery is Dr. Edon Mazwai, now the Dean of the Faculty of Medicine at UNITRA. Adekulene brought me to UNITRA to meet the Dean, who wishes to speak further with me in formalizing the HVO arrangement with GSO. This is a fortunate situation in which surgeons can solve the administrative problems in organizing something they understand.

Adekulane came from Ibadan where I have been a visiting professor. Adekulane was pleased that I knew of Ibadan and that his colleague Stola Adebonojo had received favors and guidance along the way from me. The

Deputy Chief of the Department of Surgery is Mr. Takie, another Nigerian. This deputy position is a job that I would not like here or anywhere on earth where the work of the world is done by the fellow who can never get the credit but is always available for the blame. He had worked at Al Khobar in Saudi Arabia. I know his colleagues who are still there whom I had visited as recently as ten months ago. He had started out in Dammam, and was talking longingly about the tax-free salaries of $4,000 per month each of his African colleagues had received saying that one of his friends was now the highest paid African in Saudi Arabia. Another tier higher than that are the German, UK, and US physicians. The Saudi titular chiefs are in a whole other league, even if the foreign deputies do their work.

UNITRA, A LARGE INSTITUTION OF THE "HBU" TRADITION

HBU means "Historically Black University." They were neglected before 1994, and now are worse off than the others. They had a large and bloated payroll, providing employment to many in the surrounding community. Now there is a greater fiscal accountability that is being applied to hospitals to lay off the "feather bedders" in the system. It sounds almost like the restructuring of American health care, "trimming the fat" by (if you don't mind the mixing of a half-dozen metaphors) "throwing the baby out with the bath" and gutting some effective programs. Through it all are the political necessities, such as Dr. Zuma. Behind my "cottage," here built by AMM for volunteers such as I, are the accommodations for a dozen Cuban physicians, imported by Dr. Zuma's grand plan to pay back political debts for the communist support during the long South African struggle for black majority rule.

ALISTAIR SAMMON,
MY "HOUSEMATE" FROM BRISTOL, UK

Chris MacConnachie told me that I would have lots in common with Alistair Sammon who would be arriving today. He turns out to be an asthenic fellow who looks like many British internists I have known. That initial impression turns out to be wrong. He is doing research on an epidemic of esophageal carcinoma in South Africa. This new disease had fascinated me when I was here as the James IVth Scholar in 1986. This cancer of the esophagus epidemic crawled up and over the Natal scarp and entered the Transvaal in the prior decade. It became the most common admission diagnosis at Hillbrow Hospital at Wits. Alistair thinks that it is related to introduction of maize into their diet leading to an insufficiency of certain lipids that play an indirect role in the immune response. The natives ingest a salicylate-rich herb for heartburn, which seems to offer some protection from esophageal cancer. This observation also supports his theory. Sammon thinks that supplementing maize with fish oils could prevent the disease. He is also interested in my goiter work, and points out that he agrees with my theory of intervention in vertical care programs and associated environmental degradation due to population growth.

Alistair and I went to dinner in town this evening. He worked for four years in Kenya in Chigori, where he learned to speak Kimeru and he had worked here for ten years, speaking Xhosa. Recently, he has been going back to Bristol, where he wanted to finish his research on esophageal cancer. My friend and his Chairman, John Farndon, gave him a senior lecturer appointment until he could finish his research. He has been gathering data all of today—much as I had in the anthropologic linguistics—and he will relay my own greetings back to John Farndon, a fellow endocrine surgeon, co-author, and a host for my visiting professorship in Bristol in 1990.

Sammon has an idea that disease in so prevalent in Africa not because Africa is such a germy and creepy-crawly place, but because recent dietary changes, along with population pressures, have caused decreased immune competence. This would account for the very high rates of tuberculosis, other bacterial infectious diseases, and AIDS. He thinks that the immunosuppression came first and the tropical disease came second. If he is right, relatively simple dietary supplements, e.g., fish oil, might improve the situation. Fish are widely available in Africa. Furthermore, when dried or processed into fish-meal, they could be conveniently transported to areas of need. He was justifiably proud of having helped reduce Kenya's fertility rate from 7.8% to 4%, still unsustainable, but a lot better than before.

47 UNITRA FINALE

August 4, 1998

I wanted to send some e-mail but the system is not working, for one of two reasons, depending on whom you ask. Some say that the gurus at UNITRA information systems are upgrading the whole system, and will be replacing it with newer and more powerful equipment, and that is the reason it is temporarily down. Others report that the financially-strapped university has had a budget cutback and has been told to start laying off employees. They are reluctant to do so, and as a consequence, have elected not to pay bills instead. Whatever may be the reason, I have left a message in the queue, summarizing my experience in Africa. I have gone through the long wait to see the Dean for a second time to finalize the details for establishing the HVO surgical program. Meanwhile I have been getting to know Alistair Sammon and discussing our mutual interests.

Last night, we had dinner together. He had rented a car and had driven 400 km north where he had left his wife. She has finished her qualifications as a GP, a similar situation as that of Chris MacConnachie's wife. Both surgeons are married to M.D.'s in general practice. The surgeons spent their middle years in Africa while their wives raised families as they worked in Africa in this setting along the "Wild Coast" of the Eastern Cape—described by Alistair as the most beautiful place he has ever seen anywhere on earth. He described the people of Chigori, Kenya, where he worked for three years after ten years here in Transkei, as "Scots." They are dour, hard-working, honest people who never laugh and have no fun. The Transkei Xhosa are into ceremony. Births, weddings and funerals all require a full celebration. The Kenyans with whom he worked celebrated only the funeral component. He thought the orientation of the Chigori people made it easier to work with them. There were fewer reasons for not getting anything done there. They even were able to make some inroads on the birthrate, in which Kenya was the unenviable and unsustainable world leader, with a rate of well over seven children born per woman, which he said was a recent improvement from the dozen or more being born to each woman before.

The population control efforts, largely led by expatriates concerned about Kenyan population bomb, started making some sense to the Kenyan population themselves.

All around the wards here in Umtata are messages about AIDS and its prevention. The street signs in Zambia were full of advice on how to avoid contracting any kind of sexually transmitted disease, with the kick line, "AIDS is real, and it is no joke." AIDS prevention programs are far behind in Zimbabwe, where Robert Mugabe's idea of a solution, was to rally support behind himself by pillorying homosexuals. Just before I left Zimbabwe, the newspapers were full of stories about one high-ranking military officer and a hero of the revolution who was allegedly sodomizing young soldiers. This was a bit embarrassing to the ruling party that had just played their trump card of institutionalizing homophobia. Whatever his political yield from this effort, it overlooks the fact that the transmission of HIV is mainly heterosexual and vertical (mother to child) in his country. I also think that the good "Comrade Mugabe" tried to play the communist card at the wrong time and place. Communism and Africa are a rather strange fit. He has managed, just as well as his anticommunist colleague Sese Mobutu, to accumulate vast amounts of filthy capital in accounts kept safely among the running dogs of capitalist wealth. Approximately 30% of the males in Harare are thought to be HIV-positive. The standard of living in Zimbabwe is declining because of inflation. His people are worse off from the AIDS policies and the economic theories of this hero of the revolution. It turns out that the Dean for whom I have been waiting for the "closure interview" after yesterday's enthusiastic reception for the GSO idea from HVO, has left on leave today, since he is preparing for the wedding of his son this week. I will carry on the further plans by correspondence with him particularly relating to setting up a fast track for getting credentials for volunteers.

The original correspondents and the linchpins of all the volunteer programs here at UNITRA are the Doctors MacConnachie. They head up the AMM here at Umtata, and will coordinate the accommodation and other details through the phone and fax numbers and an e-mail address that works as intermittently as all the others in this part of the world. We will probably await cellular telephone satellite world communication for my next trip to Africa. Iridium has already hung the satellites up there and all I will need to do is keep the phone well-charged and unstolen.

The final details of my work here in Umtata are falling into place. All I need to do now is implement the flow of volunteers once they know these excellent facilitates are available and the staff here are competent and very interested in receiving them. I have received important contact information on the faculty at UNITRA and will now start sending volunteers to them. The volunteers can be incorporated into the schedule of a busy surgical service that is being run increasingly like a US surgical service and less like a UK clone. My mission here has been successfully completed.

48 OUT OF AFRICA

August 4, 1998

My trip has been a rewarding and exciting excursion, once again, through all of the African regions I have explored, particularly in revisiting my friends in the remote and isolated poverty of northeast Congo. After a month of the struggles there, I had completed three objectives: 1) The delivery of medical supplies and surgical work; 2) The linguistic anthropology study completed for twenty informants in Pazande and Bangala; 3) This book, *Out of Assa: Heart of the Congo*. I returned through Nyankunde, and looked into the exciting possibilities for collaborative public health ventures when and if the situation returns to some degree of stability and the graft of the kleptocracy subsides. I made my last "run" in East Africa over the Ngong Hills by day with all night work on the discs that I mailed out of Kenya from the US Embassy. I had given away almost all my personal effects (clothing, supplies, and even my shoes) and come back with exposed film, audiotape and the raw manuscript for this book.

ZIM/ZAM: THE SAFARI FROM HARARE

The next week was filled with the bush-bashing throughout the remote National Parks of Zambia. On the way to Zambia, I was almost squashed by an enraged bull elephant at Kariba airstrip. A couple of nights were spent camped out in the Lochinvar National Park seeing herds of the endemic Kafue lechwe, and exotic bird life of the Kafue River flood plain. Then we went to Kasanka National Park, where we camped out along the Congo River's upper tributaries, only 20 km from the copper belt of southeastern Congo. Here I took long solitary bush walks, with precious finds including the last of my Southern African turacos, the Ross's Turaco, complete with a souvenir flight feather stained with the turacin. When I had left Assa, I had seen a Crowned Eagle strike and kill and carry off a Green Mamba in the jungle canopy overhead. This omen did not mean I encountered any snakes (except for a dead cobra on the road, killed by a

Yellow-billed Kite). I did see another Crowned Eagle in action at Kasanka. The huge eagle was on the ground with a new primate species for me, a yellow baboon, it had just swooped down and killed. The dead baboon's diaphragm was still twitching. It was still supple and warm, and it had a mbola plum stuck in its mouth.

I had another encounter with a bull elephant in Kasanka, which was more respectful and majestic than my last. He snorkeled and flapped his ears, and then he charged. This was a mock charge, a type to be preferred if you are given your choice. We saw quite a few beautiful bird species including the Ross's Turaco and Boehm's Bee-Eater, enough to put the birders into ecstasy, although they were prepared to blow off the reason for my pilgrimage to this remote region. I was intent on seeing the last stop of my hero David Livingstone.

SON OF DOCTOR LIVINGSTONE, I PRESUME

At each stop along the way when I had been "discovered"—for example, by Eric Sarin arriving in Nyankunde, or by guide Peter tracking me to the Machan Sitatunga Hide overlooking the Kapabi Swamp where I sat in the canopy of a giant *Khaya anthotheca* tree watching the last of my twisthorns, the sitatunga—I had heard the words of greeting: "Doctor Geelhoed, I presume!" I had been off in a pan called Lake Chisamba with a "Garden-of-Eden-like" experience solo, surrounded by puku and watching Wattled Cranes preening and prancing with African Fish Eagles overhead and a sitatunga ewe emerging from the reeds in front of me followed by twin sitatunga lambs. I went on from my naturalist Africanist ecstasy and fixed on finding the site, only 17.1 miles away on my GPS, of Chitambo, the last place of David Livingstone's long African exploration, and where he died and where his heart was buried under the mpundu tree. His salted and mummified body was carried back to the Tanzanian coast where a steamer brought it back to burial under the stone I have visited in Westminster with full honors of the great man he was, all dismissed as the ravings of a religious zealot, by my companions, who preferred the thoughts of sitting about camp in the fading light of our last day in the bush with the execrable Mosi beer.

So, off to Chitambo I went, to see the final resting-place of David Livingstone. I also signed in the book at the Chitambo Clinic, arranged to give them my antimalarials and antibiotics, and gave away what had not already been given away or pinched in the Congo. I am wearing the single bush-stained safari outfit that I had left behind in Nairobi before plunging into the Congo, including the shoes I bought in the muddy market in Nyankunde. This is all I have left with which to make an appearance introduced as a distinguished visiting professor from America here at UNITRA, probably devaluing the future short-termer visitors from the USA I am trying to arrange for HVO to be sending here!

UMTATA, TRANSKEI, UNITRA, AND AMM AT UMTATA GENERAL HOSPITAL

I am now at Umtata, awaiting a second visit with the Dean, formerly the Professor of Surgery—for which reason we understand each other very well. I met a delightful fellow, Alistair Sammon and we shared our mutual interests in improving the public health of impoverished Africans. I have finished writing this book and many serial letters and postcards. I am packing out a full brick of exposed film and a dozen audiotapes, for whomever wishes to understand the complexities of this still mysterious, but ever-fascinating "Dark Continent."

I have been to the heart of the African interior, as had David Livingstone. I came out of Africa in somewhat less dried out state than he did, and hardly expect a hero's welcome or Westminster enshrinement. Livingstone's heart was buried under the tree that bears the fruit that the yellow baboon was eating when killed by the Crowned Eagle. I too left my heart behind in the destitute African bush.

Just to convince you that this vast continent is very real, very current, and not at all to be sentimentalized, the mpundu tree under which Livingstone's heart was buried is gone, although the inscription has been saved. The rural people are always chopping and burning, and so much the worse for the environment that they must eke out a living in while others come to visit, admire the physical and animal beauty, and leave. A cutting from the original tree and a stone monument now serve as his memorial in Chitambo. This entire area has changed insignificantly from the time when he came through on his way to Lake Bangweulu, still in search of the source of the Nile River.

But Livingstone had discovered something more than a lot of interesting geography, and the stunning *"Mosi-o-Tunya"* (the name given by Zambians, which means "the smoke that thunders") he named Victoria Falls, or a dozen birds and beasts named for him. If all our exploration carried back were a few more ticks on a bird list, or a whole carton full of linguistic anthropology data, or an idea about the etiology of esophageal cancer from mealie maize, or any of the other portable microanalyses pulled from Africa for fun, fascination or profit, the dark brooding Africa would remain here with people who must chop and burn, and forage and scrounge and somehow survive.

It is a real tribute that desperately poor people buried Livingstone's heart and memorialized him. I will leave this odyssey with only dollars given away, lost, or officially pilfered, still carrying the word, image and impression of this wild, real Africa to bring back alive. Somehow, these people do survive, against all odds. They even manage to thrive, with an art, culture, faith and happiness that are common among the poorest of these poor people who have taught Livingstone—and one of his latter day followers—much, as we have both taken our leave, out of Africa.

THE END

Glenn W. Geelhoed, M.D.
Umtata, Transkei
AUGUST, 1998

1. African Inland Mission (AIM)
P.O. Box 21285
Nairobi, Kenya
Attn: Ed Morrow, or assistants Bernice or Lydia
Phone: 254-2-501-651
Fax: 254-2-501-612
AIM through AIM Serve, and AIM Air will know where to contact me, since they will have the radio for contact with the Cessna aircraft I am chartering, and would have the scheduled flights known (7/6/'98 NBO to Bunia and to CME, Nyankunde; and 7/24/'98 CME, Nyankunde to Bunia to NBO) as well as the charters 7/7--23/'98 throughout remote Zandeland, with the "ultimate destination" being Assa, DRC.

2. Centre Médical Évangélique (CME) , Nyankunde, DRC
Phone: 871-7615-8361
Fax: 871-7615-8363
E-mail cmenyan@maf.org
I will be at the CME Guest House and working with the staff at the CME Hospital, and can be reached directly, or through Dr. (Alberto) Ahuka Longombe or Dr. Hubert Kakalo.

3. Mayfield Guest House (MGH), Nairobi, Kenya
Phone: 254-2-724-582
I will be returning here on July 24, leaving on July 25, 1998. The couple now in charge of the MGH is Steve and Deborah Wolcott.

4. Bronte Hotel, Harare, Zimbabwe
Kurt Johnson has the phones and faxes for each of the above:
Phone: 703-823-9833
Fax: 703-823-9834
E-mail anakej@gwumc.edu
This will be the staging area for the next take-off into incommunicado safari throughout Southern Africa, from Zimbabwe to Zambia and return to Harare.

5. Dr. Gordon and Maeve Hersman, Johannesburg, RSA
> A 101 Riepan Hall
> 21 Riepan Avenue
> Riepan Park, JNB, RSA
> Phone: 11-783-2605, 2606
> Fax: 11-783-4868
> E-mail: 042gordo@chiron.wits.ac.za

I will be meeting them again on Sunday August 2, at JNB in transit as I go on to Umtata, Transkei, RSA later the same day.

6. Umtata, Transkei, RSA
> Dr. Chris MacConnachie at AMM (African Medical Mission)
> Private Bag X5014
> Umtata, Transkei
> Phone: 27-471-312-652 (also Fax)
> E-mail hvo@aol.com

I will be here 8/2-8/5/98 for General Surgery Overseas/Health Volunteers Overseas site visit.

7. Please distribute to the following who may want to contact me:

> msdhjt@gwumc.edu
> [Editor's Note: the list included 26 other addresses.]

8. Itinerary for Africa

Into Africa: Leave Derwod (home) through Dulles and Heathrow to Jo'burg en route through Nairobi
> 1 Jul Wed 9:35 PM BA 222 IAD to LHR 9:35 AM 2 July Thu
> 2 Jul Thu 9:00 PM BA 57 LHR to JNB 8:50 AM 3 July Fri

Jo'burg : Visit to Witwatersrand University and Hersmans in Riepan Park before transit on to East Africa
> 4 Jul Sat 3:15 PM Kenya Air 461 JNB to NBO 7:10 PM

Mayfield Guest House, staging area for Congo arrangements and last postal or e-mail service

Into the Congo, Assa, and Out of Assa to Nairobi
> 6 Jul, Mon AIM Air charter 8:00 AM from Wilson Field to Bunia, DRC 4:00 PM
> 6 Jul Mon MAF charter (following Bunia customs) from Bunia to CME, Nyankunde
> 7 Jul Tue MAF charter from Nyankunde to Nebobongo en route to Assa, Congo
> 7 Jul Tue to 22 Jul Thu Assa, Congo

Assa station: medical, surgical, linguistic, and writer's work among the frightened survivors of Assa and surrounding Congolese bush

22 Jul Thu MAF charter returns for flight from Assa via Nebobongo to Nyankunde

23 Jul Fri MAF charter 8:15 AM from Nyankunde to Bunia to connect with

23 Jul Fri AIM Air charter 10:00 AM to Nairobi's Wilson Field 4:00 PM transfer

23 Jul Fri to 25 Jul Sun Mayfield Guest House

Zim/Zam Safari from Harare for birding and bush-bashing in Zambia

25 Jul Sun 10:00 AM Kenya Air 440 NBO to HRE 12:00 PM Bronte Hotel, Harare, Zimbabwe

26 Jul Mon to 1 Aug Sun Zambian holiday safari

Surface transport via Kariba and entry into Zambia for Lochinvar NP, Lusaka, Kasanka NP, Luapula Bridge, Lake Bangweulu, Livingstone's Memorial, Zambezi Escarpment, and return to Harare

Umtata and Out of Africa

2 Aug Mon 9:00 AM Air Zim UM 361 HRE to JNB for revisit with Hersmans at Sandton Sun

2 Aug Mon 4:00 PM South African SAA JNB to MTT Umtata, Transkei, RSA

Visit Africa Medical Mission at University of the Transkei Medical Faculty at Umtata General Hospital and review opportunity for General Surgery Overseas of Health Volunteers Overseas

5 Aug Thu 9:00 AM SAA flight MTT to JNB to connect with international flights

5 Aug Thu 10:00 PM BA 035 JNB to LHR London 7:00 AM 6 Aug

6 Aug Fri 12:30 PM BA 223 LHR to IAD Washington, DC 4:30 PM

Return home to Derwood.

Geelhoed, Glenn W. (George Washington) LINGUISTIC RELATIVITY AMONG PAZANDE-BANGALA BILINGUALS: LANGUAGE AS CONTEXT FOR COGNITION Residents of Oriental Province, Democratic Republic of the Congo, are bilingual in Pazande, their household language, and Bangala, the lingua franca, distinct linguistic families. Twenty bilinguals named Munsell colors with twice as many terms in Pazande than in Bangala, suggesting they differentiate more acutely when speaking Pazande. Thus, we hypothesized: (1) bilinguals would demonstrate stronger emphasis on difference and weaker emphasis on similarity when assessing color chips in response to instructions in Pazande than when performing the same assessments in response to Bangala; (2) bilinguals would show parallel divergence of emphasis when assessing objects whose colors were identical. We conducted four experiments per individual—two in each language—by asking each person to arrange in triangle triads of color chips and triads of same-colored objects according to how different they are and, on another day, how similar they are, recording resultant distances on paper background. In response to each language, with both colors and objects, bilinguals arranged larger triangles to show difference than to show similarity, implying these judgments are differentially integral to cognition. But in every task, bilinguals arranged significantly larger triangles when instructed in Pazande than when instructed in Bangala. We conclude each language provided a context that influenced thought, defined as reciprocally weighted emphases on similarity and difference. Prior tests of the Sapir-Whorf hypothesis have correlated grammatical or lexical categories with behavior attributed to cognition, not complete language contexts with cognition attested by the same experiments. We discuss implications for linguistic relativity and the effect of context on thinking.

APPENDIX III
A SIMPLE LISTING OF COLOR NAMES IN THE TWO LANGUAGES

COLOR	PAZANDE	BANGALA
RED	zambaha	motane
ORANGE	nouvgboko	monzano
YELLOW	nouvgboke	monzano
GREEN	rangi kpe	rangi na kasa or rangi na mayotu
BLUE	ngaruyantule	rangi ya mayotu
INDIGO	ngbruglantula	hapata ya maupa
VIOLET	falala	ndunda
BLACK	bihe	moindo
WHITE	puse	pembe

PAZANDE MODIFIERS

biliki = brick. requires further adjactive
dagba = between. off (e.g.. dagba bihe = off-black)
dagba puse = off-white
gadia = cassava
gbaya = nearly. not quite. just off
gbaya ha = off-yellow
ime = water
kpe = leaf
kpe ndunda = leaf stem (purple stem. green leaf)
kure = blood-like
langi = the spoken color word
mai = cloud color
mzete = wood
naya = a kind of cucumber color
ndimo = orange (if with modifying adjective)
ndunda = the stem of the leaf
ngbanghuturu = sky
ngbunghe = bright red
nvugbehe = tan color. off-yellow
pai pai = papaya
rangi = the written color word
sende go = ground color in termite mound
sene graeyed = normal ground color
zambaha = blood-like

BANGALA MODIFIERS

mai na = water of
makasi = hard
moke = little
mwa = like, almost
pete pete = slowly

APPENDIX IV
GETTING YOUR OWN BEARINGS
FROM THE UNEXPLORED ASSA RIVER,
"THE RIVER OF MYSTERY"

If you have in mind being an explorer of the unexplored, let me tell you how to get here and how far away you are. I will start with a few bearings on the GPS of places I have marked along the way here in Central Africa. First, I will tabulate the fixes of my "marks" near my Assa base, and then I will give you distances and bearings from the fixed point of the Assa River crossing. I figure that to be a landmark that more people might know and one that will be a bit more permanent than the front door of the house at Assa station.

MARK	SITE	LONGITUDE	LATITUDE
ASSA	Assa airstrip on MAF chart	4° 37.00′ N	25° 52.00′ E
CONG	Assa airstrip, my measurement	4° 38.55′ N	25° 50.65′ E
ASS1	Front door Assa house	4° 36.88′ N	25° 50.62′ E
RIVE	Assa River bridhe	4° 34.03′ N	25° 49.21′ E
BUNI	Bunia airstrip	3° 00.00′ S	23° 00.00′ E
NEBO	Nebobongo airstrip	2° 27.12′ N	27° 37.32′ E
RIFT	Great Rift Valley	1° 16.98′ N	36° 27.46′ E
VICT	Lake Victoria, Entebbe	0° 22.80′ N	34° 30.26′ E
WILS	Nairobi, Wilson Field	1° 7.88′ S	36° 48.18′ E

MARK	"GO TO" PLACE	MILES FROM "RIVE" MARK	BEARING
ASS1	Assa front door	3.53	25°
CONG	Assa airstrip	5.34	18°
HOME	Derwood, MD	6,703	311°
JNBA	Jo'Burg Airport	2,125	176°
MART	Martheen's door Grand Rapids, MI	7,060	316°
MIKE	Michael's door, San Antonio, TX	8,060	307°
MILI	Milly's door, Jenison, MI	7,072	316°
NAIR	Mayfield, Nairobi	859	118°
NEBO	Nebobongo Airstrip	192	140°
NEED	Lake Needwood, MD	6,702	31°

REGF	Reg's door,	8,058	320°
	Denver, CO		
RIFT	Great Rift Valley	838	119°
SHIR	Shirl's door	7,063	316°
	Grand Rapids, MI		
VICT	Lake Victoria, Uganda	690	120°
WAPI	Wapiti Lodge,	8,113	321°
	Steamboat, CO		
WILS	Wilson Field, Nairobi	859	118°
WORK	GWUMC, Ross 103,	6,701	311°
	Washington, DC		

So, now, you not only know where I am, you know where you are relative to me! So, anytime you would like to come to explore, and help, just follow the bearings!

AIRSTRIP INFORMATION FOR FUTURE REFERENCE

Airstrip	Longitude Latitude	Altitude	Length	Width	Radio
Assa	4° 38.30′ N				
	24° 51.20′ E	2,000	750	30	37 8188.6L
Nebobongo	2° 27.23′ N				
	27° 38.00′ E	2,550	1,000	20	NC 3827 Coord
Nyankunde	1° 26.00′ N				
	36° 02.00′ E	3,500	1,300	30	AB 0226 Coord

APPENDIX V

ABSTRACT FOR *NUTRITION* ARTICLE

Endemic hypothyroidism has been studied in a Central African population in remote Congo (ex-Zaïre) to investigate the prevalence, severity, causes and potential control of this disorder, with questions as to why this disease is conserved, and whether it confers any adaptive advantage in this resource-constrained environment. Iodine deficiency, cassava goitrogens and selenium deficiency were found to be the factors implicated in the severe hypothyroidism expressed in congenital cretinism and high goiter incidence in this isolated population, which continues under observation following medical intervention.

Profound hypothyroidism was encountered in whole village populations as measured by serum TSH determinations ranging from very high to over 1000 IU, and thyroxin levels ranging from low to undetectable. Cretinism rates were as high as 11% and goiter incidence approached 100%. Assessment of endocrinologic status, caloric requirement, energy output, fertility and ecologic factors was carried out before and during iodine repletion by depot injection.

Hypothyroidism was corrected and cretinism eliminated in the treatment group, with goiters reduced in most instances with regrowth exhibited in some who escaped control. Some symptomatic goiter patients were offered surgical treatment for respiratory obstruction. Individual patient benefits were remarkable in development expressed in improved strength and energy output.

The social and developmental consequences observed within the collective groups of treated patients were remarkable for an increase in caloric requirement and a dramatic increase in fertility which led to quantitative as well as qualitative increase in resource consumption. Micronutrient iodine repletion was not accompanied by any concomitant increase in macronutrient supply, and hunger and environmental degradation resulted.

It may be that the highly prevalent disease of hypothyroidism is conserved in areas of greatest resource constraint, in which it happens to be found in highest incidence, because it may confer adaptive advantage in such marginal environments as an effect as well as cause of underdevelopment. It may limit energy requirements, fertility, and consumer population pressure in closed ecosystems that could otherwise be outstripped. Single factor intervention in a vertical health care program not sensitive to the fragile biologic balance and not part of a culture-sensitive development program might result in medical maladaptation.

Reprinted with permission American Elsevier Publishing, New York.

SUGGESTED READINGS

Blaikie, W. G. *The Personal Life of David Livingstone*. Fleming H. Revell, New York, 1880.

Brokken, J. *The Rainbird: A Central African Journey*. Lonely Planet, Berkeley, CA, 1997.

Conrad, J. *Heart of Darkness*. Penguin, London, 1995.

Dinesen, I. *Out of Africa*. Modern Library, New York, 1992.

Farwell, B. *Burton: A Biography of Sir Richard Burton*. Penguin, London, 1990.

Geelhoed, G. W. Medical adventures in the Nigerian bush: report of an African foreign fellowship. New Phys. *17*:348-356, 1968.

Geelhoed, G. W. Who will help the helpers? The migration of African AIDS from town to country. African Urban Quarterly, *6*: 45-52, 1991.

Geelhoed, G.W. *Natural Health Secrets from Around the World*. Keats Publishing, New Canaan, CT, 1997.

Geelhoed, G. W. Wanted: world-class surgeons. Bull. Amer. Coll. Surg. *83*: 33-42, 1998.

Geelhoed, G. W. An author's editorial: health care advocacy in world health. Nutrition *15*: 940-943. 1999a.

Geelhoed, G. W. Metabolic maladaptation: individual and social consequences of medical intervention in correcting endemic hypothyroidism in Central Africa. Nutrition *15*: 908-932. 1999b.

Geelhoed, G. W. Ed. *Surgery and Healing in the Developing World*. Landes BioScience, Austin, TX, 2000.

Geelhoed, G.W. Linguistic relativity among Pazande-Bangala bilinguals: Language as context for cognition. American Association of Anthropology, October, 1999c.

Geelhoed, G. W. and D. C. Downing. Goiter and cretinism in the Uele Zaire endemia: studies of an iodine-deficient population with changes following intervention: I. Morphologic aspects; II. Functional and behavioral aspects. In: *The Damaged Brain of Iodine Deficiency*, J. B. Stanbury, ed., Cognizant Communications, New York, 1994.

Gide, A. *Travels in the Congo*. Ecco Press, Hopewell, N.J.,1994.

Gourevitch, P. *We wish to inform you that tomorrow we will be killed with our families: Stories from Rwanda*. Farrar Straus and Giroux, New York, 1998.

Hochschild, A. *King Leopold's Ghost*. Houghton Mifflin, Boston, 1998.

Kingdon, J. *The Kingdon Field Guide to African Mammals*. Academic Press, San Diego, 1997.

Kingsolver, B. *The Poisonwood Bible*. Harper Collins, New York, 1999.

Lamb, D. *The Africans*. Vintage, New York, 1987.

Naipaul, V.S. *North of South: An African Journey*. Penguin, London, 1979.

Neuman, K. *Neuman's Birds of Southern Africa*. Southern Book Publishers, Halfway House, Republic of South Africa, 1983.

Nicholls, C.S. *David Livingstone*. Sutton Publishing, Gloucestershire, UK, 1998.

O' Hanlon, R. *No Mercy: A Journey to the Heart of the Congo*. Alfred A. Knopf, New York, 1997.

Stanley, H. M. *Through the Dark Continent*. Dover Publications, New York, 1988.

Ungar, S.J. *Africa: The People and Politics of an Emerging Continent*, ed. 3. Simon & Schuster, New York, 1989.

Wheatley, N. *Where to Watch Birds in Africa*. Princeton University Press, Princeton, NJ, 1996.

Zimmerman, D.A., Turner, D.A., and Pearson, D.J. *Birds of Kenya and Northern Tanzania*. Princeton University Press, Princeton, NJ, 1996.

Endpiece

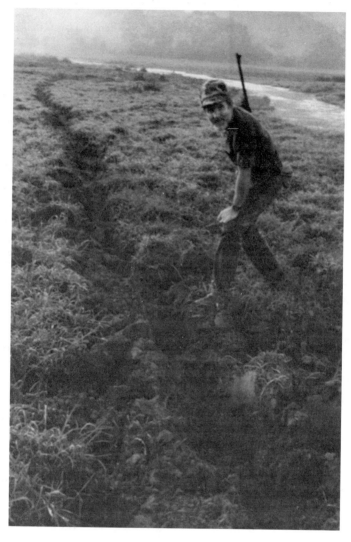

*The real tragedy of human life is not so much what men suffer,
but what they miss.*

Thomas Carlyle

Additional copies of this book can be purchased at your local bookstore, through Internet book services, or directly from Three Hawks Publishing Company, LC. You can order by phone (703-823-9833), fax (703-823-9834), e-mail (*kej@3hawks.com*), or directly from our website: *http://www.3hawks.com*, where you can also find more about this book and the author. If you indicate interest in making a purchase, please supply your shipping and billing address. We will ship the book by Priority Mail and send you a bill for $15.95 + $3.20 S&H, payable by cash, check, or money order.

Kurt E. Johnson, Ph. D., President and Publisher
Three Hawks Publishing Company, LC
1300 Bishop Lane
Alexandria, VA 22302

he